Diagnostic and Laboratory Testing in Psychiatry

CRITICAL ISSUES IN PSYCHIATRY
An Educational Series for Residents and Clinicians

Series Editor: **Sherwyn M. Woods, M.D., Ph.D.**
University of Southern California School of Medicine
Los Angeles, California

Recent volumes in the series:

ADULT DEVELOPMENT: A New Dimension in Psychodynamic Theory
and Practice
Calvin A. Colarusso, M.D., and Robert A. Nemiroff, M.D.

SCHIZOPHRENIA
John S. Strauss, M.D., and William T. Carpenter, Jr., M.D.

EXTRAORDINARY DISORDERS OF HUMAN BEHAVIOR
Edited by Claude T. H. Friedmann, M.D., and Robert A. Faguet, M.D.

MARITAL THERAPY: A Combined Psychodynamic–Behavioral Approach
R. Taylor Segraves, M.D., Ph.D.

TREATMENT INTERVENTIONS IN HUMAN SEXUALITY
Edited by Carol C. Nadelson, M.D., and David B. Marcotte, M.D.

CLINICAL PERSPECTIVES ON THE SUPERVISION OF
PSYCHOANALYSIS AND PSYCHOTHERAPY
Edited by Leopold Caligor, Ph.D., Philip M. Bromberg, Ph.D.,
and James D. Meltzer, Ph.D.

MOOD DISORDERS: Toward a New Psychobiology
Peter C. Whybrow, M.D., Hagop S. Akiskal, M.D., and
William T. McKinney, Jr., M.D.

EMERGENCY PSYCHIATRY: Concepts, Methods, and Practices
Edited by Ellen L. Bassuk, M.D., and Ann W. Birk, Ph.D.

DRUG AND ALCOHOL ABUSE: A Clinical Guide to Diagnosis
and Treatment, Second Edition
Marc A. Schuckit, M.D.

THE RACE AGAINST TIME: Psychotherapy and Psychoanalysis
in the Second Half of Life
Edited by Robert A. Nemiroff, M.D., and Calvin A. Colarusso, M.D.

DIAGNOSTIC AND LABORATORY TESTING IN PSYCHIATRY
Edited by Mark S. Gold, M.D., and A. L. C. Pottash, M.D.

CONTEMPORARY PERSPECTIVES ON PSYCHOTHERAPY WITH
LESBIANS AND GAY MEN
Edited by Terry Stein, M.D., and Carol Cohen, M.D.

A Continuation Order Plan is available for this series. A continuation order will bring
delivery of each new volume immediately upon publication. Volumes are billed only
upon actual shipment. For further information please contact the publisher.

Diagnostic and Laboratory Testing in Psychiatry

Edited by
Mark S. Gold, M.D.
and
A. L. C. Pottash, M.D.

Fair Oaks Hospital
Delray Beach, Florida and
Summit, New Jersey

PLENUM MEDICAL BOOK COMPANY
New York and London

Library of Congress Cataloging in Publication Data

Main entry under title:

Diagnostic and laboratory testing in psychiatry.

(Critical issues in psychiatry)
Includes bibliographies and index.
1. Mental illness—Diagnosis. 2. Diagnosis, Laboratory. 3. Neurologic examination.
I. Gold, Mark S. II. Pottash, A. L. C. III. Series. [DNLM: 1. Diagnosis, Laboratory. 2.
Mental Disorders—diagnosis. WM 141 D53662]
RC473.L32D5   1985   616.89′075   85-24465
ISBN 0-306-42054-6

© 1986 Plenum Publishing Corporation
233 Spring Street, New York, N.Y. 10013

Plenum Medical Book Company is an imprint of Plenum Publishing Corporation

Printed in the United States of America

Contributors

R. Michael Allen, M.D., Associate Director, Neuropsychiatric Evaluation Unit, Psychiatric Institute of Fort Worth, Fort Worth, Texas 76104, and Clinical Assistant Professor of Psychiatry, University of Texas Southwestern Medical School, Dallas, Texas 75235.

Lawrence DeMilio, M.D., Director of Adolescent Substance Abuse, Stony Lodge Hospital, Ossining-on-Hudson, New York 10562.

Todd W. Estroff, M.D., Research Facilities, Fair Oaks Hospital, Summit, New Jersey 07901.

Irl Extein, M.D., Medical Director, Fair Oaks Hospital at Boca/Delray, Delray Beach, Florida 33445.

Frederick C. Goggans, M.D., Director, Neuropsychiatric Evaluation Unit, Psychiatric Institute of Fort Worth, Fort Worth, Texas 76104, and Clinical Instructor, Department of Psychiatry, University of Texas Health Science Center, Dallas, Texas 75235.

Mark S. Gold, M.D., Director of Research, Research Facilities, Fair Oaks Hospital, Summit, New Jersey 07901, and Fair Oaks Hospital at Boca/Delray, Delray Beach, Florida 33445.

David A. Gross, M.D., Fair Oaks Hospital at Boca/Delray, Delray Beach, Florida 33445.

Cary L. Hamlin, M.D., Associate Director, Outpatient Research Unit, Fair Oaks Hospital, Summit, New Jersey 07901.

William Hapworth, M.D., Associate Clinical Director, The Regent Hospital, New York, New York 10021.

Michael H. Kronig, M.D., Chief of Affective Disorders Service, Hillside Hospital, A Division of the Long Island Jewish Medical Center, Glen Oaks, New York 11004.

David Martin, Psychiatric Diagnostic Laboratories of America, Inc., Summit, New Jersey 07901.

H. Rowland Pearsall, M.D., Clinical Director, Stony Lodge Hospital, Ossining-on-Hudson, New York 10562.

A. L. C. Pottash, M.D., Executive Medical Director, Fair Oaks Hospital at Boca/Delray, Delray Beach, Florida 33445, and Fair Oaks Hospital, Summit, New Jersey 07901.

Sheldon H. Preskorn, M.D., Departments of Psychiatry and Pharmacology, Washington University School of Medicine, St. Louis, Missouri 63110.

William S. Rea, M.D., Lake Hospital of the Palm Beaches, Lake Worth, Florida 33460, and Fair Oaks Hospital at Boca/Delray, Delray Beach, Florida 33445.

David E. Sternberg, M.D., Medical Director, Falkirk Hospital, Central Valley, New York 10917, and Lecturer in Psychiatry, Yale University School of Medicine, New Haven, Connecticut 06508.

Karl Verebey, Ph.D., Director of Clinical Pharmacology, New York State Division of Substance Abuse Services, and Associate Professor of Psychiatry, SUNY Downstate Medical School, Brooklyn, New York 11217.

Foreword

Most psychiatrists had their education at a time when the relevant knowledge about diagnostic and laboratory testing in psychiatry could easily have been reviewed in a very small monograph. Within recent years, however, we have witnessed a virtual eruption of new knowledge regarding the biological aspects of nearly every axis I diagnosis, as well as some interesting findings concerning axis II.

Laboratory methods are now available to help confirm clinical diagnostic impressions, to predict the response to treatment, to regulate dosage of medication, to improve the efficiency of therapeutic interventions, and to help in the estimation of prognosis. The sensitivity (true positives), specificity (exclusion of false positives), and confidence level (likelihood of identifying a true positive by an abnormal laboratory level) now often approach that which obtains for many of the routine tests regularly employed in medicine. Computerized axial tomography (CAT), nuclear magnetic resonance (NMR), and positron emission transaxial tomography (PETT) are likely within the near future to revolutionize our understanding of normal and pathological anatomy and physiology, and therefore diagnosis and treatment.

Doctors Gold and Pottash have succeeded in reviewing the massive and often confusing literature in this field. They have evaluated it with their extensive experience at both the research and clinical levels, and have produced succinct and practical summaries of virtually every clinical and laboratory testing procedure currently known. Particularly important is the manner in which they have correlated the procedures with known physiological mechanisms, clinical presentation, and clinical relevance.

Accurate psychiatric diagnosis and treatment have always, and will always, require educated and sensitive subjective clinical observation. State of the art now demands equally educated and sensitive utilization of those objective evaluative methods that are essential to the modern practice of psychiatry. This is a book that most of us will refer to with great frequency as we struggle to understand the complexities of diagnosis and treatment in our patients.

Sherwyn M. Woods

Preface

Diagnostic procedures and laboratory testing in psychiatry are becoming integral parts of the evaluation and treatment of the psychiatric patient. It is clear to any observer that this field is rapidly expanding. We are learning what some of the abnormalities are that occur as part of psychiatric diseases, what the implications of the abnormalities are, and also what is causing these abnormalities. Diagnostic and laboratory testing is neither limited to one test or procedure nor limited to one psychiatric syndrome or disease. Similarly, tests usually are neither simplistically good or bad, or useful or useless, but rather have limited applications in limited clinical situations, where they may add valuable data that are otherwise unavailable or provide an impartial "third-party" evaluation unbiased by placebo or transference effects. Testing can also be superfluous, as it may be when testing is ordered merely to protect against the possibility of a malpractice suit.

The laboratory evaluation of the psychiatric patient has changed dramatically over the last decade. One of the many factors that has contributed to this change is the DSM III. Logically enough, all of the axis I conditions have as an inclusion criterion "not due to any organic mental disorder" since, as any experienced clinician knows, a number of organic disturbances may have associated behavioral, cognitive, mood, and personality disturbances. As psychiatrists have begun vigorously to rule out such competing medical diagnoses, the procedures available for laboratory evaluation and diagnosis have been expanded and, in some cases, rediscovered by clinicians.

Any procedure that can lead to more accurate diagnosis, safer use of medications, or speedier clinical decision making has critical benefits in terms of patient safety and humanitarian interest in decreasing the needless suffering of the misdiagnosed patient. However, the benefit can also be financial. A procedure that decreases hospital stay by even 1 day saves the patient an expense far in excess of the cost of most tests. When, for example, an antidepressant level is found to be so low as to reveal clear non-compliance, and if the psychiatrist can cause the patient to improve compliance, consequences ranging from wasted hospital days or outpatient treatment to non-response and relapse can be avoided. Thus, laboratory procedures have the potential to improve the quality of care. Psychiatrists, like their colleagues in other medical specialties, will increasingly be able to use laboratory tests as an adjunct to their obviously crucial clinical skills.

For example, drug intoxication and most drug withdrawal diagnoses require identification of the drug in exhaled breath, blood, or urine. Routine "drug screens" may not have the sensitivity necessary to measure psychiatrically relevant quantities of these drugs, and more specific (e.g., antibody-based) tests may need to be ordered. The psychiatrist can test specifically for additional abusable substances on the basis of the patient's signs, symptoms, history, and age and the family's description of the phenomenology and the assessment of drug use/abuse. A negative history of drug use or abuse, however, is not sufficient to replace negative specific tests for drugs of abuse.

Newer urine drug abuse screens that use enzymatic assays are sensitive to concentrations of drugs in the abuse range, as opposed to the older thin-layer chromatographic assays, which are less sensitive. Gas chromatograph–mass spectroscopy (GC–MS) assays for all major drugs of abuse in blood are now available.

As soon as the patient has been interviewed and the physical examination has been performed, it is advisable to send samples of blood and urine to the laboratory for identification and quantification of the drugs of abuse. Antibody-based urine assays may be used for most drugs of abuse, including alcohol. Quantitative, capillary-column GC, or GC–MS analysis of blood for specific drugs not easily detectable in urine (e.g., glutethimide, PCP, cocaine, Δ^9-THC) are ordered when clinically indicated. When a urine sample is used to detect drug abuse, a supervised first-void morning urine is essential. Concurrent urine specific gravity is used to insure that the sample is actually the concentrated first-void morning urine.

One area of growing use of laboratory procedures is in the application of techniques of therapeutic drug monitoring to psychiatric patients. Historically, the growth in the use of psychopharmacological agents in psychiatry ultimately led to the development of methods of therapeutic drug monitoring. The desirability of such testing was obvious to psychiatrists, who could see that physicians in other branches of medicine had increasingly relied on such techniques for monitoring use of medications. Growing concern over the side effects of psychotropic medications emphasized the need for treatment with the individualized dosage regimens that therapeutic drug monitoring allows. In addition, such concerns have spurred the search for additional diagnostic procedures to supplement clinical impressions. The availability of effective and specific psychotropic treatments for major depression, manic–depressive illness, and schizophrenia have emphasized the importance of accurate diagnosis. A number of other laboratory tests useful for diagnosis have begun to allow physicians greater certainty in their evaluation of need for medications and even in their choice of a particular psychopharmacological agent. As psychiatrists have gained more clinical experience with the use of these medications, the recognition of other side effects has emphasized the need for periodic laboratory assessment of basic medical functions such as tests of renal and thyroid status in patients on lithium.

The last 10 years of basic and applied research have contributed to an unprecedented expansion of the use of the laboratory in psychiatry. Many psychiatrists now use clinical state markers such as 3-methoxy-4-hydroxyphenylglycol (MHPG) levels to predict antidepressant treatment response, the dexamethasone suppression test (DST), the diurnal cortisol test (DCT), and the thyrotropin-releasing hormone test (TRH) to confirm the presence of "neurobiologically active" major depression or identify those patients who have not responded "biologically" to treatment and who are at high risk for early relapse. Other psychiatrists are more interested in trait markers and use or would like to use tests of platelet monoamine oxidase inhibitor, cerebrospinal fluid 5-

HIAA, platelet serotonin transporter, platelet imipramine binding, lithium efflux, or fibroblast acetylcholine receptor density to identify the introvert from the extrovert, the stimulus seeker from the stimulus reducer, the patient at high risk for suicide or aggression, or the patient at high risk for developing bipolar or major depressive illness.

Other psychiatrists use antidepressant dose-prediction tests, blood levels of antidepressants, blood levels of antipsychotics, dopamine radioreceptor binding as an index of total dopamine receptor blockade in antipsychotic management, and platelet MAO inhibition as an index of MAO blocking activity in MAOI management. Some psychiatrists do not draw blood and do not have a working understanding of the laboratory and the procedures available and as a result do not order laboratory testing. Other psychiatrists refer their patients to an internist or other physician so that the patient can have a "doctor" to take care of him. Although they themselves do not order tests, these psychiatrists have the illusion that their patients are being properly evaluated or "cleared" for psychiatric treatment. Nothing, in our experience, could be further from reality than this notion, which is shared by all too many nonmedical psychotherapists and a small number of psychiatrists.

Other psychiatrists use diagnostic and laboratory testing during the evaluation of new patients or patients with the emergence of an unusual or nonresponsive syndrome. These psychiatrists have become experts in evaluation and testing procedures that can detect those patients who meet criteria for a psychiatric diagnosis but who actually have naturally occurring medical, neurological, endocrinologic, and other known diseases or diseases caused by prescribed medications, illicit drugs, or exogenous poisons. Other psychiatrists have become experts in psychopharmacology and understand the strengths, limitations, and interpretations of medication blood levels. Other psychiatrists have become experts in evaluation and use of state markers in treatment-resistant patients or in the prediction of relapse and so on.

Through a process of self-education and learning by doing, many psychiatrists have become the ultimate expert on their own patient population. A psychiatrist who treats or evaluates adolescents or children should become an expert in the detection, both clinical and laboratory, of drug intoxication and withdrawal states. Where one practices will also make a difference. For example, the number of depressed patients referred to Fair Oaks Hospital's Neuropsychiatric Evaluation Unit with hypothyroidism is 7 to 8%. We also know the number of major depressives with DST, TRH, and other neuroendocrine abnormalities, the number of DSM-III-qualifying depressives with underlying medical illnesses, and so on. In short, we know the false positives and false negatives, the specificity and sensitivity of each test, and the yield or usefulness in our population. The experience of Fair Oaks as a tertiary center evaluating patients who did not respond to a crisis or a previous brief admission to a general hospital would be expected to be greatly different than the experience of the NIMH, which usually receives very severely ill and atypical treatment nonresponders who meet diagnostic criteria. The typical Fair Oaks patient would also be different from the general hospital depressives who meet criteria and who almost immediately respond to antidepressants. For psychiatric tests to have meaning in their present state, and for the appropriate panel of tests to be ordered by the psychiatrist, the setting and the patients who are typically seen must be taken into consideration. After understanding the available tests and their strengths and limitations, the psychiatrist who is ready to incorporate these tests into his or her practice should take a step back and compare the setting and the issues addressed by the tests to determine whether the particular test or procedure is an appropriate use of resources.

Laboratory tests in clinical use vary with regard to both sensitivity and specificity. The sensitivity of a test as we use the term here describes the ability of the test to correctly identify through an abnormal or positive result a percentage of patients with a given syndrome (true positives). The remaining, unidentified patients are the false negatives. Specificity is related to the ability of a test to exclude false-positive patients. The confidence level describes the likelihood that an abnormal laboratory result in a given population will identify a true positive patient. For a test to be useful in laboratory medicine, neither 100% sensitivity, 100% specificity, nor 100% confidence level is necessary or even expected. Of course, it is important to become familiar with the limitations of each particular test.

For these and other reasons, laboratory tests can never replace physicians. Diagnosis in laboratory medicine is often based on the review of the results derived from a number of tests, each with a different sensitivity and specificity. The best example of this is the use of the laboratory in the diagnosis of various autoimmune diseases. Some of the commonly used laboratory tests in these medical syndromes have very low sensitivities or specificities, although the results of such tests can still contribute to the process of diagnosis. It is our hope that this book will aid the practicing clinician in doing just this. All of us should have a working knowledge of the state of the art in the field of diagnostic and laboratory testing.

Diagnostic and laboratory testing in psychiatry is becoming so important that it can no longer be ignored by any psychiatrist. Rather than proposing that a new subspecialty of psychiatry emerge to integrate the new information into the framework of traditional psychiatry, we believe that the new tests and procedures are not difficult to understand, especially after supervised hands-on experience and the opportunity to use the testing procedures in clinical practice. We hope that this book with its description of the major diagnostic procedures and emphasis on the "how to's" (how to use, how to interpret, how to choose which patient will benefit from . . .) will be useful as a review of the state of the art at the present time and as a reference manual.

Emerging understanding of brain function at the membrane and neurotransmitter levels is creating new approaches to diagnosing and treating psychiatric disorders. The approaches discussed here are likely to become a part of psychiatry in the 1980s. Over the next decade, we expect continued expansion of our knowledge and understanding of pathophysiology and prognostic markers, with the result being improvement in treatment response.

Mark S. Gold
A. L. C. Pottash

Summit, New Jersey

Contents

1

Introduction and Overview

Mark S. Gold, M. D., and A. L. C. Pottash, M.D.

1. Introduction

Psychiatry is in the midst of a number of changes that are now being felt by clinicians, researchers, and patients. With the return of the internship to residency training came the return of the notion that psychiatry was a medical specialty and not an extension of psychology. With the Research Diagnostic Criteria and the DSM III came the return of the notion that diagnosis matters and that syndromal consistency and reliability were important. After 10 years of research and the National Collaborative Study on Depression, a body of information about the dexamethasone suppression test, the thyrotropin-releasing hormone test, MHPG levels, and antidepressant blood levels was developed. Tertiary-care psychiatric facilities began using psychiatric laboratory testing procedures to confirm clinical impressions, predict treatment response, reduce side effects of medications, improve efficacy, and estimate prognosis.

As testing slowly enters routine psychiatric practice, numerous issues arise. Among these are questions of what tests are available, what the uses and limitations are of these tests, and which tests might improve the standard care of which patients. From the early list of testing procedures have come tests to predict violence and even likelihood of suicide (CSF 5-hydroxyindoleacetic acid), tests that predict which patients might be stimulus seekers or risk takers or prone to need psychiatric care or to abuse drugs and alcohol (platelet MAO). Other tests enable clinicians and researchers to see the brain at work in schizophrenia and other pathological mood states (positron emission scan), to detect recent and even not so recent drug use (gas chromatography/mass spectroscopy), and to confirm the diagnosis of panic disorder (lactate infusion). Recent tests can begin to distinguish bipolar depression from other depressive states and may even be able to determine in advance who has the propensity to develop a manic–depressive disorder (skin fibroblast). Although the list of new procedures and tests is increasing rapidly, there has not been an effort made to put together the state of the art for each of the tests and procedures and to describe the possible clinical uses at this point in their development.

Mark S. Gold, M.D. • Research Facilities, Fair Oaks Hospital, Summit, New Jersey 07901, and Fair Oaks Hospital at Boca/Delray, Delray Beach, Florida 33445.   *A. L. C. Pottash, M.D.* • Fair Oaks Hospital at Boca/Delray, Delray Beach, Florida 33445, and Fair Oaks Hospital, Summit, New Jersey 07901.

In this volume, we review the major tests and procedures by testing type, organ system, and clinical usefulness. Testing and evaluation protocols for various disease states and diagnoses are given for the most frequent clinical problems encountered in the clinical practice of psychiatry. Controversies that exist regarding the various markers are discussed but do not dominate this book, as they have overshadowed much of the good work reported in the psychiatric literature over the past few years. We focus on neuropsychiatric evaluation unit programs that are state of the art and the type of clinician who has remained current. These programs and clinicians in many cases have taken a leadership position in developing clinical uses for procedures and tests. Psychiatrists as medical subspecialists are in a unique position to make important diagnoses. Many of the patients with psychiatric complaints turn out to have a causative or precipitating medical illness. A psychiatrist who is interested in examination and evaluation procedures makes a differential diagnosis and systematically rules out of active consideration all competing illnesses with the help of the laboratory and his understanding of the strengths and limitations of the various testing measures.

Deciding on the usefulness of evaluation procedures should not be limited to the analysis of the value of a single test such as an electroencephalogram (EEG). Although the EEG is an example of a test often blindly used on all patients by clinicians who at the same time consider themselves ''conservative'' and ''antitest,'' in many settings the EEG has not been studied from the point of view of yield. What is the yield of the EEG for eliciting a new nonpsychiatric diagnosis or treatment (how often do EEG results cause the physician to order a different treatment)? What is the yield for different types of patient (does the test do better with different patients)? It is probably not controversial to say that a patient who has failed in outpatient treatment should be evaluated and treated more invasively. However, would many first-episode outpatients who received a similar but earlier invasive evaluation have had life-saving earlier diagnoses and rapid return to full productivity? The demand in a first-episode presentation for a full work-up is voiced most commonly by the well-informed patient.

2. Terminology

Laboratory tests in medicine vary with respect to sensitivity and specificity. The sensitivity of a test, as we use the term here, describes the ability of the test to correctly identify a percentage of patients with a given syndrome (true positives) through an abnormal or positive result. The remaining unidentified patients are the false negatives. Specificity is a measure of the test's ability to exclude false-positive patients. The confidence level describes the likelihood that an abnormal laboratory result in a given population will identify a true-positive patient. Contrary to beliefs held by many psychiatrists, for a test to be useful in clinical practice or laboratory medicine, neither perfect (i.e., 100%) sensitivity and specificity nor confidence level is necessary or even expected. What would be the sensitivity, specificity, or diagnostic confidence of a particular test for a specific chief complaint (e.g., depression) or working descriptive syndromal diagnosis (e.g., major depression)? It is the physician's responsibility to become familiar with the uses and limitations of each laboratory test in every specific psychiatric syndrome. For these and other reasons, laboratory tests can never replace physicians. Diagnosis in laboratory medicine is often based on the review of the results derived from a number of unrelated tests, each with a different sensitivity and specificity. The best example of this is the use of the laboratory in the diagnosis of various endocrinopathies or autoimmune diseases. Some of the most commonly used laboratory tests in these diseases have very low sensitivities or specificities, although the results of sequential, provocative, or additive tests can make important contributions to the diagnostic process.

3. Types of Procedures

Some procedures can be important in making a diagnosis of an underlying or precipitating illness, whereas others improve treatment efficacy and/or reduce risks. Still another group of tests can identify stable traits of the person that bias behavior and can be used to predict suicide, impulsivity, or stimulus seeking. Finally, a new group of tests is appearing that even enables the physician to make a diagnosis of a medical illness at a time when the illness is not obvious from the clinical presentation. In allowing the physician to make not only the overt diagnoses but also the subclinical or covert diagnoses, tests allow patients with partial clinical syndromes and confusing clinical presentations and history to be evaluated, given the appropriate diagnosis, and treated. When the particular subclinical state of the disease has a predilection for a behavioral change or psychiatric presentation, it is extremely important that a diagnosis of a subclinical disease be made. Thyroid dysfunction, B_{12} deficiency, and folate deficiency are diagnoses that can be made before their classical presentations as myxedema or anemia, at a time when they only present with depression or other behavioral disturbance. Diabetes, especially the autoimmune form, other endocrinopathies, and subclinical forms of epilepsy will be very important diagnoses for the psychiatrist of the future to make. These diagnoses will be possible as the laboratory tools and provocative testing protocols for uncovering covert disease become available.

With the incidence of thyroid failure in depressed patients at least 7%, it is very important for the psychiatrist to fully understand the thyroid axis, the examination of the thyroid, the tests of thyroid function, and the evolution of thyroid disease from normal thyroid function to myxedema. The psychiatrist should also understand the importance of thyroid hormone in the brain as a neuromodulator and be able to explain to his skeptical endocrinologist colleagues why it is important to treat a depressed patient with a ΔTSH of 100 on the TRH test and high titers of thyroid autoantibodies with thyroid hormone rather than following the patient for the emergence of myxedema.

Finally, the psychiatrist must make peace with the notion that he or she will see more subclinical and incomplete disease states than other specialists since the brain is not a very forgiving organ. Its needs are great when it comes to the regulation of normal mood and behavior. Most overt diagnoses are usually made by the primary physician and readily treated. In medicine, as the diagnosis and treatment of overt disease states become more objective and less complex, changes seem to occur in the patient flow. In the case of diabetes or overt hypothyroidism, the family physician has replaced the endocrinologist. The psychiatrist sees in consultation the difficult patient, the atypical patient, the patient the primary physician thinks has a psychiatric problem on the basis of behavioral complaints and the absence of overt, easily diagnosed medical disease. This fact of medical life explains why it is that sending a psychiatric patient to an internist to vaguely rule out nonpsychiatric disease is a particularly bad idea. The psychiatrist who specializes in and actively practices in a neuropsychiatric evaluation setting has the theoretical background and volume of actual cases to be the ideal diagnostician when it comes to behavioral presentations. If consultations with other medical specialists are indicated, the psychiatrists should know the exact questions they are looking for answers to, so that a highly focused and successful consultation is the result.

4. Biopsychiatry Today

Unraveling the intricacies of the human brain is the last frontier of medicine. With the emergence of both basic science and clinical biopsychiatric research, a new medicine of the mind has been developed. Psychiatric diseases—diseases of the brain cells and the neurotransmitters—can now be understood and treated with new technologies.

The concept of biopsychiatry is not new. Hippocrates, the father of medicine, felt that mental anguish or melancholia resulted from the presence of "black bile." Sigmund Freud, the father of psychoanalysis, suspected that depression arose from changes in the brain. Although the technologies of their day did not allow them to prove their theories, both knew that limited approaches to mental illness would not last. Although medical research provided insights into all other areas of medicine, the workings of the brain in the major psychiatric diseases remained out of reach until the 1970s. Since then, research has uncovered the neurotransmitters, receptors, and brain neurotransmitter systems that have led to a chemical understanding of depression, mania, schizophrenia, and even drug addiction.

With the steady progress toward understanding how the brain sends and receives mood, thought, and other complex messages have come new insights into the biochemical basis of psychic disorders. The new psychiatry goes well beyond subjective psychiatric interviews and psychotherapy. Diagnosis and treatment are based on objective findings in the patient's history, physical, psychiatric, or neurological examination, and psychiatric laboratory testing. The new psychiatry's approach promotes more specific and individualized treatment and more rapid recovery. The modern psychiatrist retains all of his clinical insights and personal sensitivity but now can also call on modern science and the psychiatric laboratory.

Just as all who wheeze do not have asthma, and everyone with chest pain does not suffer from angina or even heart disease, all who are depressed do not have the medical illness we call depression. What appears to be true depression can actually result from a host of medical illnesses ranging from thyroid disease and diabetes to mononucleosis, anemia, or cancer. Depression is often the first sign or clue to the presence of subtle or evolving medical illness. Drug and alcohol abuse can also mimic depression, misleading both patients and physicians. Such "secondary" depressions are not cured by psychotherapy or antidepressants but rather by treatment of the underlying illness. The modern psychiatrist, a practicing medical doctor and specialist in the new medicine of the mind, finds secondary depressions by appropriate interpretation of physical examination, X ray, and laboratory results.

In contrast, "primary" depression can be confirmed by new blood tests. The two most commonly utilized tests, the DST (dexamethasone suppression test) and TRH (thyrotropin-releasing hormone) test, are neuroendocrine tests that measure hormonal responses to chemical probes or challenges. Since these tests are at least one step away from the abnormalities in depression—they diagnose the chicken by testing the egg— they will most certainly be replaced by newer, more specific tests. This is the history of medical progress. But in the meantime, these tests confirm that the depressed person has active neurobiological disease that should be treated with antidepressant medication until both the patient and the tests are normalized. Thus, today's technology supports Hippocrates, Freud, and others who thought that depression was a chemical imbalance or physical disturbance.

Results from the psychiatric laboratory can also help the physician decide which type of therapy to employ and how long medical treatment should be continued. The cardiologist looks to the patient's progress, EKG, cardiac enzymes, and other laboratory procedures when a heart attack victim says he feels fine and wants to walk, leave the coronary care unit, or leave the hospital. Similarly, changes in the patient and these neuroendocrine tests assure the biopsychiatrist that the patient is indeed improving when he says he feels much better. Failure of the testing to return to normal, even in a person who sounds and acts completely cured, suggests that the depression will be present at full force within 6 months.

Once treatment has begun, tests that accurately measure the level of the antidepressant medication in the blood enable the physician to individualize prescription and dosage. Before such testing was available, psychiatrists started patients on the same dose and increased or decreased the dose depending on whether the patient said he or she felt the same or better or complained of side effects. These tests also help to overcome the common problem of failure to take the medication: the depressed person's sense of helplessness, despair, and negativism, which often meant that they did not take their medication (they believe "It wouldn't help me anyway") or forgot (concentration and memory problems are part of the illness). Now that dosage can be tailored to each person's illness and metabolism, risks and side effects are minimized, and benefits of the antidepressant can be maximized.

5. Biopsychiatry Tomorrow

Most of the tests and treatments discussed so far are now available to practitioners across the country. On the horizon are tests that can answer some of the most important questions in biopsychiatry. With the increasing data on familial patterns of the major psychiatric disorders and clear evidence of genetic factors in many disorders, biopsychiatrists have recently developed a skin test that identifies those people who have been born with the biological vulnerability or program to develop manic–depressive disease. This test and tests like it offer great promise for families in which someone has a manic–depressive or depressive disease. Another laboratory test has been developed that identifies those people who are at great risk for suicide. However, since it relies on measuring a breakdown product of the neurotransmitter serotonin in the spinal fluid, its present uses have been limited, although its promise is tremendous. Tests that identify people who may be at high risk of developing alcoholism or drug addiction are promising as well. By identifying potential victims, these skin, spinal fluid, and blood tests may allow biopsychiatrists to actually prevent the development of illness and in some cases prevent disability and death.

Positron emission tomography (PET scanning), a radiological technique even more advanced than CAT scanning, allows us actually to see the working brain's neurotransmitters and receptors in action. Biopsychiatrists are evaluating the use of PET to see the brain neurotransmitter disease in depression, schizophrenia, and other mental illnesses. Newer tests of brain electrical activity or brain waves have shown promise in uncovering forms of epilepsy in which the "seizure" manifests itself in abnormal thinking, feeling, behavior, or mood. With all of these advances, biopsychiatrists will have to become accomplished psychiatrists, internists, neurologists, neuroradiologists, neurochemists, and psychopharmacologists after finishing medical school. Mental illness is not a figment of the imagination or in the head but in the brain.

6. Testing as an Interim Measure

As part of their formal training and through the experience of trial and error, nonpsychiatric physicians learn about laboratories and testing and have realistic expectations. They do not find a laboratory test useless or suspect if it fails to have accuracy of 99% or more. They learn that laboratory testing is one component in the diagnostic and treatment process. Discussions about utility of a particular test in a particular disease result in a constant state of evolution with regular improvement and progress. Understanding the limitations of a particular test, these physicians use the test results in the context of other signs and symptoms. They considered the neurological examination before the spinal fluid examination was sufficiently improved, then, in order, the EEG, the brain scan, the arteriogram, and the CAT scan or NMR or PET scan. All this occurred because of an underlying bias that one cannot "smell syphilis," and the addition of an important third party to mediate clinical inconsistencies and disputes is necessary even when the mediator is imperfect.

Recognition of imperfections led to the next diagnostic refinement and step. Some psychiatrists have never learned, or they fail to remember, these basic principles of laboratory medicine, and they express nihilistic views suggesting that a lack of sensitivity is proof of the uselessness of a test. In addition, as some types of specialized laboratory testing are a relatively new area, psychiatrists need to learn the concept of interim measures *vis à vis* these tests. Jarvik did not expect to devise the perfect artificial heart. Barney Clark got a Jarvik 7, and the valves needed replacing. William Schroeder got an improved heart and new generation pump. With experience the necessary improvements become obvious. Cardiologists would never have defined the uses and limitations of the cardiac enzymes unless they were widely used by clinicians. Just so, psychiatrists need to have hands-on experience with the full spectrum of psychiatric laboratory tests to find out what syndromes they have been missing and to improve their patient evaluation and treatment as well as to impact on the use and improvement of such procedures. Finally, psychiatrists need to remember that medicine has, as part of its tradition, new tools and techniques that have been developed since their residency, which often necessitate additional postresidency training. Just imagine the consequences of a surgeon not learning the newer techniques of laparoscopy or arthroscopy. Some psychiatrists feel that they have learned enough and nothing "that" important has happened to force them to take an in-depth training program or to change the way they practice. This is unfortunate, since the psychiatrist is the logical physician candidate to master neurobiology and the new medicine of the mind.

Dramatic changes in the self-identity of psychiatrists and the perception of psychiatrists by other physicians and prospective psychiatrists are likely to follow the reintegration of psychiatry into medicine and incorporation of technological advances into the practice of psychiatry. However, it is important always to keep in mind that laboratory tests and procedures are interim measures and will never be able to replace psychiatrists. As adjuncts, the tests will be changing constantly as their widespread use reveals missing pieces and as new needs are identified. Psychiatrists with the most experience with these new technologies will be their master rather than slaves to them. It is our hope that this book will make the future more understandable and less threatening and at the same time encourage realistic expectations about today's most widely used tests and procedures.

Medical Evaluation of the Psychiatric Patient

Todd W. Estroff, M.D., and Mark S. Gold, M.D.

1. Low Response Rates

A recent study of the long-term outcome of patients presenting with Research Diagnostic Criteria (RDC) major depressive episodes treated with medication and psychotherapy reveals some startling statistics.[1] Twenty-one percent of the patients were still severely depressed 2 years later, and an additional 14% patients had had an "incomplete recovery." Only 65% of the patients experienced a complete recovery despite the fact that they had been treated at five top-notch academic psychiatric centers, Harvard, Columbia, the University of Chicago, Washington University in St. Louis, and the University of Iowa.

2. Misdiagnosis Is Common

These statistics are quite disturbing, but they are not unusual.[1,2] Most doctors and patients feel that the response rates could and should be higher.[3-9] One major barrier to improving these response rates is the fact that many treating psychiatrists, psychologists, and social workers do not have much information about medical illnesses that present psychiatrically. Therefore, they do not evaluate their patients for these disorders. If they could, many patients would not receive any psychiatric treatment at all but would instead be treated for an underlying causative medical problem. This problem of misdiagnosis could be avoided if the evaluating psychiatrist tried to detect and rule out medical illnesses before instituting psychiatric treatments. Unfortunately, even when treating psychiatrists are aware of these disorders, diagnostic errors can occur because many physicians are not able to adequately work up their patients. This sad state of affairs does not exist because psychiatrists are sloppy or do not care about their patients.[7,10] Many psychiatrists once possessed the necessary skills as medical stu-

Todd W. Estroff, M.D. • Research Facilities, Fair Oaks Hospital, Summit, New Jersey 07901. *Mark S. Gold, M.D.* • Research Facilities, Fair Oaks Hospital, Summit, New Jersey 07901, and Fair Oaks Hospital at Boca/Delray, Delray Beach, Florida 33445.

dents, interns, and residents to look for these disorders, but the skills have been lost or actively avoided. They want to help their patients as much as possible, but they often allow their medical skills to atrophy. Medical training and skills are often deemphasized once the future psychiatrist enters a psychiatric residency.

2.1. Psychiatrists Allow Their Medical Skills to Atrophy

Frequently, supervising psychiatrists have less medical skills than the residents they teach. They are thus incapable of imparting any new knowledge about the interface and overlap between medical and psychiatric illnesses to their trainees. Often residents are instructed not to touch their patients for fear of ruining the transference. They are then encouraged to allow other specialists to take over the physical examination of their patients. The result is a rapid loss of their own skills of physical examination. By the time they reach practice, fewer than 35% of all psychiatrists attempt to examine their patients.[11] Thirty-two percent of psychiatrists in one survey said they were "incompetent" to perform any physical examination at all.

This deemphasis of medical skills reached its zenith when the requirement for an internship prior to entering psychiatric residency was eliminated in the early 1970s. It was fortunately reinstituted in 1978.

2.2. Inadequate Medical Clearance

The consequence of all these pressures is that psychiatrists begin to rely more and more heavily on other specialists to medically certify that their patients do not have a medical illness that might be causing the psychiatric symptoms. This is a grave mistake that leads to continued underdiagnosis of all kinds of medical disorders in psychiatric patients.[12,13]

The demand on other specialists to clear psychiatric patients medically is a consultation that other specialists are not fully prepared to perform. It was initially embraced and later rejected by both Hall[3,4] and Koranyi[5] because it provided "a false sense of security for the treating psychiatrist." Koranyi[5] states "My early practice consisting of a referral for routine medical consultation proved to be insufficient and unsatisfactory." He goes on to say,

> a thorough and unprejudiced physical examination (by the treating psychiatrist) with the appropriate biochemical screening is a singularly important act to be performed with the greatest thoroughness on all patients. . . . The examiner must continually entertain the question what "other than the obvious" might be the cause or contributing factor to the presenting symptoms?

Unfortunately, few psychiatrists or internists think or act along these lines when confronted with a patient who has psychiatric symptoms.

2.3. Widespread Lack of Knowledge

The process of referring out to other specialists is unsatisfactory because of a variety of other factors.[7] Almost no physician, psychiatric or nonpsychiatric, has any specific training in this broad and confusing area between psychiatry and medicine.[9]

The knowledge has not diffused well through the psychiatric community, so it is not surprising that it has not spread into other fields of medicine. As a result, the non-psychiatric physician asked to medically clear a patient with psychiatric symptoms does not know exactly which diseases, signs, or symptoms will yield clues to the proper diagnosis. The physical examination becomes routinized, perfunctory, superficial, and cursory. The laboratory tests ordered are generalized routine screens and are not directed toward finding the diseases mentioned later in this chapter. Many of these diseases can only be diagnosed by specific chemical or biochemical testing, which are not part of routine screens.

2.4. Personality Factors

Psychological and personality factors also play a large part in the non-psychiatrist's lack of contact with and attention to psychiatric patients. Godwin *et al.* [14] showed that many physicians have an unusual ability to single out and label as "most disliked" all the patients demonstrating psychiatric symptoms. This dislike obviously leads to less attention, less careful examination, and less precise laboratory testing of these patients. When the routine examination and testing are declared "normal," the patients are "medically cleared," and many diseases actually present are missed. The patient is rapidly passed on to a psychiatrist, who may inappropriately treat for a nonexistent psychiatric disorder. When psychiatric treatment fails, these patients are then labeled as refractory.

3. Psychiatric Symptoms Are Nonspecific

In order to avoid similar diagnostic disasters, it is essential for all physicians to learn and remember that psychiatric and behavioral symptoms are nonspecific. [3–5,7,9,12,13] Other causes must be ruled out first, before any psychiatric treatment begins. One of the best examples of this is the symptom of catatonia.

For many years the symptom of catatonia was considered the pathognomonic hallmark of catatonic schizophrenia. However multiple studies and case reports have repeatedly documented that catatonia is nonspecific. [17–20] Its presence demands that causative physical or metabolic disorders must be ruled out first and foremost. The differential diagnosis is extensive and continues to grow with new reports emerging each month.

Gelenberg, [18] in his classic article in 1976, listed the following possibilities: arteriosclerotic parkinsonism and lesions of the basal ganglia, viral encephalitis, akinetic mutism, vascular lesions of the temporal lobes, tumors of the septum pellucidum infringing on the fornix, tumors and traumatic hemmorhage in the region of the third ventricle, focal lesions of the thalamus, frontal lobe tumors and lesions, anterior cerebral arterial aneurysms, AV malformations of the posterior cerebral circulation, diffuse brain trauma, diffuse encephalomalacia following closed head injuries, *petit-mal* epilepsy, status epilepticus, the postictal phase of epilepsy, Wernicke's encephalopathy, tuberous sclerosis, general paresis of syphilis, narcolepsy, acute phase of encephalitis lethargica, and cerebral macular degeneration. Many metabolic conditions are associated with catatonia: diabetic ketoacidosis, hypercalcemia from parathyroid adenomas, pellagra, acute intermittent porphyria, homocystinuria, membranous glomeruloephritis, and hepatic encephalopathy. It has also been associated with poisoning with organic fluorides, illuminating gas, mescaline, large quantities of ethyl alcohol, chronic intoxication with amphetamines, and acute phencyclidine (PCP) intoxication. It has also been associated with medications such as aspirin overdoses, ACTH, and antipsychotic medications. All of these possibilities and more must be ruled out before a psychiatric diagnosis is made. Even then, the catatonia is probably associated with an affective rather than a schizophrenic disorder.[19] In order to make a diagnosis of a catatonic schizophrenic under DSM III, the patient must meet full criteria for both catatonia and schizophrenia simultaneously.[15] Over 100 different nonpsychiatric disorders have been noted to induce depression, with at least 24 causing it frequently[12,13]

There are at least eight causes of mania, 21 causes of depersonalization, 56 causes of delusions, 12 causes of hyperventilation, 28 causes of auditory hallucinations, and 26 causes of euphoria that also must be ruled out before any psychiatric diagnosis is indicated.[7,12,13]

A clue to a nonpsychiatric illness is the presence of visual hallucinations. They are almost never found in primary psychiatric illness and are frequently found accompanying medical illnesses with psychiatric symptoms.[3] Other clinical signs suggesting a nonpsychiatric illness are weight loss (20 pounds or more), failure to respond to a well-organized antidepressant trial, and a progressive course.

4. Relationship between Medical and Psychiatric Disorders

The relationships between physical and psychiatric illnesses are wide-ranging and varied. It is therefore helpful to clarify how they are related by subclassifying them into causative, exacerbating, coexistent, or reactive to physical illness or psychiatric illness with secondary physical symptoms.[5,7]

4.1. Causative Physical Illness

Another problem in underdiagnosis is that many psychiatrists and physicians do not believe that causative medical illness is a common occurrence. Causative physical illness where no psychiatric illness is present was demonstrated by both Hall *et al.* and Koranyi to be present in between 7.7% and 9.1% of psychiatric outpatients and in 5% to 43% of psychiatric inpatients.[3-6]

4.2. Exacerbating Physical Illness

Physical illness may also be classified as exacerbating when it precipitates psychiatric symptoms in already vulnerable individuals. Treatment of exacerbating medical disorders may lead to substantial improvement or elimination of the psychiatric symptoms.

4.3. Coexistent Physical Illness

Coexistent medical disorders have no relationship to the patient's psychiatric illness. Treatment of the medical disorder has no effect on the psychiatric symptoms and *vice versa*.

4.4. Reactive Psychiatric Illness

Some very severe or chronic illnesses may weigh so heavily on a patient that they produce a reactive secondary psychiatric illness such as depression in reaction to the physical illness. Improvement of the illness may lead to less psychiatric illness, but this is not certain or predictable, and the patient may require independent psychiatric treatment.

4.5. Psychiatric Illness with Physical Symptoms

There is even a class of pure psychiatric illness that has physical symptoms as its chief presentation. These psychiatric disorders are often mistaken for and treated as a physical illness. Panic disorder is the best example of this class of illness. Medical treatment is ineffective, whereas psychiatric treatment is the treatment of choice.

5. Differential Diagnosis

The illnesses most likely to cause psychiatric symptoms are called "the great mimickers" in psychiatry and are reviewed in greater detail elsewhere.[7] They must always be kept in the differential diagnostic formulation whenever a patient presents with psychiatric or behavioral symptoms.

5.1. Endocrine Disorders

The most common category of diseases that cause psychiatric symptoms in involuntary inpatients are the endocrine disorders.[4] They include hypothyroidism,[16] hyperthyroidism,[4,21,22] diabetes mellitus,[4,5] hypoglycemia,[23] especially from tumors[24,25] or exogenous insulin administration,[25] hyper-[26-34] and hypoadrenalism[31] (Cushing's and Addison's diseases), hyper-[31,35] and hypoparathyroidism, pheochromocytoma,[36-39] carcinoid,[36] abnormalities of sexual hormones including birth control medications[40,41] and panhypopituitarism.[27,30]

5.2. Central Nervous System Disorders

The second most common organ system affected is the central nervous system. Diseases that must carefully be ruled out include narcolepsy,[36,42-47] epilepsy of all forms, especially partial complex seizures,[48-67] normal-pressure hydrocephalus,[68-70] Huntington's chorea,[71,72] multiple sclerosis,[73,74] Parkinson's disease,[75]

Post-concussion syndrome,[76,77] Pick's disease, strokes, and brain and spinal cord tumors.[78,79]

5.3. Medication, Drug Abuse, and Toxin Disorders

Toxic disorders and withdrawal states are next most common. Precipitating factors can include over-the-counter medications and a wide spectrum of prescribed medication, which are reviewed extensively elsewhere.[80-82] Drug abuse and dependence are also major causes of psychiatric symptoms and are covered in much more detail later in this chapter.[83-87]

Heavy metals[4,36,88-91] including magnesium, copper, zinc, manganese, lead, mercury, thalium, bismuth, aluminum, arsenic, and bromides as well as other environmental toxics such as organometal complexes,[92] volatile hydrocarbons,[93,94] and anticholinesterase insecticides are being increasingly recognized as producing psychiatric symptoms.

5.4. Nutritional Disorders

Nutritional disorders and infectious diseases cause about equal amounts of psychiatric dysfunction. Nutritional disorders include malnutrition, dehydration, and deficiencies of B_{12}, niacin (nicotinic acid), zinc, B_6, and thiamine.[4,36,95-108]

5.5. Infectious Disease

Infectious diseases affecting mood behavior and thought processes include the once-prevalent tertiary syphilis,[109,110] viral hepatitis,[111] infectious mononucleosis,[112-114] malaria, bacterial and viral pneumonia, *brucella*, tuberculosis, and some severe viremias.[3-5]

5.6. Metabolic Diseases

Some unusual metabolic disorders occur more frequently in psychiatric populations than in general populations. Diseases that must be ruled out are hepatolenticular degeneration (Wilson's disease),[115,116] acute intermittent porphyria,[36,117-119] G6-PDase deficiency, and systemic lupus erythematosis.[120-125]

5.7. Cancer

Cancers cannot be overlooked as a cause of psychiatric symptoms,[126] Depression is a frequent presentation, especially in pancreatic carcinoma,[127-130] but any kind of tumor, especially of the brain, spinal cord,[78,79] or endocrine system, can cause behavioral or mood disturbance.[126]

6. Systematic Evaluation

In light of such a confusing situation, the question arises as to how the patient is best evaluated.

6.1. History

The most important requirement is for all treating physicians to remember that psychiatric symptoms are nonspecific and to keep the differential diagnosis of all the previously mentioned diseases constantly in mind. Next, a drug-free washout period is indicated unless severe medical or psychiatric decompensation would occur. If this is not possible, a change to less potent acceptable substitute medication may prove useful. The importance of a compulsive, thorough, complete, and integrated medical history, psychiatric examination, and appropriate laboratory testing cannot be overestimated. It is a good idea to have these examinations repeated again by other psychiatrists, residents, and interns as well as by highly trained masters-level nurse clinicians. Many times the repetition uncovers new symptomatic historical, physical, or biochemical clues that lead to the proper diagnosis.

6.2. Physical Examination

During a thorough complete physical examination that is directed towards finding "the great mimickers of psychiatric disease," particular attention is directed towards but not limited to discovering abnormalities of the thyroid, carotid arteries, retinal vasculature, heart, and abdominal aorta. The skin and nails are carefully examined for indications of collagen vasular diseases. Of course, a careful neurological examination is of particular importance.

6.3. Consultations

If any abnormalities are found, appropriate specialty consultation is requested from a group of consulting physicians who are sensitive to the problem of medical illness with a psychiatric presentation.

6.4. Laboratory Testing

Appropriate laboratory testing is indicated, but good sound clinical judgment combined with full awareness of the differential diagnosis is critical.[131,132] Routine admission lab testing should include a CBC, sedimentation rate, SMA 22 (which includes total protein albumin, globulin, A/G ratio, calcium, inorganic phosphates, triglycerides, BUN, uric acid, creatinine, total bilirubin, bilirubin, alkaline phosphatase, L.O.H., SGOT, glucose, SGPT, GGTP, sodium, potassium, chloride, iron), R.P.R., urinalysis, EKG, chest X ray, and an EEG that is sleep deprived with nasopharyngal leads. A comprehensive supervised urine screen for drug abuse using antibody immuno assay methods is mandatory for all patients.[86,87] It includes tests for opiates, methadone, amphetamine, barbiturates, cocaine, benzodiazepines, phencyclidine (PCP), THC (marijuana, hashish), alcohol, propoxyphene, and methaqualone. Since glutethimide, ethchlorvinyl, and LSD are not picked up in this urine screen, serum testing may be indicated if abuse of these substances is suspected.[87]

Blood levels of psychiatric medication and antiepileptic medications, if the patient has had them prescribed, are indicated and easily help determine if the patient was compliant with prescribed treatment. They may also reveal overdose situations that were either unintentional but produced psychiatric symptoms or were part of a suicide attempt.[7,131,132]

Specific testing for unusual diseases may be indicated to diagnose SLE, porphyria, Wilson's disease, vitamin deficiencies, or toxic disorders caused by heavy metals or other environmental pollutants. A 24-hr EEG or a CAT scan may be indicated if the patient has an abnormal EEG or neurological examination.[5,7,34,131,132]

6.5. Neuroendocrine Testing

If all of this examination and testing results in no medical diagnosis, then a psychiatric disorder is almost certain. Confirmatory neuroendocrine testing, especially in disorders with an affective component, is indicated. Diurnal cortisol, dexamethasone suppression testing (DST), and TRH/TSH thyroid testing should be performed. These tests can also help to reveal endocrinological diseases such as Addison's or Cushing's disease or subclinical hypo- or hyperthyroid states.[7,131,132]

Some clinicians may disagree with this approach, but if it is ignored, many of the "great mimickers" will be missed if they are not actively searched for in a complete systematic and compulsive manner.

The psychiatry of the 1980s and 1990s will change to take this new knowledge into account. It will lead to better detection of medical illness and improved treatment of all patients with psychiatric or behavioral symptoms. Improved response rates will automatically follow.

7. Evaluation of Drug-Abusing Patients

This already complicated and confusing situation becomes even more so when drug- or alcohol-abusing patients are treated. Many patients have the dual problem of simultaneous psychiatric and drug-abuse disorders for which no clear distinction can be made. In these cases, it is very helpful if the treating physician is both a psychiatrist who possesses all the knowledge and skill mentioned earlier in the chapter as well as a physician who is thoroughly familiar with the evaluation, medical complications, and treatment of substance-abusing patients.[87]

7.1. Environmental Controls

Major additions are needed to evaluate and care for drug-abusing individuals. They start with a locked evaluation unit, which permits total control of the drug abuser's environment. This procedure along with thorough searching of the patient's belongings and any packages, flowers, or mail sent to the patient prevents drugs from entering the hospital, while the locked doors prevent the patient from leaving and finding drugs to abuse. The patient is kept on the unit and is constantly observed so that emergency care can be given immediately if the patient has either overdosed, starts to have severe withdrawal problems, or develops any other emergent medical problems.

Drug-abusing patients are usually more medically unstable than psychiatric patients. It is therefore important for the admitting psychiatrist to interview and examine the patient as rapidly as possible. This should occur within a half hour of admission.

7.2. History

The initial interview is focused on what drugs were abused, how much and how often they were abused, and when the last dose was taken. Questions about possible medical diseases are asked to determine if the patient has had or might have bacterial endocarditis, tuberculosis, hepatitis, cellulitis, or pneumonia. A preliminary psychiatric examination elicits information about past non-drug-related psychiatric symptoms and illness as well as drug-induced depression, paranoia, delusions, or psychosis. A current mental status examination must also be performed to assess dangerousness related to psychosis or suicidal and homicidal ideation. It must be emphasized however that the mental status exam can be highly fluctuant over time and must be periodically reassessed throughout the hospital stay.

7.3. Pressures and Leverage

Finally, it is important to ask about the pressures that finally led to hospitalization. The answers may provide a source of future leverage to help the patient remain in treatment should his commitment to recovery decrease. The pressures may include those from family members, job, debts, or legal problems.

7.4. "Tanking Up"

Many addicts are afraid they will be forced into a prolonged and extremely uncomfortable detoxification. As a consequence, they may take any and all drugs available immediately prior to admission. This can result in an emergency overdose situation necessitating emergency transfer to a general hospital. This possibility must also be assessed during the interview and physical examination.

7.5. Physical Examination

A thorough, complete physical examination is mandatory and must first be directed to looking for signs of the infections that drug-abusing patients are so prone to develop, such as abcesses, cellulitis, hepatitis, endocarditis, arrhythmias, and pneumonia.

7.6. Laboratory Testing Is Mandatory

The patient's own self-reports of which substances are being abused and to what extent cannot be relied on for a variety of reasons. It is therefore mandatory that confirmatory urine or blood testing be performed. The urine tests should be first-void morning specimens, and they must be supervised. A simultaneous specific gravity helps to insure the specimen's integrity.

Thin-layer chromatographic (TLC) tests are much less sensitive than antibody-based or gas chromatography/mass spectometry (GC/MS) tests, which are approximately 100 and 1000 times more sensitive, respectively, than TLC. These more sensitive tests can provide an objective historical record of which drugs were ingested up to 1 week prior to admission.[85,131,132]

8. Stabilization

Even before the results of this testing have been returned, the patient must be stabilized on some medication to prevent withdrawal. Medications are only given if the patients demonstrate objective signs of withdrawal. Complaints alone without physical signs of withdrawal are not treated under any circumstances. Dually addicted patients present a particularly challenging problem, which is best dealt with using the least-risk technique.

The "least-risk" approach to patients who are dually addicted to sedative hypnotics or alcohol and opiates is to treat the sedative hypnotic or alcohol withdrawal aggressively with benzodiazepines and undertreat the opiate withdrawal. The reasons for this are that overdose with benzodiazepines is safe, whereas undertreatment can lead to DTs, seizures, and status epilepticus. In addition, opiate withdrawal is not dangerous, whereas overdose can be lethal, especially in combination with the benzodiazepines. All of this leads to the conclusion that it is best to overtreat with benzodiazapines and underutilize opiates if there is any doubt which medication to use. When the results of the drug screening are reported, the medications can be further adjusted to provide for a safe comfortable detoxification.[87]

9. Medical Complications of Drug Abuse

The medical and dental complications that drug abusers—especially i.v. abusers—develop can affect almost any organ system and produce severe disease.[133-137] Because they occur frequently, it is important for the treating physician to be fully conversant with the following complications.

Dental disease is common and so severe that extraction is often necessary.[138-141] Infections of the skin include cellulitis and abcesses[142,143] and can lead to endocarditis,[144-146] pneumonia, osteomyelitis,[147] endophthalmitis,[148,149] and septic arthritis.[150,151] Systemic infections that may develop are malaria,[133] tetanus,[133] and tuberculosis.[152] Infectious hepatitis of all forms can develop from hepatitis A, hepatitis B, Epstein–Barr, cytomegalo- or δ-agent viruses and may progress into chronic active and chronic persistent forms.[153-160]

Diseases of the lungs can produce chemical, bacterial, interstitial, and granulomatous pneumonitis[161] as well as pulmonary edema and pulmonary hypertension. Neurological disorders include strokes,[162-165] seizures,[166] encephalopathies,[167] abcesses, and meningitis. Ophthalmologic problems include infections and granulomas and can lead to retinal detachments and macular ischemia.[168-172] Renal disease and failure may develop as a consequence of endocarditis, hepatitis B, rhadomyolysis, or polyarteritis nodosa acquired because of drug abuse.[173-183] Endocarditis, myotic aneurysms, coronary artery disease, hypertension, myocardial infarction, and sudden death can also occur.[184,185] Opiates may cause hypoadrenalism,[186–188] and marijuana lowers testosterone levels and sperm motility.[189,190] Heavy metal, toxin, vitamin, and amino acid disorders and deficiencies can be found in this population.[87] Drug abuse during pregnancy in many cases is not teratogenic but can have persistent behavioral effects later in the child's life.[105] Acquired immunodeficiency disease (AIDS) is always a risk among drug abusers, especially intravenous users. Any unusual signs of infection, shortness of breath, oral thrush (*Candida*), unusual skin lesions, or generalized lymphadenopathy may be signs of developing AIDS.[190,191]

10. Detoxification

Once the patient has been stabilized and all associated medical illnesses have been treated, the detoxification is relatively straightforward and without problems.

Patients stabilized on sedative hypnotics, usually benzodiazepines, are reduced 5–10%/day starting from their stabilization dose. Opiate-abusing patients have their methadone stopped entirely and are detoxified using clonidine 0.2–0.3 mg every 2 hr as needed and as long as the systolic blood pressure holds above 70 mm Hg. In a dually addicted patient, the benzodiazapines are reduced first, then the opiates.

11. Treatment Decisions

When both psychiatric and drug-abusing patients are evaluated on the same unit, improved treatment can result, since many drug abusers have psychiatric problems and many psychiatric patients abuse drugs.

If the evaluation determines that the initial problem causing admission is not the primary problem, the patient can be transferred to the most appropriate treatment unit, adult psychiatry, adolescent psychiatry, or the drug abuse treatment unit. This triage to the most appropriate treatment unit will also add to an overall improvement in treatment response and prevention of relapse.

12. Conclusion

Deviation from the systematic and somewhat rigid protocols outlined in this chapter has often resulted in a treatable illness or condition being overlooked or ignored. Such a framework makes the often complicated and confusing evaluation and treatment of psychiatric patients who may have a causative physical illness or drug abuse as well as the evaluation of drug abusers with medical or psychiatric diseases easier to understand. It is then easier to arrive at the most rational and effective treatment possible for the individual patient.

The psychiatrist is the medical subspecialist who practices biobehavioral medicine by treating mood, behavioral, and cognitive diseases of the brain. The ability to formulate a differential diagnosis after an evaluation of the patient's "psychiatric" complaints and rigorously exclude from active consideration by testing and examination competing medical illnesses is a function ideally suited for the psychiatrist. To perform this function well, a standard intake model and procedures for major syndromes should be developed and repeatedly assessed for accuracy and cost effectiveness.

References

1. Keller MB, Klerman, GL, Lavori PW, et al: Long term outcome of episodes of major depression. *JAMA* 252:788–792, 1984.
2. Hamilton M: The effect of treatment on the melancholias (depressions). *Br J Psychiatry* 140:223–230, 1982.
3. Hall RCW, Popkin MK, Devaul RA, et al: Physical illness presenting as psychiatric disease. *Arch Gen Psychiatry* 35:1315, 1978.
4. Hall RCW, Gardner, ER, Popkin MK, et al: Unrecognized physical illness prompting psychiatric admission: A prospective study. *Am J Psychiatry* 138:629, 1981.
5. Koranyi EK: Morbidity and rate of undiagnosed physical illness in a psychiatric clinic population. *Arch Gen Psychiatry* 36:414–419, 1979.
6. Herridge CF: Physical disorders in psychiatric illness: A study of 209 consecutive admissions. *Lancet* 2:949–951, 1960.
7. Estroff TW, Gold MS: Psychiatric misdiagnosis, in Gold MS, Lydiard RB, Carman JS (eds): *Advances in Psychopharmacology: Predicting and Improving Treatment Response.* Boca Raton, CRC Press, 1984, pp 34–66.
8. Hoffman RS: Diagnostic errors in the evaluation of behavioral disorders. *JAMA* 248:964–967, 1982.
9. Teitelbaum ML: Toward better integration of medical and psychiatric care. *JAMA* 248:977, 1982.
10. Klein DF, Gittelman R, Quitkin F, et al: *Diagnosis and Drug Treatment of Psychiatric Disorders: Adults and Children.* ed 2. Baltimore, Williams & Wilkins, 1980.
11. McIntyre JW, Romano J: Is there a stethoscope in the house (and is it used)? *Arch Gen Psychiatry* 34:1147–1151, 1977.
12. Giannini AJ, Black HR, Goettsche RL: *Psychiatric, Psychogenic, and Somatopsychic Disorders Handbook.* New York, Medical Examination Publishing, 1978.
13. Hall RCW (ed): *Psychiatric Presentations of Medical Illness.* New York, SP Medical and Scientific Books, 1980.
14. Goodwin JM, Goodwin JS, Kellner R: Psychiatric symptons in disliked medical patients. *JAMA* 241:1117–1120, 1979.
15. American Psychiatric Association: *Diagnostc and Statistical Manual of Mental Disorders,* ed. 3. Washington, American Psychiatric Association, 1980.
16. Gold MS, Pottash ALC, Extein I: Hypothyroidism and depression. *JAMA* 245:1919–1922, 1981.
17. Sripada P: Catatonia: A non-specific syndrome. *Resident Staff Physician* 28:41–44, 1982.
18. Gelenberg A: The catatonic syndrome. *Lancet* 1:1339–1341, 1976.
19. Abrams, R, Taylor MA: Catatonia, a prospective clinical study. *Arch Gen Psychiatry* 33:579–581, 1976.
20. Weddington WW, Marks RC, Verghese JP: Disulfiram encephalopathy as a cause of catatonia syndrome. *Am J Psychiatry* 137:1217–1219, 1980.
21. Kronfol Z, Greden JF, Condon M: Application of biological markers in depression secondary to thyrotoxicosis. *Am J Psychiatry* 139:1319–1322, 1982.
22. Carney MWP, Macleod S, Sheffield BF: Thyroid function screening in psychiatric in-patients. *Br J Psychiatry* 138:154–156, 1981.
23. Ford CV, Bray GA, Swerdloff RS: A psychiatric study of patients referred with a diagnosis of hypoglycemia. *Am J Psychiatry* 133:290–294, 1976.
24. Gorden P, Hendricks CM, Kahn CR, et al: Hypoglycemia associated with non-islet-cell, tumor and insulin-like growth factors. *N Engl J Med* 305:1452–1455, 1981.
25. Service FJ, Dale AJD, Elveback LR, et al: Insulinoma, clinical and diagnostic features of 60 consecutive cases. *Mayo Clin Proc* 51:417–429, 1976.

26. Haskett RF, Schteingart DE, Starkman MN: Use of psychiatric research diagnostic criteria in Cushing's syndrome, in: *10th Congress of International Society of Psychoneuroendocrinology, Program Abstracts*. Park City, UT, International Society of Psychoneuroendocrinology, 1979, p. 12.
27. Tonks CM: Psychiatric aspects of endocrine disorders. *Practitioner* 218:526–531, 1977.
28. Haskett RF, Rose RM: Neuroendocrine disorders and psychopathology. *Psychiatr Clin North Am* 4:239-252, 1981.
29. Devaris DP, Mehlam I: Psychiatric presentations of endocrine and metabolic disorders. *Primary Care* 6:245–265, 1979.
30. Brown GM: Psychiatric and neurologic aspects of endocrine disease, in Krieger DT, Hughes JC (eds): *Neuroendocrinology*. Sunderland, MA, Sinauer Associates, 1980, pp 185–193.
31. Ettigi, PG, Brown GM: Brain disorders associated with endocrine dysfunction. *Psychiatr Clin North Am* 1:117–186, 1978.
32. Popkin MK, Mackenzie TB: Psychiatric presentations of endocrine dysfunction, in Hall RCW (ed): *Psychiatric Presentations of Medical Illness: Somatopsychic Disorders*. New York, Spectrum Publications, 1980, pp. 139–156.
33. Lichtenstein BW: Nervous and mental manifestations of parathyroid and thyroid disorders: Hyperparathyroidism, hypoparathyroidism, hyperthyroidism, and hypothyroidism. *Otolaryngol Clin North Am* 13:137–145, 1980.
34. Sachar EJ, Asnis G, Halbreich U, et al: Recent studies in the neuroendocrinology of major depressive disorders. *Psychiatr Clin North Am* 3:313–326, 1980.
35. Petersen P: Psychiatric disorders in primary hyperparathyroidism. *J. Clin Endocrinol* 28:1491–1495, 1968.
36. Jefferson JW, Marshall JR: *Neuropsychiatric Features of Medical Disorders*. New York, Plenum Press, 1981.
37. Nanger WM, Gifford RW: *Pheochromocytoma*. New York, Springer-Verlag, 1977, pp 141–142.
38. Thomas EJ, Rooke ED, Kvale WF: The neurologist's experience with phenochromocytoma. *JAMA* 197:754–758, 1966.
39. Engleman K: Pheochromocytoma, in Beeson PB, McDermott W (eds): *Textbook of Medicine*. Philadelphia, WB Saunders, 1975, pp 1787–1795.
40. Kolodny RC, Masters WH, Kolodner RM, et al: Depression of plasma testosterone levels after chronic intensive marijuana use. *N Engl J Med* 290:872–874, 1974.
41. Klaiber EL Broverman DM, Vogel W, et al: Estrogen therapy for severe persistent depressions in women. *Arch Gen Psychiatry* 36:550–554, 1979.
42. Roth B: Narcolepsy and hypersomnia, in Williams RL, Karacan I (eds): *Sleep Disorders: Diagnosis and Treatment*. New York, John Wiley & Sons, 1978, pp. 29–59.
43. Dement WC, Baird WP: *Narcolepsy: Care and Treatment*. Stanford, CA, The American Narcolepsy Association, 1977.
44. Zarcone V: Narcolepsy. *N Engl J Med* 288:1156–1166, 1973.
45. Parkes JD, Baraitser M, Marsden CD, et al: Natural history, symptoms, and treatment of the narcoleptic syndrome. *Acta Neurol Scand* 53:337–353, 1975.
46. Bonduel M, Degos C: Symptomatic narcolepsies: A critical study, in Dement WC, Guielleminault C, Passouant P (eds): *Proceeding of the First International Symposium on Narcolepsy*. Montpelier, France, 1976, pp 313–332.
47. Roth B: Functional hypersomnia, in Dement WC, Guielleminault C, Passouant P (eds): *Proceeding of the First International Symposium on Narcolepsy*. Montpelier, France, 1976, pp 333–349.
48. Schukla GD, Srivastava ON, Katiyar BC, et al: Psychiatric manifestation and temporal lobe epilepsy: A controlled study. *Br J Psychiatry* 135:1411–1417, 1979.
49. Flor-Henry P: Ictal and interictal psychiatric manifestation in epilepsy: Specific or non-specific. *Epilepsia* 13:773–783, 1972.
50. Waxman SG, Geschwind N: The interictal behavior syndrome of temporal lobe epilepsy. *Arch Gen Psychiatry* 32:1580–1586, 1975.
51. Stevens JR: Interictal clinical manifestations of complex partial seizures, in Penry JK, Daly DD (eds): *Advances in Neurology*, vol II. New York, Raven Press, 1975, pp 85–112.
52. Taylor DC: Mental state and temporal lobe epilepsy: A correlative account of 100 patients treated surgically. *Epilepsia* 13:727–765, 1972.

53. Rodin E, Katz M, Lennox K: Differences between patients with temporal lobe seizures and those with other forms of epileptic attacks. Epileptic attacks. *Epilepsia* 17:313–320, 1976.
54. Rodin EA: Psychiatric disorders associated with epilepsy. *Psychiatr Clin North Am* 1:101–115, 1978.
55. Toone BK, Garralda ME, Ron MA: The psychoses of epilepsy and the functional psychoses: A clinical and phenomenological comparison. *Br J Psychiatry* 141:256–261, 1982.
56. Blummer D: Temporal lobe epilepsy and its psychiatric significance, in Benson BF, Blummer D (eds): *Psychiatric Aspects of Neurological Disease.* New York, Grune & Stratton, 1975, pp 171–197.
57. Blummer D, Benson BF: Personality changes with frontal and temporal lobe lesions, in Benson BF, Blummer D (eds): *Psychiatric Aspects of Neurological Disease.* New York, Grune & Stratton, 1975, pp 151–169.
58. Dreifuss FE: The differential diagnosis of partial seizures with complex symptomatology, in Penry JK, Daly DD (eds): *Advances in Neurology,* vol II. New York, Raven Press, 1975, pp 187–199.
59. Levine DM, Finklestein S: Delayed psychosis after right temporoparietal stroke or trauma: Relation to epilepsy. *Neurology (NY)* 32:267–273, 1982.
60. Delgado-Escuata AV, Mattson RH, King L, et al: The nature of aggression during epileptic seizures. *N Engl J Med* 305:711–716, 1981.
61. Pincus JH: Violence and epilepsy. *N Engl J Med* 305:796–798, 1981.
62. Klass DW: Electroencephalographic manifestation of complex partial seizures, in Penry JK, Daly DD (eds): *Advances in Neurology,* vol II. New York, Raven Press, 1975, pp 113–140.
63. Kirkpatrick B, Hall RCW: Seizure disorders, in Hall RCW (ed): *Psychiatric Presentations of Medical Illness: Somatopsychic Disorders.* New York, Spectrum Publications, 1980, pp 243–258.
64. Booker HE: Management of the difficult patient with complex partial seizures, in Penry JK, Daly DD (eds): *Advances in Neurology,* vol II. New York, Raven Press, 1975, pp 369–382.
65. Sigal M: Psychiatric aspects of temporal lobe epilepsy. *J Nerv Ment Dis* 163:348–351, 1976.
66. Rasmussen T: Surgical treatment of patients with complex partial seizures, in Penry JK, Daly DD (eds): *Advances in Neurology,* vol II. New York, Raven Press, 1975, pp 415–449.
67. Treffert DA: The psychiatric patient with an EEG temporal lobe focus. *Am J Psychiatry* 120:765–771, 1964.
68. Price TRP, Tucker GJ: Psychiatric and behavioral manifestations of normal pressure hydrocephalus. *J Nerv Ment Dis* 164:51–55, 1977.
69. Benson DF, LeMay M, Patten DH, et al: Diagnosis of normal-pressure hydrocephalus. *N Engl J Med* 283:609–615, 1970.
70. Rice E, Gendelman S: Psychiatric aspects of normal pressure hydrocephalus. *JAMA* 223:409–412, 1973.
71. Huntington G: On chorea. *Med Surg Rep* 56:317–321, 1872.
72. Caine ED, Shoulson I: Psychiatric syndromes in Huntington's disease. *Am J Psychiatry* 140:728–733, 1983.
73. Peselow ED, Fiebe RR, Deutsch SI, et al: Coexistent manic symptoms and multiple sclerosis. *Psychosomatics* 22:824–825, 1981.
74. Gross DA: Medical origins of psychiatric emergencies: The systems approach. *Int J Psychiatry Med* 11:1–24, 1981.
75. Vogel HP: Symptoms of depression in Parkinson's disease. *Pharmacopsychiatria* 15:192–196, 1982.
76. Sisler GC: Psychiatric disorder associated with head injury. *Psychiatr Clin North Am* 1:137–152, 1978.
77. Brown G, Chadwich O, Shaffer D, et al: A prospective study of children with head injuries: III. Psychiatric sequelae. *Psychol Med* 11:63–78, 1981.
78. Malamud N: Psychiatric disorder with intracranial tumors of limbic system. *Arch Neurol* 17:113–123, 1967.
79. Epstein BS, Epstein JA, Postel PM: Tumors of spinal cord simulating psychiatric disorders. *Dis Nerv Syst* 32:741–743, 1971.
80. Boston Collaborative Drug-Related Programs: Psychiatric side effects of non-psychiatric drugs. *Semin Psychiatry* 3:406–420, 1971.
81. Hall RCW, Stickney SK, Gardner ER: Behavioral toxicity of nonpsychiatric drugs, in Hall RCW (ed): *Psychiatric Presentations of Medical Illness: Somatopsychic Disorders.* New York, Spectrum Publications, 1980, pp 337–349.

82. *Medical Letter:* Drugs that cause psychiatric symptoms. *Med Lett* 23:9–12, 1981.
83. Bloodworth RC: Detection of drug abuse presenting as a psychiatric illness. *Psychiatr Hosp* 13:60–64, 1982.
84. Wilford BB: *Drug Abuse: A Guide for the Primary Care Physician.* Chicago, American Medical Association, 1981.
85. Yago KB, Pitts FN, Burgoyne RW, et al: The urban epidemic of phencyclidine (PCP) use: Clinical and laboratory evidence from a public psychiatric hospital emergency service. *J Clin Psychiatry* 42:193–196, 1981.
86. Estroff TW, Dackis CA, Gold MS, et al: Drug abuse and bipolar disorder. *Int J Psychiatr Med* 15:37–40, 1985.
87. Gold MS, Estroff TW: The comprehensive evaluation of cocaine and opiate abusers, in Hall RCW, Beresford TP (eds): *Handbook of Psychiatric Diagnostic Procedures,* vol 2. New York, Spectrum Publications, 1985, pp 213–233.
88. Edwards N: Mental disturbances related to metals, in Hall RCW (ed): *Psychiatric Presentations of Medical Illness: Somatopsychic Disorders.* New York, Spectrum Publications, 1980, pp 283–308.
89. Elliott HL, Dryburgh F, Fell GS, et al: Aluminum toxicity during regular hemodialysis. *Br Med J* 1:1101–1103, 1978.
90. Dunea G, Mahurkar SD, Mandani B, et al: Role of aluminum in dialysis dementia. *Ann Intern Med* 88:502–504, 1978.
91. Gold MS, Estroff TW, Pottash ALC: Substance induced organic mental disorders, in Yudofsky SC (ed): *Psychiatry Update,* vol 4. Washington, American Psychiatric Press, 1985, pp 223–236.
92. Ross WD, Emmett EA, Steiner J, et al: Neurotoxic effects of occupational exposure to organotins. *Am J Psychiatry* 138:1092–1095, 1981.
93. Struwe G, Knave B, Mindus P, et al: Neuropsychiatric symptoms in workers exposed to jet fuel—a combined epidemiological and casuistic study. *Acta Psychiatr Scand* 67:55–67, 1983.
94. Struwe G, Wennberg A: Psychiatric and neurological symptoms in workers occupationally exposed to organic solvents—results of a differential epidemiological study. *Acta Psychiatr Scand* 67:68–80, 1983.
95. Strickland GT, Frommer D, Leu ML, et al: Wilson's disease in the United Kingdom and Taiwan. *Q J Med* 42:619–638, 1973.
96. Anonymous: Reversible neuropsychiatric disease related to folate deficiency. *RI Med J* 64:545–546, 1981.
97. Coppen A, Abou-Saleh MT: Plasma folate and affective morbidity during long term lithium therapy. *Br J Psychiatry* 141:87–89, 1982.
98. Thornton WE, Thornton B: Folic acid, mental function and dietary habits. *J Clin Psychiatry* 39:315–319, 1978.
99. Carney MWP, Sheffield BF: Associations of subnormal serum folate and vitamin B_{12} values and effects of replacement therapy. *J Nerv Ment Dis* 150:404–412, 1970.
100. Roos D: Neurological complications in patients with impaired vitamin B_{12} absorption following partial gastrectomy. *Acta Neurol Scand [Suppl]* 69:1–7, 1978.
101. Kolhouse JF, Kondon H, Allen NC, et al: Cobalamin analogues are present in human plasma and can mask cobalamin deficiency because current radioisotope dilution assays are not specific for true cobalamin. *N Engl J Med* 299:785–792, 1978.
102. Strain GW: Nutrition, brain function and behavior. *Psychiatr Clin North Am* 4:253–268, 1983.
103. Whitehead VM, Cooper BA: Failure of radiodilution assay for vitamin B_{12} to detect deficiency in some patients. *Blood* 50(Suppl 1):99, 1977.
104. Hutchings DE: Neurobehavioral effects of prenatal origin: Drugs of use and abuse, in Schwarz RA, Yaffe SJ (eds): *Drug and Chemical Risks to the Fetus and Newborn.* New York, Alan R. Liss, 1980, pp 109–114.
105. Hutchings DE: Behavioral teratology: A new frontier in neurobehavioral research. in Johnson EM, Kochlar DM (eds): *Handbook of Experimental Pharmacology.* Berlin, Springer-Verlag, 1983.
106. Strauss ME, Lessen-Firestone JK, Chavez GJ, et al: Children of methadone treated women at five years of age. Presented at the satellite meeting of the Committee on Problems of Drug Dependence on Acute and Protracted Effects of Perinatal Drug Dependence, Philadelphia, June 7, 1979.

107. Chasnoff IG, Hatcher R, Burns WJ: Polydrug- methadone-addicted newborns: A continuum of impairment. *Pediatrics* 7:210–213, 1982.
108. Eriksson M, Larsson G, Zetterstrom R: Amphetamine addiction and pregnancy. *Acta Obstet Gynecol Scand* 60:253–259, 1981.
109. Gruenberg EM, Turns DM: Epidemiology; disappearing conditions, in Freedman AM, Kaplan HI, Sadock BJ (eds): *Comprehensive Textbook of Psychiatry,* ed 2. Baltimore, Williams & Wilkins, 1975, pp 398–399.
110. Hoffman BF: Reversible neurosyphilis presenting as chronic mania. *J Clin Psychiatry* 43:338–339, 1982.
111. Apstein MD, Koff E, Koff RS: Neuropsychological dysfunction in acute viral hepatitis. *Digestion* 19:349–358, 1979.
112. Hendler N, Leahy W: Psychiatric and neurologic sequeli [sic] of infectious mononucleosis. *Am J Psychiatry* 135:42–44, 1978.
113. Pezke MA, Mason WM: Infectious mononucleosis and its relationship to psychological malaise. *Conn Med* 33:260–262, 1969.
114. Cadie M, Nye FJ, Storey P: Anxiety and depression after infectious mononucleosis. *Br J Psychiatry* 128:559–561, 1976.
115. Cartwright GE: Diagnosis of treatable Wilson's disease. *N Engl J Med* 298:1347–1350, 1978.
116. Wilson SAK: Progressive lenticular degeneration: A familial nervous disease associated with cirrhosis of the liver. *Brain* 34:296–488, 1912.
117. Popkin MK: Psychiatric presentations of hemotologic disorders, in Hall RCW (ed): *Psychiatric Presentations of Medical Illness: Somatopsychic Disorders.* New York, Spectrum Publications, 1980, pp 223–241.
118. Weterberg L: *A Neuropsychiatric and Genetic Investigation of Acute Intermittent Prophyria.* Stockholm, Scandinavian University Books, 1967.
119. Becker DM, Kramer S: The neurological manifestations of porphyria: A review. *Medicine (Baltimore)* 56:411–423, 1977.
120. Bresnihan B, Hohmeister R, Cutting J, et al: Neuropsychiatric disorder in systemic lupus erythematosus, evidence for both vascular and immune mechanisms. *Ann Rheum Dis* 38:301–306, 1979.
121. Feinglass EJ, Arnett FC, Dorsch CA, et al: Neuropsychiatric manifestation of systemic lupus erythematosus: Diagnosis, clinical spectrum, and relationship to other features of the disease. *Medicine (Baltimore)* 55:323–339, 1976.
122. Gurland BJ, Hoff, Ganz V, et al: The study of the psychiatric symptoms of systemic lupus erythematosus: A critical review. *Psychosom Med* 34:199–206, 1972.
123. Guze SB: The occurrence of psychiatric illness and systemic lupus erythematosus. *Am J Psychiatry* 123:1562–1570, 1967.
124. Carr RI, Sucard DW, Hoffman SA, et al: Neuropsychiatric involvement in systemic lupus erythematosus. *Birth Defects* 14:209–235, 1978.
125. Hall RCW, Stickney SK, Gardner ER: Psychiatric symptoms in patients with systemic lupus erythematosus. *Psychosomatics* 22:15–24, 1981.
126. Peterson LG, Popkin MK, Hall RCW: Psychiatric presentation of cancer and sequelae of treatment. *Psychiatr Med* 1:79–92, 1983.
127. Fras I, Litin EM: Comparison of psychiatric manifestations in carcinoma of the pancreas, retroperitoneal malignant lymphoma and lymphoma in other locations. *Psychosomatics* 8:275–277, 1967.
128. Fras I, Litin EM, Pearson JS: Comparison of psychiatric symptoms of carcinoma of the pancreas with those in some other intraabdominal neoplasms. *Am J Psychiatry* 123:1553–1562, 1967.
129. Perlas AP, Faillance LA: Psychiatric manifestations of carcinoma of the pancreas. *Am J Psychiatry* 121:182, 1964.
130. Yaskin JC: Nervous symptoms as earliest manifestations of carcinoma of the pancreas. *JAMA* 96:1664–1668, 1931.
131. Pottash ALC, Gold MS, Extein I: The use of the clinical laboratory, in Sederer LI (ed): *Inpatient Psychiatry Diagnosis and Treatment.* Baltimore, Williams & Wilkins, 1982, pp 205–221.
132. Gold MS, Pottash ALC, Carman JS, et al: The role of the laboratory in psychiatry, in Gold MS, Lydiard RB, Carman JS (eds): *Advances in Psychopharmacology: Predicting and Improving Treatment Response.* Boca Raton, CRC Press, 1983, pp 307–317.

133. Ostor AG: The medical complication of narcotic addiction. *Med J Aust* 1:410–415,448–451,497–499, 1977.
134. Becker CE: Medical complications of drug abuse. *Adv Intern Med* 24:183–202, 1979.
135. Sapira JD: The narcotic addict as a medical patient. *Am J Med* 45:555–558, 1968.
136. Kurtzman RS: Complications of narcotic addiction. *Radiology* 96:23–30, 1970.
137. Geelhoed GW, Joseph WL: Surgical sequelae of drug abuse. *Surg Gynecol Obstet* 139:749–755, 1974.
138. Carter EF: Dental implications of narcotic addiction. *Aust Dent J* 23:308–310, 1978.
139. Rosenstein DI: Effect of long-term addiction to heroin on oral tissues. *J Public Health Dent* 35:118–122, 1975.
140. Rosenstein DI, Stewar AV: Dental care for patients receiving methadone. *J Am Dent Assoc* 89:356–359, 1974.
141. Colon PG: Dental disease in the narcotic addict. *Oral Surg* 33:905–910, 1972.
142. Webb D, Thadepalli H: Skin and soft tissue poly-microbial infections from intravenous abuse of drugs. *West J Med* 130:200–204, 1979.
143. Meislin HW, Lerner SA, Graves MH, et al: Cutaneous abscesses: Anaerobic and aerobic bacteriology and outpatient management. *Ann Intern Med* 87:145–149, 1977.
144. Sobel JD, Carrizosa J, Ziobrowski TF, et al: Poly-microbial endocarditis involving *Eilenella corrodens*. *Am J Med Sci* 282:41–44, 1981.
145. Andy JJ, Sheikh MU, Ali N, et al: Echocardiographic observations in opiate addicts with active infective endocarditis. *Am J Cardiol* 40:17–23, 1977.
146. Child JA, Darrell JH, Rhys Davis N, et al: Mixed infective endocarditis in a heroin addict. *J Med Microbiol* 2:293–299, 1969.
147. Holzman RS, Bishko F: Osteomyelitis in heroin addicts. *Ann Intern Med* 75:693–696, 1971.
148. Masi RJ: Endogenous endophthalmitis associated with *Bacillus cereus* bacteremia in a cocaine addict. *Ann Ophthalmol* 10:1367–1370, 1978.
149. Getnick RA, Rodriques MM: Endogenous fungal endophthalmitis in a drug addict. *Am J Ophthalmol* 77:680–683, 1974.
150. Gifford DB, Patzaus M, Ivler D, et al: Septic arthritis due to *Pseudomonas* in heroin addicts. *J Bone Joint Surg* 57A:631–635, 1975.
151. Ross GN, Baraff LJ, Quismorio FP, et al: *Serratia* arthritis in heroin users. *J Bone Joint Surg* 57:1158–1160, 1975.
152. Reichman LB, Felton CP, Edsall JR: Drug dependence, a possible new risk factor for tuberculosis disease. *Arch Intern Med* 139:337–339, 1979.
153. Norkrans G, Frosner G, Hermodsson S, et al: Multiple hepatitis attacks in drug addicts. *JAMA* 243:1056–1058, 1980.
154. Arthurs Y, Doyle DG, Fielding JF: The effects of drug abuse on the natural history and progression of chronic active and chronic persistent hepatitis. *Ir J Med Sci* 150:104–112, 1981.
155. Estroff TW, Extein IL, Malaspina D, et al: Hepatitis in suburban cocaine and opiate users. Presented at 136th Annual Meeting American Psychiatric Association, New York, April 29–May 6, 1983, pp 307–308.
156. Boughton CR, Hawkes RA: Viral hepatitis and the drug cult: A brief socioepidemiological study in Sydney, Australia. *NZ Med J* 10:157–161, 1980.
157. Blanck RR, Ream N, Conrad M: Hepatitis B antigen and antibody in heroin users. *Am J Gastroenterol* 71:164–167, 1979.
158. Serow SSW: Hepatitis in drug dependents. *Aust Fam Physician* 10:294–298, 1981.
159. Cherubin CE, Schaefer RA, Rosenthal WS, et al: The natural history of liver disease in former drug users. *Am J Med Sci* 272:244–253, 1976.
160. Raimondo G, Gallo L, Ponzetto A, et al: Multicentre study of prevalence of HBV-associated delta infection and liver disease in drug addicts. *Lancet* 1:249–251, 1982.
161. Waller BF, Brownlee WJ, Roberts WC: Self-induced pulmonary granulomatosis. *Chest* 78:90–94, 1980.
162. Delaney P, Estes M: Intracranial hemorrhage with amphetamine abuse. *Neurology (Minneap)* 30:1125–1128, 1980.

163. Dau PC, Weiner HL: Intracranial hemorrhage associated with amphetamine use. *Neurology (NY)* 31:922–923, 1981.
164. Shukla D: Intracranial hemorrhage associated with amphetamine use. *Neurology (NY)* 32:917–918, 1982.
165. Brust JCM, Richter RW: Stroke associated with addiction to heroin. *Neurol Neurosurg Psychiatry* 39:194–199, 1976.
166. Allister C, Lush M, Oliver JS: Status epilepticus caused by solvent abuse. *Br Med J* 283:1156, 1981.
167. King MD, Day RE, Oliver JS, et al: Solvent encephalopathy. *Br Med J* 283:663–665, 1981.
168. Tse DT, Ober RR: Talc retinopathy. *Am J Ophthalmol* 90:624–640, 1980.
169. Friberg TR, Gragoudas ES, Regan CDJ: Talc emboli and macular ischemia in intravenous drug abuse. *Arch Ophthalmol* 97:1089–1091, 1979.
170. Krseca LJ, Goldbert MF, Jampol LM: Talc emboli and retinal neovascularization in a drug abuser. *Ophthalmology* 87:334–339, 1979.
171. Michelson JB, Whitcher JP, Wilson S, et al: Possible foreign body granuloma of the retina associated with intravenous cocaine addiction. *Am Ophthalmol* 87:278–280, 1979.
172. Atlee WE Jr: Talc and corn starch emboli in eyes of drug abusers. *JAMA* 219:45–51, 1972.
173. Olivero J, Bacque F, Cartlon CE, et al: Renal complications of drug addiction. *Urology* 8:526–530, 1976.
174. Kohler PF, Cronin RE, Hammond WS: Chronic membranous glomerulonephritis caused by hepatitis B antigen–antibody immune complexes. *Ann Intern Med* 81:448–451, 1974.
175. Combes B, Shorey J, Barrere A: Glomerulonephritis with deposition of Australia antigen–antibody complexes in glomerular basement membrane. *Lancet* 2:234–237, 1971.
176. Gutman RA, Striker GE, Gilliland BC: The immune complex glomerulonephritis of bacterial endocarditis. *Medicine* 51:1–23, 1972.
177. Friedman EA, Rao TKS, Micastri AD: Heroin associated nephropathy. *Nephron* 13:421–426, 1974.
178. McGinn JT, McGinn TG, Cherubin CE, et al: Nephrotic syndrome in drug addicts. *NY State J Med* 74:92–95, 1974.
179. Eknoyan G, Gyorkey F, Dichoso C, et al: Renal involvement in drug abuse. *Arch Intern Med* 132:801–806, 1973.
180. Kilcoyne MM, Gocke DJ, Meltzer JI: Nephrotic syndrome in heroin addicts. *Lancet* 1:17–20, 1972.
181. Schreiber SN, Liebowitz MR, Bernstein LH, et al: Limb compression and renal impairment (crush syndrome) complicating narcotic overdose. *N Engl J Med* 284:368–369, 1971.
182. Richlim DM, Saltzman DB, Willis J: Necrotizing angiitis and hepatitis in an amphetamine abuser. *Del Med J* 49:469–477, 1977.
183. Citron BP, Halpern M, McCarron M: Necrotizing angiitis associated with drug abuse. *N Engl J Med* 283:1003–1011, 1970.
184. Coleman DR, Ross TF, Naughton JL: Myocardial ischemia and infarction related to recreational cocaine use. *West J Med* 136:444–446, 1982.
185. Yellin AE: Ruptured mycotic aneurysm a complication of parenteral drug abuse. *Arch Surg* 112:981–986, 1977.
186. Gold MS, Pottash ALC, Extein I: Evidence for an endorphin dysfunction in methadone addicts: Lack of ACTH response to naloxone. *Drug Alcohol Depend* 8:257–262, 1981.
187. Dackis CA, Gurpegui M, Pottash ALC, et al: Methadone induced hypoadrenalism. *Lancet* 2:1167, 1982.
188. Lafisca S, Bolelli G, Franceschetti F, et al: Hormone levels in methadone-treated drug addicts. *Drug Alcohol Depend* 8:229–234, 1981.
189. Kolodny RC, Masters WH, Kolodner RM, et al: Depression of plasma testosterone levels after chronic intensive marijuana use. *N Engl J Med* 290:872–874, 1974.
190. Hong CY, Chaput De Saintonge DM, Turner P: Δ^9-Tetrahydrocannabinol inhibits human sperm notility. *J Pharm Pharmacol* 33:746–747, 1981.
191. Centers for Disease Control: Epidemiologic aspects of the current outbreak of Kaposi's sarcoma and opportunistic infections. *N Engl J Med* 306:248–252, 1982.

Neurological Evaluation of the Psychiatric Patient

David A. Gross, M.D., and Mark S. Gold, M.D.

1. Essentials of the Neurological Evaluation

1.1. Introduction

The evaluation of the psychiatric patient is enhanced by the use of a general systems approach.[1] Biological, psychological, and sociological systems variables should be identified and their interaction assessed. A central part of this evaluation concerns the role that the nervous system plays in the expression of mental and behavioral disorders. Our understanding of "functional" psychiatric illness has been irrevocably influenced by the prevalence in our patients of causative or contributory central nervous system (CNS) dysfunction.[2]

The performance and interpretation of the neurological examination become an essential part of the psychiatrist's diagnostic repertoire. As a prerequisite, the examiner must have an understanding of the structure and function of the nervous system. For example, a systemic illness that eventually influences the central nervous system may present initially with a peripheral nervous system sign and a nonspecific mental state change. This change in behavior may be ignored, whereas in actual fact it represents a focal central neurological finding.

In addition to the division of the nervous system into central and peripheral anatomic components, a functional division into voluntary (skeletal) and involuntary (autonomic) can be made. Traditionally, conversion syndrome diagnoses have been based on functional voluntary nervous system symptoms, sometimes ignoring the subtle neurological signs that would confirm the presence of central nervous system disease. Multiple sclerosis has been the "great masquerader" for functional psychiatric illness and is commonly misdiagnosed as conversion reaction. Similarly, involuntary nervous system dysfunction may not necessarily indicate parasympathetic or sympathetic neuropathology because we now know that both classical and operant

David A. Gross, M.D. • Fair Oaks Hospital at Boca/Delray, Delray Beach, Florida 33445.   *Mark S. Gold, M.D.* • Research Facilities, Fair Oaks Hospital, Summit, New Jersey 07901, and Fair Oaks Hospital at Boca/Delray, Delray Beach, Florida 33445.

conditioning paradigms affect autonomic nervous system function. Thus, involuntary autonomic signs can exist as a result of learned reaction rather than tissue dysfunction. Autonomic nervous system activity is constantly monitored and interpreted by higher cortical centers. These cortical centers, especially those in the temporal lobe, modulate affect production and consequently shape the organism's behavioral response. For example, an individual with inherently hyperactive autonomic tone[3] may respond differently to a life crisis than an individual with less reactive autonomic tone. Likewise, the myxedematous brain may be the critical factor responsible for the patient's depressive syndrome and not the patient's psychosocial milieu.

The neurological evaluation of the psychiatric patient requires that the clinician utilize specific functional tests to evaluate the intactness of the nervous system. A systematic study of function that is based on an anatomic organization is most helpful. Table 3-1 provides an introduction to the systems covered by the neurological examination.

1.2. The Psychiatrist as Neurological Clinician

The neurological evaluation of the psychiatric patient requires an alteration of the psychiatrist's mental set utilized in the approach to the clinical interview. The psychiatric consultation model provides a good paradigm. The interview must be active, focused, and often problem oriented. The development of a "psychotherapeutic rapport" is not ignored but must take a back seat to the initial relationship elicited by the implicit message, "I am your doctor, and my task is to determine what is wrong." This approach requires the clinician to be actively in control of the interview.

The neurological examination that follows the interview requires a "hands-on" evaluation. Quite often, the patient is better prepared for this examination than the psychiatrist. The former expects this contact from the physician, whereas the latter may have to adjust attitudes acquired during specialty training in which psychotherapy may have been emphasized.

Table 3-1. Functional and Anatomic Aspects of the Neurological Examination

Pyramidal system: The frontal lobe motor regions provide executive control of complex motoric acts via descending tracts impinging on motor neurons.

Extrapyramidal system: The basal ganglia and pathways in conjunction with the influence of cerebellum and vestibular apparatus allow for effective gait, station, balance, and motor power.

Cerebellar system: The cerebellum integrates cortical motor, basal ganglia, vestibular, and spinal cord function and allows for balance, effective posture, gait, and complex coordinated motor activity.

Somesthetic system: The parietal cortex in concert with multisensory skin, joint, and visceral receptors provides continuous assessment of position, movement, pain, temperature, touch, and vibration.

Bulbar system: The brainstem with its variety of special sensory and motor cranial nerves, nuclei, and vegetative control centers (respiration, blood pressure, heart rate, sleep, etc.) provides for the automatic functioning of the activities that are essential to life.

Higher cortical systems: The cortical lobes with their primary, secondary, and tertiary association areas and intra- and extracortical tracts provide integration and execution of organismic function at the highest level. Problem solving is accomplished through the use of language and affective and spatially mediated activities.

1.2.1. Neurological History

The neurological history should isolate critical data from the patient's presenting illness. Target signs and symptoms will emerge from this information. Target signs and symptoms are best described using the following variables: intensity, duration, frequency, and location. Factors that provoke or alleviate symptoms must be sought. Have the patient use as much descriptive language as possible during the history. Quite often, a compilation of adjectives can be of more help in painting a clinical picture than a "pathognomonic" symptom.

1.2.2. Neurological Review of Systems

This historical neurological review should cover the systems outlined in Table 3-2. Questions should be repetitive to elicit as much information as possible. Quite often, the minor rephrasing of a question can facilitate clearer understanding on the patient's part and lead to a more meaningful report.

Table 3-2. Review of Neurological Systems

A. Motor coordination review
  1. Questions concerning changes or problems with station, gait, and posture
  2. Questions concerning the adequacy or change in coordinated acts utilizing the upper and lower extremities, e.g., writing, using utensils, pressing down on an automobile brake
  3. Questions concerning unilateral, bilateral, proximal, or distal changes in strength
B. General sensory review
  1. Questions concerning pain experience
  2. Questions concerning adequacy or alteration of temperature sensation
  3. Questions concerning adequacy and symmetry of light touch
C. Special sensory review
  1. Questions concerning auditory acuity, discrimination, and symmetry
  2. Questions concerning visual acuity, visual fields, and visual perception, special reference made to *de novo* visual experience
  3. Questions concerning vestibular adequacy
  4. Questions concerning olfactory acuity or distortion, special reference to *de novo* olfactory experience
  5. Questions concerning tactile adequacy, discrimination, and recognition
D. Higher cortical review
  1. Investigation of spheres of orientation
  2. Questions concerning difficulties with attention and concentration
  3. Questions concerning experienced difficulty with memory: immediate, short- and long-term
  4. Questions concerning intactness of language expression and comprehension
  5. Questions concerning problems with spatial–visual integration: sense of direction, geometric perception, part–whole comparisons, eye–hand coordination
  6. Questions concerning difficulties with abstract thinking and multipart problem solving
  7. Questions concerning problems with social judgment
  8. Questions concerning the presence and appropriateness of affective modulation
  9. Arithmetic competency: questions concerning problems with making change and keeping a checkbook
  10. Maintenance of usual state of basic knowledge: questions concerning the adequacy of current events, job skills, cooking skills, etc.

1.2.3. Neurological Past Medical and Family History

The construction of an adequate neurological history and review of systems are limited by the expressive abilities of the patient. Quite often we miss valuable information because our patient sometimes cannot or will not supply this information. Factors such as sophistication, psychological denial of illness, or cognitive impairment hamper our investigation. A careful review of past medical history can often reveal important clues and directions to follow in the development of the diagnostic formulation. Table 3-3 can serve as a checklist in the search for neurological dysfunction.

1.2.4. Neurological Family History

Neurological family history taking requires an intensive search for the "skeletons in the closet," the illnesses or maladies of family members hidden from view because of denial and/or suppression. Lengthy or terminal institutionalization of a family member raises clinical suspicions concerning Huntington's disease, dementia, and mental retardation. As in all history taking, redundancy and patience are critical elements. In addition to asking about family history in family members, qualify your

Table 3-3. Past Medical History Review

A. Complications of:
  1. Pregnancy (hyperemeis, toxemia, infection, diabetes, injury, toxin exposure, medication use)
  2. Labor (protracted, premature rupture of membranes, fetal distress)
  3. Delivery (premature or late, induced, general anesthesia utilization, problematic cesarian section, breech, cord around neck, problematic forceps, multiple birth, fetal cyanosis, or distress of any kind)
B. Apgar score if available
C. Childhood milestones: Any developmental observation that differentiates patient from siblings may be significant
D. Childhood behavioral anomalies:
  1. Somnambulism
  2. Motor hyperactivity
  3. Dysattention, absence episodes
  4. Enuresis
  5. Behavioral dyscontrol
  6. Cruelty to animals
  7. Firesetting
  8. Affective bizarreness
  9. Other sleep disturbances including night terrors, unusual nightmares, and narcoleptic syndromes
  10. Breath holding
E. Toxin exposure history
F. Childhood illnesses: Look for the presence of protracted febrile illnesses complicated by delirium and/or convulsions
G. Head injury history with or without loss of consciousness: Note the presence of concussive symptoms after head injury
H. Drug abuse: Special attention to hallucinogen abuse, intravenous substance administration, and alcohol use
I. Psychosocial history including sexual, educational, and interpersonal relatedness history

questions with declarations such as "on your mother's side or father's side," "aunts, uncles, cousins, grandparents, siblings," etc. Get your patient to ponder the question. Be patient.

1.3. The Neurological Physical Examination

Mastery of the neurological physical examination requires a good instructor and a great deal of practice. The psychiatrist wishing to improve on this examination should seek out a neurologist and spend an hour or two a week observing and then performing neurological examinations. For didactic study, the reader is referred to several excellent reviews.[4-7]

An emphasis on visual observation can often require a change in the clinical set of the psychiatrist, who has for so long paid attention to verbal language. Sometimes it is helpful to consciously ignore language and affective cues and concentrate on the visual array presented by the patient. Areas of concentration are outlined in Table 3-4.

2. Neurological Diseases with Psychiatric Presentations

2.1. Approaches

Chapter 2 of this book considered the "great mimickers" of psychiatry, medical illnesses with psychiatric presentations. Neurological disease can also be responsible

Table 3-4. Patient Observation

A. Body symmetry: Observe the stationary and moving patient for symmetry of gait, posture, limbs, face. These data provide clues to muscle tone, strength, and coordination.
B. Movement: Look for signs of rigidity, bradykinesia, dyskinesia, dysdiadochokinesia, stereotypy, and other adventitial movements.
   1. Rule out the presence of paucity, excess, or bizarreness of spontaneous movements.
   2. Are eye movements consensual?
   3. Quality and quantity of spontaneous speech. Is the patient dysphonic?
C. Behavior: Is the patient's behavior appropriate to the clinical setting? Describe how the behavior is inappropriate.
D. Modulation of affect: Is affective modulation observed to be appropriate to the stimuli of the interview? Be specific in describing affective changes.
E. Vigilance and task orientation:
   1. Is the patient hypervigilant and perhaps paranoid?
   2. Can the patient concentrate attention to a task at hand?
   3. The eyes give clues to attentiveness.
F. Higher cortical function observation: Much valuable mental state data can be gleaned from the observation during history taking of:
   1. Abstract language use, comprehension, and expression
   2. Problem-solving abilities
   3. Memory intactness
   4. Spatial abilities, e.g., does the patient bump into the door jamb walking into your office?
   5. Adequacy of grooming and dress
   6. Social poise

---

for false-positive psychiatric diagnoses. After all, the same organ system responsible for focal neurological signs produces the signs of psychiatric syndromes. Mental state change that results from brain pathology is influenced by (1) the location and function of the affected neural tissue, (2) the dynamic interaction between the dysfunctional tissue and the intact normal functioning tissue, and (3) the cumulative effects of cell loss on brain function.

It is absolutely critical that the psychiatric clinician consider mental state changes as focal neurological signs. A diagnostic conclusion that the patient's presenting signs and symptoms are psychiatric and nonneurological may arise from the confounding influence of the patient's personality style on the clinician's objectivity. Likewise, the personality dynamics of the clinician may influence what we attend to, downplay, or emphasize in the evaluation of our patients. Thus, neurological disease may "present" as psychiatric illness (1) because we are fooled by the symptom complexes themselves and base psychiatric diagnosis on so-called pathognomonic signs or the impressive bizarreness of the clinical picture, (2) because of the intermittent or stuttering course of the symptoms, (3) because our inability to adequately present a neurologically based explanation for the symptoms results in the conclusion that the cause must be functional, (4) because our cultural belief in free will and invincibility leads the clinician to deny the presence of illness, or (5) because we are all too often distracted by the presenting state of the patient rather than the wealth of information supplied by the course of the illness.

Ambrosino[8] provides a helpful approach to the problem of psychiatric misdiagnosis of neurological disease when he divides the clinical presentation of neurological dysfunction into (1) the release phenomena responsible for motoric, sensory, and cognitive disinhibition, (2) catastrophic, confabulatory, or referential reactions to higher cortical deficits, and (3) the direct tissue effect of the central nervous system lesion as exemplified by the dreamy states of partial complex seizure disorder. In addition, the presence of a poor historian, denial of illness, previous psychiatric history, and the reliance on history for symptom description if the patient is asymptomatic at the time of examination further complicate the neurological interview. The clinician who adopts an evaluative position that places the burden of proof on ruling out neurological or other organ system dysfunction performs a service for his patients. The clinician who rules in psychiatric disease after one or more traditional psychiatric interviews may, despite all good intentions, preclude a more comprehensive differential diagnostic understanding of the patient's presenting complaints.

2.2. Clinical Examples

2.2.1. The Alcoholic Brain Syndromes

The toxic effects of acute and chronic alcohol abuse on brain function produce a diversity of mental state changes. The alert clinician will notice aberrations throughout the entire higher cortical examination of Table 3-5. Representative alcohol syndromes are included in Table 3-6.

2.2.2. Central Nervous System Collagen-Vascular Disease

The cerebral vasculitis of systemic lupus erythematosus (SLE) can produce a myriad of "psychiatric" mental state symptoms ranging from depressed mood to frank psychosis. The nature of symptoms and clarity of the sensorium may depend on the cerebral location and extent of the vasculitis.

Psychiatric misdiagnosis may be made when the underlying collangenosis is quiescent or the diagnosis is based on negative laboratory testing and a non-central-nervous-system review of systems. At such times, the patient's symptoms are often ascribed to environmental events or to the individual's psychological adjustment to chronic disease. Rudin,[9] however, presents a challenging model for the development of a spectrum of "functional" psychiatric disorders ranging from schizophrenia to neuroses. Rudin postulates a covert immune complex disease of the choroid plexus resulting in membrane transport dysfunction of the limbic system. It is this tissue dysfunction that produces the personality change.

The clinical dictum that mental state symptoms in a patient with SLE are psychiatric if they present in the absence of "lupus cerebritis" should be revised to allow for a more intensive search for central nervous system dysfunction in this disease. Future use of positron emission tomography in these disorders will serve to enlighten this controversial issue.

2.2.3. Dementia

2.2.3a. Alzheimer's Dementia. Dementia of the Alzheimer's type is the principal degenerative brain disease encountered in psychiatric practice. Because these patients rarely complain of dementia or its deficits, their indifference may be misinterpreted as indicative of a psychiatric process. Early in the course of the disease, the presence of facetiousness, defensive humor, and confabulation in the face of generally intact personality function erroneously supports a psychiatric formulation. In addition, the loved ones accompanying the patient are themselves in a state of emotional disrepair because of the demands in caring for the Alzheimer patient. Family pressure may lead the psychiatrist to conclude that there are conscious or unconscious mechanisms at work in the patient and/or family responsible for the apparent emotional distress. With progression of the disease and the development of more apparent focal neurological deficits, the Alzheimer diagnosis is more easily made.

2.2.3b. Progressive Supranuclear Palsy. Subcortical brain failure presents us with another diagnostic dilemma because of the subtlety of symptoms present. To complicate matters, psychiatrists are not always attuned to evaluate subcortical brain function. Patients with progressive supranuclear palsy often look psychomotorically depressed, complain of dysmnesia, new knowledge utilization, and social indifference.[1,10] The dramatic inappropriateness of affective incontinence provides further false proof of an "emotional disorder."

2.2.3c. Binswanger's Dementia. The slow stuttering development of midlife cognitive deterioration, episodic psychiatric symptomatology, and signs of pseudo-

Table 3-5. The Neurological Physical Examination

A. Observation: See Table 3-4
B. Basic motor system testing
  1. Motor strength and motility should be tested in a systematic fashion starting at the head and working down the body to the feet with attention paid to differentiating proximal from distal motor function and upper from lower motor neuron dysfunction
    a. Passive range of motion of extremities provides valuable motor tone data. Look for the presence of clonus
    b. Deep tendon reflexes provide a more objective method of assessing muscle tone and the integrity of stretch receptor circuitry
  2. A brief screening examination is often helpful and includes having the patient
    a. Perform a deep knee bend
    b. Walk on toes and heels
    c. Negotiate getting into and out of a chair
    d. Grip examiner's hand
C. Coordinated motor system testing involves cerebellar, extrapyramidal, and pyramidal systems. Coordination difficulties in the face of intact pyramidal system testing suggest cerebellar and/or extrapyramidal pathology.
  1. Tandem gait: heel to toe
  2. Romberg test: In addition to the traditional "crucifixion" pose, have the patient touch the tip of his nose with the forefinger of each hand simultaneously.
  3. Rapid alternating movements of hands and feet
  4. Sequential rhythmic movements
    a. Heel to contralateral knee and down the shin
    b. Elbow to contralateral antecubital fossa and down the arm
    c. Apposition of thumb to fingers of the same hand
  5. Speech articulation
  6. Handwriting
D. Somesthesia testing: look for symmetry
  1. Light touch—use a wisp of cotton
  2. Position sense
    a. Up-and-down movement at a joint
    b. Two-point discrimination—requires parietal lobe function in addition
    c. Face–hand test (double simultaneous stimulation)
  3. Pain, pin prick
  4. Temperature, warm and cold test tubes
E. Bulbar integrity
  1. Cranial nerves of the medulla
    a. Hypoglossal (12): tongue motility
    b. Accessory (11): sternocleidomastoid and trapezius cervical muscles, joins vagus to innervate larynx: Shrug shoulders, turn head to resistance
    c. Vagus complex (10):
      i. Autonomic nervous system regulation of cardiac, pulmonary, gastrointestinal, and renal function
      ii. Visceral sensory innervation of pharynx, larynx, trachea, esophagus, and thoracic–abdominal viscera
      iii. Motor to pharynx to larynx
      iv. General sensory innervation of part of ear and auditory meatus.
    d. Glossopharyngeal (9):
      i. Sensory innervation of posterior one-third of tongue; taste
      ii. Motor to pharynx: gag reflex, symmetry of posterior pharynx, voice quality, fluid–swallowing ability; overlaps with cranial nerve 10
      iii. Sensory from carotid sinus: valsalva maneuver; overlaps with cranial nerve 10

(continued)

Table 3-5. (*Continued*)

  e. vestibulocochlear (acoustic, 8):
    i. Auditory acuity: watch ticking
    ii. Equilibrium: Romberg, gait
 2. Cranial nerves of the midbrain and pons
  a. Facial (7):
    i. Facial expression: spontaneous and instructed facial expression, observe resting symmetry of face
    ii. Motor to upper eyelid: open eyes against resistance
  b. Abducens (6): lateral rectus muscles of eye, lateral eyeball movements
  c. Trigeminal (5):
    i. Motor to muscles of mastication: clench jaw and teeth, chew
    ii. Motor to palate: swallowing
    iii. Motor to middle ear muscles
    iv. Sensory to three anatomic division of face: facial sensation, corneal reflex
  d. Trochlear (4): motor to superior oblique muscles of eye, downward gaze
  e. Oculomotor (3):
    i. Motor to medial rectus and inferior oblique eye muscles: medial and upward gaze, respectively
    ii. Autonomic motor to muscles of pupillary constriction to light and accommodation: swinging flashlight test, internal convergence test
    iii. Motor to upper eyelid
  f. Optic nerve (2): visual acuity, Snellen chart; visual field integrity, visual fields to confrontation
  g. Olfactory nerve (1): olfaction
F. Autonomic nervous system testing
 1. Vital signs including postural pulse and blood pressure
 2. Unusual skin rubor, pallor, or cyanosis
 3. Valsalva maneuver
 4. Pupillary response to light and accommodation
G. Higher cortical testing
 1. Orientation to time of day, place, person, and the present environment (doctor's office, hospital, nursing home, etc.)
 2. Attention and concentration
  a. Eye contact and vigilance
  b. Aphasia screen: note that the validity of the mental status examination depends on intact receptive and expressive langue function
    i. Comprehension of commands
    ii. Repetitive speech, "no if, ands, or buts"
    iii. Part–whole naming
    iv. Intact written language
  c. Serial 7s from 100 and/or serial 3s from 25
  d. Repetition of digits forwards and backwards
  e. Spelling a five-letter word forwards and backwards
  f. Memory: immediate, short-term, long-term
  g. Calculation
  h. Praxis: constructional, idiomotor
  i. Gnosis: tactile, body part and location, word
  j. Graphesthesia
  k. Frontal lobe release signs: palmomental, snout, suck, root, grasp
  l. Temporal lobe screen: episodic disturbance of:
    i. Perception: macropsia, hallucinosis, equilibrium
    ii. Reality experience: depersonalization, *déjà vu*, dreamy states
    iii. Affect: rage, attacks, giddiness
    iv. Attention: concentration, absence
    v. Autonomic function—tachycardia, vascular headache, syncope
    vi. Language: word-finding difficulties

Table 3-6. Alcoholic Brain Syndromes

A. Alcohol withdrawal with delirium tremens, alcoholic paranoia, and/or alcoholic hallucinosis: The presence of autonomic excitation, dysphoria, central nervous system excitation (increased reflexes, tremulousness, startle reactions, heightened sensory acuity), referential thinking, sleep disturbance with change in dreaming, and multisensory hallucinosis may lead to the following psychiatric misdiagnoses:
   1. Anxiety syndromes with or without panic or phobic components
   2. Affective syndromes, especially agitated depression
   3. Schizophrenic disorders with major paranoid or catatonic (excited) components
   4. Other psychotic states, e.g., reactive psychosis
   5. Paranoid disorders
   6. Dissociative syndromes
   7. Somatoform syndromes
B. Wernicke–Korsakoff syndrome: This well-known syndrome often presents the patient in a "bad light" because of the presence of confabulation, poor memory, and indifference in an individual with an otherwise relatively intact mental state. These patients can be mistaken for malingerers or diagnosed as having personality disorders.

---

bulbar palsy typify the subcortical multiple-infarct dementia of Binswanger. This diagnosis is not easily made from the clinical course of the illness. These unfortunate patients often seek psychiatric treatment before a computerized axial tomography (CAT) scan reveals periventricular density change.

2.2.4. Focal Degenerative Brain Disease

2.2.4a. Huntington's Disease. Once the dyskinesia and/or genetic pedigree of this disorder are obvious, psychiatric misdiagnosis is avoided. However, these patients can present with a veritable diagnostic manual of psychiatric signs and symptoms. Caine and Shoulson[11] take us through a differential description of mental state changes found in Huntington patients. It is no surprise that their findings are not dissimilar from the array of changes noted in other forms of degenerative brain disease and include dysfunction of arousal and attentional mechanisms, abnormalities of affective control and expression, perceptual and ideational disturbances, cognitive higher-order deficits, and general personality changes.

2.2.4b. Parkinson's Disease. Parkinson's disease is an example of a disorder that has become more complex and less well understood the more it has been studied. What appeared to be a circumscribed basal ganglia degenerative process with well-defined extrapyramidal symptoms has become a neuropsychiaric disorder with depressive signs, dementia, delirium, and formal visual hallucinosis.[12] Cummings and colleagues[13] reviewed the nonextrapyramidal symptoms in patients with idiopathic basal ganglia calcification and suggested that this type of subcortical pathology can result in a schizophreniform or dementia syndrome depending on age of presentation.

2.2.5. Central Nervous System Infections: Herpes Simplex Encephalitis

Viral central nervous system infections have a proclivity for the temporal lobes. Therefore, it is no surprise that the initial manifestations of viral encephalitis include more striking personality alterations than constitutional signs. The mortality and morbidity risk of herpes simplex encephalitis is such that rapid diagnosis of this condition is critical[14] A schizophreniform mental state may be quite prominent and serve as a "red herring" for the diagnostic process.

2.2.6. Demyelinating Disease: Multiple Sclerosis

Clinical lore has it that one of the most difficult differential diagnoses in neurology or psychiatry is between the diagnosis of multiple sclerosis and hysteria/conversion syndromes. The diverse effects of multiple, widespread, and apparently unrelated demyelination of the central nervous system produce a puzzling clinical picture that is further obscured by the recurrent remitting nature of the disease. Psychopathological complaints may be more impressive than motor or sensory complaints when the former include affective dyscontrol (e.g., hypomania, depression, temper outbursts, and labile emotionality), psychosis, or nonspecific personality change.

2.2.7. Epilepsy: Partial Complex Seizure Disorder

Partial complex seizure disorder, the new term for temporal lobe epilepsy, provides one of the best examples of a neurological process easily mistaken for psychiatric disease. A previous publication[1] reviews the diverse clinical appearance of this disorder, including perceptual, ideational, affective, ideomotor, and autonomic nervous system phenomena. The presence of interictal higher-order mental state changes, including obsessive-compulsiveness, difficulty with interpersonal closeness and intimacy, hypo- or hypersexuality, religiosity, mystical and existential preoccupation, affective constriction and aloofness, and schizophreniform states compound the problems in establishing the clinical diagnosis of epilepsy. Electroencephalography may be of variable assistance depending on the availability of video–telemetric monitoring and sphenoidal or nasopharyngeal leads.

2.2.8. Traumatic Brain Injury: Postconcussion Syndrome

Postconcussion syndrome is highlighted in this section. The diagnosis of postconcussion syndrome is difficult (1) because of the nonspecific and vague nature of subjective complaints such as "mild contusion," "fuzzy-headedness," "concentrating difficulties," "I don't feel like myself," "I've lost all drive and motivation," etc.; (2) because symptom onset may be delayed by hours to days; (3) because of the episodic and fluctuant nature of the symptoms; (4) because patients often complain of musculoskeletal problems and ignore or deny subtle changes in cognition; (5) because the complaint may appear to be out of proportion to the head injury itself; (6) because litigation and compensation aspects may color the clinical picture; and (7) because the syndrome may persist for as long as 2 or more years after the traumatic event.

Repeat awake, sleep, and sleep-deprived electroencephalograms, neuropsychological testing, and comprehensive neuropsychiatric examination are a must in this disorder. The presence of adequate premorbid psychosocial functioning often offers clues to this neurological diagnosis.

2.2.9. Central Nervous System Mass Lesions

Cerebral neoplasms, cerebrovascular thrombi or hemorrhage, subdural hematomas, third-ventricle colloid cysts, cerebral abscesses, and gummae produce neuropsychiatric symptoms based on (1) the function(s) of the tissue the mass resides in, (2) how adjacent and/or distant cerebral functional centers "perceive" the dysfunctional tissue, and (3) the generalized effects of the increased cranial pressure that results from a growing tissue mass. The latter can be catastrophic, as in uncal herniation, or insidious, as exemplified by slowly developing hydrocephalus.

The effects of mass lesions in "silent" cortical areas reveal themselves to be not so silent when careful neuropsychological testing is employed. A working understanding of a higher cortical neuropsychological screening examination (D. A. Gross and M. S. Gold, unpublished work) is an essential part of the clinician's evaluative repertoire. This implies the ability to differentiate dominant versus nondominant hemispheric function, anterior versus posterior cortical functions, and cortical versus subcortical functions. A clinician cannot rest easy because the patient does not demonstrate classic focal neurological signs. As mentioned previously, changes in the display of complex behavior, affect, and ideation that we term mental state often represent focal neurological signs.

References

1. Gross DA: Medical origins of psychiatric emergencies: The systems approach. *Int J Psychiatry Med* 11:1–24, 1981.
2. Rickler KC: Neurological diagnosis in psychiatric disease. *Psychiatr Ann* 13:408–411, 1983.
3. Malmo RB: Anxiety and behavioral arousal. *Psychol Rev* 64:276–287, 1957.
4. Mancall EL: *Alpers and Mancall's Essentials of the Neurologic Examination,* ed 2. Philadelphia, F A Davis, 1981.
5. Van Allen MW, Rodnitzky RL: *Pictorial Manual of Neurologic Tests,* ed 2. Chicago, Year Book Medical Publishers, 1981.
6. DeJong RN: *Tne Neurologic Examination,* ed 4. New York, Harper & Row, 1979.
7. Strub RL, Black FW: *The Mental Status Examination in Neurology.* Philadelphia, F A Davis, 1977.
8. Ambrosino SJ: Neurological signs and symptoms that pose as psychiatric problems. *Resident Staff Physician* 56–62, 1973.
9. Rudin DO: The choroid plexus and system disease in mental illness. I. A new brain attack mechanism via the second blood–brain barrier. *Biol Psychiatry* 15:517–539, 1980.
10. Albert ML, Feldman RG, Willis AC: The subcortical dementia of progressive supranuclear palsy. *J Neurol Neurosurg Psychiatry* 37:121–130, 1974.
11. Caine ED, Shoulson I: Psychiatric syndromes in Huntington's disease. *Am J Psychiatry* 140:728–733, 1983.
12. Rabins PV: Psychopathology of Parkinson's disease. *Comp Psychiatry* 23:421–429, 1982.
13. Cummings JL, Gosenfeld LF, Houlihan JP, et al: Neuropsychiatric disturbances associated with idiopathic calcification of the basal ganglia. *Biol Psychiatry* 18:591–601, 1980.
14. Lauter CB: Herpes simplex encephalitis: A great clinical challenge. *Ann Intern Med* 93:696–698, 1980.

Tests of the Hypothalamic–Pituitary–Adrenal Axis

Mark S. Gold, M.D., and Michael H. Kronig, M.D.

1. The Hypothalamic–Pituitary–Adrenal Axis

Circulating glucocorticoids are released and regulated by the hypothalamic–pituitary–adrenal (HPA) axis. This axis is of importance in psychiatry because abnormalities in cortisol production are the most extensively studied and the most robust neuroendocrine findings in depressive disorders. In essence, the hypothalamus stimulates the pituitary, which in turn stimulates the adrenals to produce cortisol.[1,2]

Corticotropin-releasing factor (CRF) was the first hypothalamic releasing factor recognized. It is a neurohormone whose structure has not yet been determined. Axons from the limbic system impact on the cells in the hypothalamus that release CRF. The process is known as neuroendocrine transduction, whereby neuronal (electrical) signals are changed into hormonal (blood-borne) messages. Although experimental data in humans are incomplete and somewhat controversial, it appears that CRF secretion is stimulated by serotonin (5-HT) and acteylcholine (ACh) and inhibited by norepinephrine (NE).

Corticotropin-releasing factor is released into the hypophyseal portal blood system and is carried to the anterior pituitary, where it stimulates the release of adrenocorticotropic hormone (ACTH), a polypeptide with 39 residues. ACTH is the major regulator of glucocorticoids (cortisol) and those sex steroids that are produced by the adrenals (androsterone and androstenedione). The half-life of injected ACTH is about 10 min, and its biological activity seems to be similarly transient.

ACTH is released in bursts into the peripheral circulation, where it binds to specific cells in the adrenal cortex. Via a cAMP "second messenger" system, it stimulates the production and release of steroids. For our purposes we focus on the principal glucocorticoid, cortisol, as the other steroids are of lesser importance in the study of psychiatric disorders. The cortisol response to a burst of ACTH is detectable within 3 min; it continues to rise to a peak at about 10 min and then declines over the

Mark S. Gold, M.D. • Research Facilities, Fair Oaks Hospital, Summit, New Jersey 07901, and Fair Oaks Hospital, at Boca/Delray, Delray Beach, Florida 33445.   *Michael H. Kronig, M.D.* • Hillside Hospital, A Division of the Long Island Jewish Medical Center, Glen Oaks, New York 11004.

next 10 min or so. Cortisol has a half-life of about 60–90 min. It is about 75% bound to transcortin, 15% bound to albumin, and 10% free.

In normals, plasma cortisol has a diurnal variation with lowest levels in the late evening and highest levels shortly before awakening. There are about eight or nine secretory bursts during the day, for a total of about 16 mg cortisol released per day. Feedback loops exist whereby cortisol interacts both at the pituitary and hypothalamus, and perhaps even at the limbic level, to inhibit the HPA axis.

2. Cortisol Production in Psychiatric Illness

Since the mid-1960s there have been reports of increased cortisol production in patients with depressive disorders.[3,4] Although studies are methodologically different, there is general agreement that cortisol is elevated in CSF, plasma, and urine.[5] The CSF measures of cortisol are of research interest only, as it is not feasible to perform routine lumbar punctures on psychiatric patients in the usual outpatient or hospital setting. As Carroll and colleagues[6] note, 24-hr urinary collections for cortisol are in some ways superior to base-line plasma cortisol determinations because the urinary measures give an indication of cortisol release over time. Since cortisol production is pulsatile, plasma measures in the base-line condition are variable, depending on whether one happens to draw blood during a peak or a trough in production.

Carroll's group refined previous work in this area by measuring 24-hr urinary free cortisol (UFC) in 95 patients, 60 with depressive illness and 35 with other diagnoses. The UFC is a more accurate reflection of cortisol secretion than urinary measures of 17-hydroxycorticosteroids (17-OHCS) or 17-ketogenic steroids (17-KGS). Bipolar and unipolar patients had significantly elevated UFC as compared to patients diagnosed as depressive neurosis or other psychiatric diagnosis. In many patients, the elevation in UFC was into the range seen in patients with Cushing's disease. Eleven patients were restudied following treatment with electroconvulsive therapy (ECT). Their 24-hr UFC fell significantly compared with pretreatment values, although posttreatment values were still greater than those seen in patients without unipolar or bipolar depression.[6] A later study by another team of investigators confirmed Carroll's pretreatment results.

Sachar and colleagues[7] studied cortisol secretory patterns in seven depressed patients and 54 normals. They used an indwelling venous catheter and drew blood samples every 30 min for 24-hr. Depressed patients had elevated cortisol levels at all times. This increase was statistically significant from 12 noon through the evening and night and until about 4 a.m. In addition to elevated cortisol levels, depressed patients had a flattened curve with a loss of some of the circadian pattern of normals.

There are methodological problems if one attempts to use either the 24-hr UFC or catheter studies routinely. The test that is most frequently used to identify abnormalities of the HPA in depressed patients is the dexamethasone suppression test (DST). As is discussed below, it is methodologically simple, is well tolerated by patients, and, when administered correctly, has high predictive value.

3. The Dexamethasone Suppression Test

Dexamethasone is a synthetic glucocorticoid that is widely used in medicine. In normal individuals, dexamethasone exerts negative feedback on the HPA at the pituitary and probably also at the hypothalamic level. It acts much in the same way as endogenous cortisol to "turn off" the HPA and thereby reduce cortisol secretion. In normals, a 1-mg dose of oral dexamethasone given at 11 p.m. will reduce plasma cortisol levels to less than 5 μg/dl for the next 24 hr. By way of contrast, normal cortisol values without dexamethasone are up to 25 μg/dl in the morning and less than 6 μg/dl around midnight. The DST was first used to diagnose patients with Cushing's disease, who were found to be resistant to dexamethasone. That is, plasma cortisol remains elevated despite dexamethasone. Since some depressed patients exhibited overactivity of the HPA, the DST was then used to study psychiatric populations.

The DST has been studied by many groups of investigators. Carroll and colleagues[8] began by studying a group of patients with "endogenomorphic depression" (by DSM III criteria, these patients would fit most closely into the category of major depression, with melancholia, except for some bipolar patients, depressed type, who also had features of melancholia). They found that approximately 50% of such patients had elevated postdexamethasone cortisol values, which is called "positive DST" or "dexamethasone nonsuppression." Only about 4% of normals or patients with other psychiatric diagnoses had a positive DST. The most common pattern of positive DST is "early escape": patients suppress normally the morning after dexamethasone but escape from suppression later in the day.[9]

Many other investigators have studied the DST in endogenous depression. Although there is some variability in sensitivity and specificity, probably as a result of technical and diagnostic differences, there is a remarkable consensus that the DST is abnormal in approximately 50% of endogenously depressed patients and is positive in no more than 10% of controls.[10–17]

Does a positive DST identify cortisol hypersecretors as defined by elevated 24 hour plasma cortisol? Asnis and colleagues[18] compared DST results (using 2 mg dexamethasone) with mean 24-hr plasma cortisol (obtained from an indwelling catheter). About half of the hypersecretors (mean 24-hr cortisol 8 μg/dl) were also dexamethasone nonsuppressors. Only one patient with a normal mean 24-hr cortisol had a positive DST. Therefore, the 2-mg DST is fairly specific for cortisol hypersecretion but "misses" about half the patients with elevated mean 24-hr cortisol. The 1-mg DST, which results in more positive tests (nonsuppression), may be more sensitive.

3.1. Clinical Correlates

Many psychiatric patients present with a chief complaint of "depression"; their diagnoses include just about the full range of psychiatric disorders. Just whom does the DST identify? The answer is not 100% straightforward because of the various diagnostic systems in use. Carroll found the DST to be highly specific for melancholia, which is similar to the concept of "endogenous depression."[19] Schlesser and colleagues[20] had essentially similar results when dividing patients into primary unipolar depression (patients with no other psychiatric diagnosis, 65/146 DST-positive) versus secondary unipolar depression (preexisting nonaffective psychiatric disorder, 0/42 DST-positive). Most investigators have found the DST equally sensitive for both unipolar and bipolar depression. An exception is Rothschild and colleagues,[21] who found DST to have low sensitivity in bipolar depression. There is disagreement about whether a positive DST correlates with severity of depression. Overall, the data point toward a positive correlation between symptom severity and rate of positive DST. In one small sample, there was an indication that DST nonsuppression was correlated with later suicide.[22]

3.2. Standardization and Technical Considerations

Many of the discrepant results reported by different groups can be explained on the basis of different testing procedures. For example, the 1-mg DST will result in more positive tests than will the 2-mg DST. The more postdexamethasone blood samples one draws, the higher is the probability of obtaining an elevated cortisol.

Carroll and colleagues[19] have standardized the DST by experimenting with different doses, time points, and cut-off criteria for a "positive" cortisol value. This standard procedure is as follows: 1 mg dexamethasone is given at about 11 p.m. The next day, blood is drawn for cortisol at 4 p.m. and 11 p.m. (The 8 a.m. blood draw used in early studies was found to add little additional information, since many melancholic patients show normal 8 a.m. suppression but "escape" from suppression later on.) No dietary or activity restrictions are necessary. The cortisol values must be determined in a laboratory equipped to accurately measure cortisol in the lower ranges. It is usually done by competitive protein binding or radioimmunoassay. A positive test is defined as any postdexamethasone cortisol > 5 µg/dl.

3.3. Exclusion Criteria

There are no absolute contraindications to performing a DST. However, there are many factors that interfere with the interpretation of test results. A high percentage of abnormal DSTs are found in patients with alcoholism, anorexia nervosa, malnutrition, obesity, tumors that secrete ACTH, Cushing's syndrome, renovascular hypertension, chronic hemodialysis, and acute medical illnesses or major trauma.[23] Weight loss itself may cause dexamethasone nonsuppression in nondepressed subjects.[24]

Many drugs also interfere with interpretation of the DST. In depressed patients, dexamethasone half-life is similar to that found in normals; therefore, the abnormal DST in depressed patients is not caused by differences in dexamethasone metabolism. Drugs such as phenytoin, barbiturates, carbamazepine, and rifampicin increase corticosteroid catabolism. Dexamethasone is cleared faster, and the result is a false-positive DST. Patients on steroids, including topical and nasal preparations, may show cortisol suppression and therefore false-negative tests. Whether oral contraceptives in the usual doses also cause false negatives is unclear. By an unknown mechanism, high-dose benzodiazepines may also result in false-negative tests. Most psychotropics do not seem to affect directly interpretation of the DST including tricyclic antidepressants, MAO inhibitors, lithium, neuroleptics, and low-dose benzodiazepines. It is thought that psychotropics may normalize the DST, but only as a result of their successfully treating depression. However, there is a paucity of controlled studies in this area. Since antidepressants affect 5-HT, NE, and ACh, all of which regulate CRF release, it is certainly possible that they would alter DST results even without reversing depression.

3.4. Indications for DST

3.4.1. Diagnosing Major Depression

The main indication for performing the DST is for the confirmation of suspected major depression.[23] A positive test is excellent confirmatory evidence of the diagnosis. Using Carroll's figures and methods (blood drawings at 4 p.m. and 11 p.m.), one assumes a 50% prevalence of melancholia in a given population. A positive test then carries a diagnostic confidence of 94%, whereas a negative result carries a 74% diagnostic confidence for ruling out melancholia. Thus, the clinician has hard evidence for his diagnosis and increased certainty that somatic treatment is warranted. Whether a positive DST is a good predictor of favorable response to somatic treatment remains controversial. Some studies are limited by lack of controlled[10] or adequate treatment.[25] In other treatment studies, there are differences in the diagnostic mix of DST-positive and DST-negative group.[11] Kane *et al.*[26] treated a homogeneous group of patients with desipramine up to 300 mg daily (mean 227 mg daily) and found an identical 78% response rate among suppressors and nonsuppressors. Using a lower dose of desipramine (125–200 mg daily), Ettigi found that a positive DST did correlate with favorable response.[17]

In addition to providing the clinician with objective evidence of major depression, a positive DST also confirms for the patient that he/she has an illness, often making it easier for him/her to accept treatment. We have seen several depressed patients, among them scientists, engineers, and physicians, who had resisted and refused antidepressant treatment until they could be shown that they had a major depression with biochemical changes.

3.4.2. Following Course of Treatment

For patients with an initially positive DST, repeat DSTs can be used to monitor treatment response.[27] The DST should normalize in association with full clinical recovery. If a patient has apparently improved but clinically the DST remains abnormal, early relapse is likely to occur if treatment is discontinued.[28] In the inpatient setting, we recommend repeat DSTs prior to discharge in patients with an initial abnormal result; we feel that continued nonsuppressors must be watched especially closely and will consider alternative somatic therapy if clinical improvement is less than complete. We strongly advise repeat DSTs prior to discontinuing antidepressants and would not discontinue medication if the DST were positive. The DST also normalizes in patients who respond to ECT, and frequently this normalization occurs quite early in those who eventually respond, even before observable clinical improvement. Thus, the DST can be used to monitor treatment response much in the same way that the patient with a myocardial infarction is monitored with serial EKGs and cardiac enzymes. Note that repeat DSTs should be performed at least 1 week apart to prevent contamination from the prior tests. Also, there is little indication for repeat DSTs in patients who are initially dexamethasone suppressors unless their clinical condition deteriorates.

3.4.3. Diagnostic Dilemmas

Several groups of patients regularly present as diagnostic problems. The first is the group of schizoaffective disorders. Schizoaffective patients have abnormal DSTs in about the same percentage as patients with major depression.[29] The DST can therefore be used to rule in an "affective component" to the clinical picture. Although it has not been studied double blind, we feel that dexamethasone-resistant schizoaffective patients should guide the psychiatrist toward somatic treatment for depression.

Patients with schizophreniform disorders are first-break patients with less than 6 months' duration of symptoms. They are often later recategorized as schizophrenic or as affective disorder. Both fluphenazine and lithium have been shown effective in schizophreniform patients. It seems important to identify those patients who have primarily affective disease as opposed to schizophrenia, since that may guide the choice of maintenance treatment. So far there are no reliable clinical indicators to tease apart these two groups. Targum[30] reports that an abnormal DST can help in this distinction. What remains to be studied is whether schizophreniform patients with abnormal DSTs actually do better on lithium or tricyclic maintenance as opposed to neuroleptics.

It has long been postulated that some alcoholics and substance abusers are actually self-medicating for depression. Depressive affect is certainly common among these groups, and identification of endogenous depression would be useful. Alcohol itself can cause false-positive results on the DST,[31] with one group reporting that 62% of patients undergoing withdrawal exhibit dexamethasone nonsuppression.[32] Most of these patients switch to dexamethasone suppression within 3–4 weeks after completion of withdrawal. In this study, 28% were DST positive after 3–6 weeks of abstinence.[32] This group may represent a subset of alcoholics who would respond favorably to antidepressants. This question has not been studied in double-blind fashion, but anecdotal reports are encouraging. The same questions exist in substance abusers and need further study. Dackis and colleagues[33] report that among opiate addicts abstinent for 2 weeks, the DST was abnormal in 15 of 42 patients. Twelve of the 15 patients were diagnosed as depressed. Only two of 27 addicts without depression had a positive DST.

3.4.4. Major Depression in Children and Adolescents

This is being recognized with greater frequency, with these groups being symptomatically similar to their adult counterparts. Extein and colleagues[34] have found that the 1-mg DST identifies major depression in adolescents with reliability similar to that obtained in adults: 53% sensitive and 92% specific. A positive DST may predict good response to antidepressants in the group.

Other diagnostic problems for which the DST may be useful include the depression presenting as catatonia,[35] depressive pseudodementia versus true dementia,[36] reversible depression in stroke victims,[37] and severe character disorders with coexisting major depression.[29]

3.5. Caution in Interpretation of the DST

As has just been reviewed, the DST is sensitive and specific for the diagnosis of major depression with melancholia provided that patients are carefully screened for medical illness and use of drugs that interfere with the DST. Most importantly, patients need to be screened for depressive symptoms. This seemingly obvious statement is often overlooked. If one administers the DST more or less randomly, the absolute number of false positives will increase, and the diagnostic confidence of a positive test will fall dramatically. Patients should have clinical signs and symptoms that at least point towards a major depression, or the DST results will be uninterpretable.

4. Summary

Cortisol secretion is evaluated in a significantly large subgroup of patients with major depression. The mechanism appears to be hyperactivity of the HPA axis at the level of the hypothalamus, probably as a result of alterations in neurotransmitter turnover. Many research strategies have been used to measure cortisol in psychiatric illness, but the major clinical tool is the 1-mg dexamethasone suppression test. The DST can be used to confirm the diagnosis of major depression, to follow the course of treatment, and as an aid in differential diagnosis. Although abnormal in 30–70% of patients with major depression and schizoaffective disorder, depressed, the DST is abnormal in only 0–10% of patients with other psychiatric disorders or with no psychiatric diagnosis. Care must be taken to exclude from study patients with certain medical illness or who use certain drugs or alcohol.

References

1. Liddle GW: The adrenal cortex, in Williams RH (ed): *Textbook of Endocrinology.* Philadelphia, W B Saunders, 1974, pp 233–282.
2. Martin JB, Reichlin S, Brown GM: *Clinical Neuroendocrinology.* Philadelphia, F A Davis, 1977.
3. Gibbons JL: Cortisol secretion rate in depressive illness. *Arch Gen Psychiatry* 10:572–575, 1964.
4. Sachar EJ, Hellman L, Fukushima DK, et al: Cortisol production in depressive illness. *Arch Gen Psychiatry* 23:289–298, 1970.
5. Carroll BJ, Curtis GC, Mendels J: Cerebrospinal fluid and plasma free cortisol concentrations in depression. *Psychol Med* 6:235–244, 1976.
6. Carroll BJ, Curtis GC, Davies BM, et al: Urinary free cortisol excretion in depression. *Psychol Med* 6:43–50, 1976.
7. Sachar EJ, Hellman L, Roffwang HP: Disrupted 24-hour patterns of cortisol secretion in psychotic depression. *Arch Gen Psychiatry* 28:19–24, 1973.
8. Carroll BJ, Curtis GC, Mendels J: Neuroendocrine regulation in depression: II. Discrimination of depressed from non-depressed patients. *Arch Gen Psychiatry* 33:1051–1058, 1976.
9. Carroll BJ, Curtis GC, Mendels J: Neuroendocrine regulation in depression: I. Limbic system–adrenocortical dysfunction. *Arch Gen Psychiatry* 33:1039–1044, 1976.
10. Brown WA, Johnston R, Mayfield D: The 24-hour dexamethasone suppression test in a clinical setting: Relationship to diagnosis, symptoms, and response to treatment. *Am J Psychiatry* 136:543–547, 1979.
11. Brown WA, Shuey I: Response to dexamethasone and subtype of depression. *Arch Gen Psychiatry* 37:747–751, 1980.
12. Brown WA, Qualls CB: Pituitary–adrenal disinhibition in depression: Marker of a subtype with characteristic clinical features and response to treatment? *Psychiatry Res* 4:115–128, 1981.
13. Schatzberg AF, Rothschild AJ, Stahl JB, et al: The dexamethasone suppression test: Identification of subtypes of depression. *Am J Psychiatry* 140:88–91, 1983.
14. Stokes PE, Pick GR, Stoll PM, et al: Pituitary–adrenal function in depressed patients: Resistance to dexamethasone suppression. *J Psychiatr Res* 12:271–281, 1975.

15. Gold MS, Pottash ALC, Extein I, et al: Diagnosis of depression in the 1980's. *JAMA* 245:1562–1564, 1981.
16. Evans DL, Nemeroff CB: Use of the dexamethasone suppression test using DSM-III criteria on an inpatient psychiatric unit. *Biol Psychiatry* 18:505–511, 1982.
17. Ettigi PG, Hayes PE, Narasimhaehari N, et al: *d*-Amphetamine response and dexamethasone suppression test as predictors of treatment outcome in unipolar depression. *Biol Psychiatry* 18:499–504, 1983.
18. Asnis GM, Sachar EJ, Halbreich U, et al: Cortisol secretion and dexamethasone response in depression. *Am J Psychiatry* 138:1218–1221, 1981.
19. Carroll BJ, Feinberg M, Greden JF, et al: A specific laboratory test for the diagnosis of melancholia: Standardization, validation and clinical utility. *Arch Gen Psychiatry* 38:15–22, 1981.
20. Schlesser MA, Winokur G, Sherman BM: Hypothalamic–pituitary–adrenal axis activity in depressive illness: Its relationship to classification. *Arch Gen Psychiatry* 37:737–743, 1980.
21. Rothschild AJ, Schatzberg AF, Rosenbaum AH, et al: The dexamethasone suppression test as a discriminator among subtypes of psychotic patients. *Br J Psychiatry* 141:471–474, 1982.
22. Coryell W, Schlesser MA: Suicide and the dexamethasone suppression test in unipolar depression. *Am J Psychiatry* 138:1120–1121, 1981.
23. Kalin NH, Risch SC, Janowsky DS, et al: Use of the dexamethasone suppression test in clinical psychiatry. *J Clin Psychopharmacol* 1:64–69, 1981.
24. Edelstein CK, Roy-Byrne P, Fawzy FI, et al: Effects of weight loss on the dexamethasone suppression test. *Am J Psychiatry* 140:338–341, 1983.
25. Nelson WH, Orr WW, Stevenson JM, et al: Hypothalamic–pituitary–adrenal axis activity and tricyclic response in major depression. *Arch Gen Psychiatry* 39:1033–1036, 1982.
26. Green HS, Kane JM: The dexamethasone suppression test in depression. *Clin Neuropharmacol* 6:7–24, 1983.
27. Albala AA, Greden JF, Tarika J, et al: Changes in serial dexamethasone suppression tests among unipolar depressives receiving electroconvulsive treatment. *Biol Psychiatry* 16:551–560, 1981.
28. Greden JF, Albala AA, Haskett RF, et al: Normalization of dexamethasone suppression test: A laboratory index of recovery from endogenous depression. *Biol Psychiatry* 15:449–458, 1980.
29. Carroll BJ: The dexamethasone suppression test for melancholia. *Br J Psychiatry* 140:292–304, 1982.
30. Targum SD: Neuroendocrine dysfunction in schizophreniform disorder: Correlation with six-month clinical outcome. *Am J Psychiatry* 140:309–313, 1983.
31. Newsom G, Murray N: Reversal of dexamethasone test non-suppression in alcohol abusers. *Am J Psychiatry* 140:353–354, 1983.
32. Abou-Saleh MT, Merry J, Coppen A: Dexamethasone suppression test in alcoholism. *Acta Psychiatr Scand* 69:112–116, 1984.
33. Dackis CA, Pottash ALC, Gold MS, et al: The dexamethasone suppression test for major depression among opiate addicts. *Am J Psychiatry* 141:810–811, 1984.
34. Extein I, Rosenberg G, Pottash ALC, et al: The dexamethasone suppression test in depressed adolescents. *Am J Psychiatry* 139:1617–1619, 1982.
35. Greden JF, Carroll BJ: The dexamethasone suppression test as a diagnostic aid in catatonia. *Am J Psychiatry* 136:1199–1200, 1979.
36. McAllister TW, Ferrell RB, Price TRP, et al: The dexamethasone suppression test in two patients with severe depressive pseudodementia. *Am J Psychiatry* 139:479–480, 1982.
37. Finklestein S, Benowitz LI, Baldessarini RJ, et al: Mood, vegetative disturbance, and dexamethasone suppression test after stroke. *Ann Neurol* 12:463–486, 1982.

Thyroid Testing in Psychiatric Patients

Michael H. Kronig, M.D., and Mark S. Gold, M.D.

1. The Hypothalamic–Pituitary–Thyroid Axis

The thyroid gland is one link in the neuroendocrine system known as the hypothalamic–pituitary–thyroid (HPT) axis.[1–3] Within this axis, circulating thyroid hormones are tightly regulated by both central nervous system input and peripheral feedback control. The hypothalamus secretes thyrotropin-releasing hormone (TRH) into the portal system of the adenohypophysis; TRH stimulates the pituitary thyrotrope cells to release thyroid-stimulating hormone (thyrotropin, TSH), which in turn increases the rates of iodide uptake, hormone synthesis, and release of thyroxine (T_4) and triiodothyronine (T_3).

Input from the hypothalamus is essential for normal thyroid function.[2,3] Experimental lesions that destroy or disconnect the hypothalamus from the pituitary result in hypothyroidism.[4] Thus, it appears that the major hypothalamic input is stimulatory. Blood from the hypophyseal portal system stimulates the pituitary to release TSH.[5] The active substance, TRH, is a tripeptide hormone.[6] By a variety of techniques such as microlesions, biopsies, electrical stimulation, and, finally, immunoassay, TRH was found in the highest concentrations in specific areas of the hypothalamus.[2,7,8] Of theoretical interest, TRH is widely distributed throughout the brain and spinal cord.[7,8] It is estimated that as much as 80% of TRH is extrahypothalamic; this extrahypothalamic TRH may act as a peptide neurotransmitter.

The release of TRH is controlled at least in part by monoamine neurotransmitters.[2,3,6,9] Animal studies indicate that dopamine (DA) and norepinephrine (NE) increase TRH release, whereas serotonin (5-HT) inhibits TRH release. The acetylcholine (ACh) analogue carbachol has no effect.[9] There is little human data available at this time, except for one study that tends to support the fact that serotonin inhibits TRH release.[10] Of course, alterations in these same neurotransmitters—NE, 5-HT, DA, and, more recently, ACh—are thought to be involved in the pathophysiology of a variety of psychiatric disorders.

Thyrotropin is found in specific basophilic (thyrotrope) cells of the anterior pitui-

Michael H. Kronig, M.D. • Hillside Hospital, A Division of The Long Island Jewish Medical Center, Glen Oaks, New York 11004.   *Mark S. Gold, M.D.* • Research Facilities, Fair Oaks Hospital, Summit, New Jersey 07901, and Fair Oaks Hospital at Boca/Delray, Delray Beach, Florida 33445.

tary, which are discrete from those cells that secrete gonadotropins and ACTH.[1-3] It is a glycoprotein (molecular weight 28,000) with two subunits. Once released into the blood, it circulates unbound and has a half-life of 50–60 min.[11] Thyrotropin levels in man have a circadian rhythm with the highest levels from 4 a.m. to 8 a.m.[12]

Thyrotropin-releasing hormone interacts with specific high-affinity receptors at the pituitary[13] to stimulate the release of TSH, probably via a cAMP "second messenger" system.[14] The TRH-induced TSH response is altered by other hormones. Estrogen enhances TSH release, whereas glucocorticoids, growth hormone, and somatostatin inhibit TSH release.[2,15,16]

In addition to control from hypothalamic centers, the release of TSH is under negative feedback from circulating thyroid hormones. Circulating T_3 and T_3 made locally (within the thyrotrope) from the monodeiodination of T_4 interact with a receptor on the cell nucleus. Presumably, a protein is synthesized that competitively interferes with the thyrotrope's responsiveness to TRH. The TSH release is suppressed, and stimulation of the thyroid gland decreases.

The thyroid gland secretes primarily T_4 but also T_3.[17,18] Thyroxine is deiodinated by the liver, kidneys, and other peripheral tissues to T_3.[19] Most of the thyroid hormone bioactivity is provided by T_3.[13,18] Only a small percentage of T_3 and T_4 circulate free, with the major part bound to proteins such as thyroid-binding globulin (TBG) and thyroid-binding prealbumin (TBPA). The presence of dietary iodide (I^-) is crucial for the production of thyroid hormones. Insufficient iodide leading to hypothyroidism and goiter was previously common in certain sections of the United States but is now rare because of the addition of iodide to salt and packaged foods.

2. Base-Line Thyroid Testing

In the past, the only laboratory methods available were the measurement of circulating thyroid hormones. This situation has changed, and the clinician should be familiar with the newer thyroid tests.

2.1. Triiodothyronine, T_4, and T_3 Resin Uptake

Circulating thyroid hormones used to be measured by protein-bound iodine (PBI) or T_4 by column chromatography. These methods lack sensitivity and specificity and are of historical interest only. The most widely used assays for T_4 are the competitive protein-binding assay and the radioimmunoassay. Because both of these techniques measure total T_4, they are influenced by changes in the number of binding sites. Binding capacity is increased in conditions such as pregnancy and hepatitis and with the use of certain medications (estrogens, perphenazine). It is decreased in major illness, nephrotic syndrome, and with other medications (salicylate, phenytoin).[18]

To help correct for these changes in binding capacity, the T_3 resin uptake (T_3RU) determination is performed. This is a measurement of the number of thyroid hormone binding sites available. A standard amount of the patient's serum is mixed with radioactively labeled T_3 (T_3^*) and with a resin that absorbs thyroid hormones. The T_3^* that is not absorbed by binding sites in the patient's serum is absorbed by the added resin, which is then measured. If the patient has an excess of thyroid hormone (hyperthyroidism) or a decrease in binding sites, most of the patient's binding sites are already filled, and there is a surplus of T_3* absorbed by the resin. The opposite is true in hypothyroidism or when binding sites are increased. Interpretation of the T_3RU, then, is as follows: increased T_3RU indicates a decrease in available binding sites, and decreased T_3RU indicates an increase in available binding sites.

2.2. Other Measures

Other measures are free T_4 by a dialysis technique, T_3 by radioimmunoassay, and free T_3 by dialysis. The free thyroxin index (FTI) is the product of total T_4 and T_3RU. It is a calculated value that generally correlates well with free T_4 as measured by dialysis.

2.3. Reverse T_3

Thyroxine is deiodinated to T_3 by removal of an iodine atom from the "outer" (phenol) ring. However, as much as 30–40% of T_4 is deiodinated on the "inner" (tyrosine) ring to form reverse T_3 (RT_3). This is an apparently inactive form of T_3 that can be measured by radioimmunoassay.[17] Its importance is just being investigated. One theory is that an abnormal increase in deiodination to RT_3 rather than T_3 would result in hypothyroid states.

2.4. Thyrotropin

Circulating levels of TSH are now measured routinely by radioimmunoassay. The TSH level yields a measure of compensatory pituitary function and responsiveness to feedback.[17,18] If circulating free T_4 and T_3 decrease for any reason, the pituitary loses its T_3-induced inhibition. It becomes more sensitive to TRH, and the release of TSH increases relative to the person's previous base line or to normal. The thyroid gland is then stimulated in an attempt to maintain output in the normal range. If the thyroid fails to produce sufficient hormone, this cycle continues, and eventually the clinical picture of hypothyroidism emerges. At this point the laboratory data will reveal decreased T_4 and elevated TSH. An elevated TSH is present only when the thyroid is failing or with rare TSH-secreting tumors.

3. Thyrotropin-Releasing Hormone Thyroid Test

The TRH stimulation test is a provocative test of the HPT axis at the pituitary level that can also shed light on the state of the thyroid gland itself.[18,20] In this test, the responsiveness of the thyrotrope to a TRH challenge is measured. Our technique is as follows. The patient is fasted overnight. At about 8:30 a.m., the patient is asked to lie in a comfortable position, and a butterfly needle is inserted in standard fashion. The vein is kept patent by a slow drip of normal saline. Blood is drawn for TSH, T_4, T_3RIA, and T_3RU at 8:59. Then, a 500-mg bolus of synthetic TRH (protirelin) is injected over 30–60 sec. Side effects noted are transient and include a feeling of warmth, desire to urinate or defecate, nausea, metallic taste, headache, dry mouth, chest tightness, and a pleasant genital sensation. Blood is drawn for TSH 15, 30, 60, and 90 min after the TRH is infused. The base-line TSH value is subtracted from the peak TSH to give the ΔTSH. In normals, ΔTSH is 7–15 μIU/ml. Hypothyroid patients have supersensitivity to the TRH and, therefore, an elevated ΔTSH; hyperthyroid patients are subsensitive and have a decreased or "blunted" ΔTSH. The TRH test in psychiatric patients is discussed more fully below.

4. Thyroid Autoantibodies

The immune system, under certain circumstances, makes antibodies directed against thyroid substances.[21] Two commonly measured substances are antimicrosomal (anti-M) and antithyroglobulin (anti-T) antibodies. High titers, which may be transient or permanent, are evidence of autoimmune disease. In one Australian study of a "random" population of 2838 subjects, the prevalence of anti-M antibodies was 9.8% in women and 2.8% in men. Women in the sixth decade had a prevalence of 15%.[22] The presence of anti-M antibodies was related to thyroid disease as determined by thyroid biopsy and elevated TSH levels. It is notable that antibodies are most prevalent in older women, which is also the high-risk group for unipolar major depression.

5. Hypothyroidism and Depression

It has long been known that many signs and symptoms of overt thyroid disease, such as anergia, constipation, and appetite and weight changes, overlap with those of depression.[17,23–25] Because both thyroid disease and depression carry a good prognosis when treated correctly, it is crucial to make an accurate diagnosis prior to treatment. Psychiatric diagnostic systems such as the DSM III[26] and RDC[27] emphasize differential diagnosis among psychiatric syndromes and stress the importance of ruling out organic causes.[28] The DSM III category of organic affective syndrome is described by the same clinical features as major depressive episodes except that in addition to mood disturbance only two "associated features" are needed instead of four.

Most psychiatrists routinely include hypothyroidism in the differential diagnosis of depressive states. Although this has not been studied systematically, the average workup probably comprises a T_4 and T_3RU, and a base-line TSH may be ordered. These tests will certainly pick up patients with overt thyroid failure and some with lesser degrees of thyroid dysfunction but will not detect mild degrees of hypothyroidism. Recent evidence, which is reviewed below, indicates that this latter group is highly represented in psychiatric patients presenting with depression.

5.1. Grades of Hypothyroidism

Endocrinologists no longer describe hypothyroidism as an "all-or-nothing" phenomenon. Rather, thyroid dysfunction is seen as a spectrum illness with various grades of disease.[29-33] Testing for TRH has been a major tool in this conceptual development and in the early diagnosis of hypothyroidism.

Grade 1 hypothyroidism is overt hypothyroidism. These patients have the classical signs and symptoms of hypothyroidism that are found in any medical text: lethargy, weakness, slowed mentation, sluggish reflexes, constipation, weight gain, and hair and skin changes. Laboratory values show decreased T_4, elevated TSH, and increased ΔTSH.

Grade 2 hypothyroidism is mild hypothyroidism. Grade 2 patients have a few clinical symptoms such as lethargy and early skin or hair changes or more numerous nonspecific complaints. The T_4 is normal, but base-line TSH is marginally elevated. The TRH test reveals an increased ΔTSH.

Grade 3 hypothyroidism is also known as "subclinical" hypothyroidism, which may be a misnomer. These patients have few clinical symptoms, and laboratory testing is normal except for an increased ΔTSH on TRH stimulation.

5.2. The Blunted ΔTSH: An Unexpected Finding

The TRH test has been used in psychiatric settings for about a decade. Prange and associates, studying the relationship of thyroid status to antidepressant response, tested ten unipolar depressed women with the TRH test. Two of the initial ten patients had a blunted TSH response ($\downarrow \Delta$TSH) to TRH.[34] This finding has been replicated by many investigators, with about 20–40% of patients with major depression having a blunted ΔTSH.[35-40] Further studies by Gold *et al.*[41] and Extein *et al.*[42] but not Linkowski *et al.*[43] have shown that the decreased ΔTSH is generally confined to unipolar depressed patients.

The finding of a blunted TSH response to TRH infusion contradicts the notion that depressed patients may be hypothyroid. If anything, mild hypothyroidism would render the pituitary supersensitive to TRH, with a resulting augmentation of TSH response ($\uparrow \Delta$TSH). The reason for this finding is unclear. One theory is that the decreased ΔTSH is secondary to alterations in monoaminergic systems at the hypothalamic level. Studies of this have been inconclusive. Another postulate is that the blunted ΔTSH in the unipolar depressive is secondary to elevated glucocorticoid levels; this has not been found in two separate studies.[35,41] Regardless of the mechanism, the finding of blunted ΔTSH is approximately 40% sensitive and 85% specific for unipolar major depression.

5.3. The Augmented ΔTSH in Depressed Patients

Gold and colleagues[44] at Fair Oaks Hospital evaluated a large series of 250 patients with the TRH test. All patients were referred for depression and/or anergia. None was referred specifically for thyroid evaluation or replacement, nor had any been treated with thyroid hormones for at least 12 months. Patients were medication-free for 1 week. Of these patients, 20 (8%) had some degree of hypothyroidism as evidenced by TRH testing. As defined above, grade 1 (overt) hypothyroidism was present in two patients (<1%), grade 2 (mild) hypothyroidism in eight patients (3.2%), and grade 3 (subclinical) hypothyroidism in ten patients (4.0%). This is a much higher percentage of thyroid disease than has been previously reported. What is also impressive is that, in open trials, some refractory patients had an excellent response to thyroid replacement. Sternbach and colleagues[45] followed the inpatient study with a series of 44 outpatients evaluated at Fair Oaks Hospital for complaints of depression and/or anergia. Of these patients, six (13.5%) had an augmented TSH response to TRH infusion consistent with thyroid dysfunction. Five of these six patients had other evidence of thyroid disease (elevated base-line TSH and/or positive antithyroid antibodies). Similar results have been found in other centers.

5.4. Etiology of Hypothyroidism

An important question is the etiology of the thyroid dysfunction. A well-recognized entity in the endocrinologic literature is called symptomless autoimmune thyroiditis (SAT).[46] This entity affects 5–15% of the general population and is especially prevalent in elderly women; it is defined by the presence of lymphoplasmocytic infiltration of the thyroid and the presence of antithyroid antibodies. A high proportion (65%) of patients with SAT have elevated ΔTSH on TRH testing. Gold *et al.*[47] tested 100 consecutive patients complaining of depression and/or anergia; in this study, 15% had some degree of hypothyroidism. Of these 15 patients, nine (60%) were positive for anti-M antibodies. From these studies, the conclusion is that many psychiatric patients presenting with depression and/or anergia are hypothyroid and that the most common etiology is SAT. In other words, thyroid failure that is "symptomless" to the endocrinologist may be "depression" to the psychiatrist.

5.5. Treatment Implications

Clearly, all patients with grade 1 (overt) disease need thyroid replacement. Recent reports in the endocrinologic literature indicate that patients with grade 2 (mild) hypothyroidism should be treated routinely with thyroid replacement. It is felt that hypothyroidism is progressive, and there are some reports that patients with mild hypothyroidism are at increased risk for cardiac disease and myocardial infarction.[48] There are proven beneficial cardiac reponses to thyroid replacement in patients with grade 2 hypothyroidism.[49] It is likely although unproven in large trials, that thyroid replacement will improve mood in patients with mild hypothyroidism who present with depression and/or anergia. At this time, we recommend thyroid replacement in all such patients, with the addition of antidepressants if response to thyroid hormone alone is incomplete. Treatment for depressed patients with grade 3 (subclinical) hypothyroidism is less clear. At this point, patients should be treated on an individualized basis; certainly, those who do not respond to 21 consecutive days at therapeutic blood levels of an antidepressant should be tried on thyroid hormone in addition to the antidepressant. We have generally used T_3 (liothyronine sodium, Cytomel®) for replacement, beginning with a daily dosage of 25 µg, and closely monitor the patient's clinical condition. A good biochemical endpoint for thyroid replacement is normalization of the TRH stimulation test.

6. Hyperthyroidism and Psychiatric Illness

The classic psychiatric presentation of hyperthyroidism is generalized anxiety.[23,24] When other clinical signs such as weight loss with increased appetite, tachycardia, fine tremor, and exophthalmos are present, the diagnosis is self-evident. What is not clear is the prevalence of hyperthyroidism among patients presenting with a chief complaint of anxiety.

Manic and schizophrenic syndromes have also been associated with thyroid hormone. In one series of 100 committed inpatients,[50] three patients were hyperthyroid and met RDC for manic depressive illness, and three were hyperthyroid and met RDC for schizophrenia. In another series of 191 inpatients,[51] seven were hyperthyroid: five presented as affective psychosis, one as neurotic depression, and one as schizophrenia. There are recent cases reported in the literature of mania following the administration of exogenous thyroid. In reviewing the literature, Josephson and MacKenzie[52] found 25 cases of ''mania'' following thyroid replacement for hypothyroidism. They analyzed 18 case reports and determined that 15 of these patients were psychotic prior to thyroid replacement; the significance of this is not clear. Hyperthyroidism can also present as depression. There is a case report of thyrotoxicosis presenting as a delusional depression that resolved only on treatment of the endocrine disorder.[53]

Bipolar, lithium-free manics have a blunted TSH response to TRH infusion.[43,54,55] Acute mania is often difficult to distinguish from an acute schizophrenic episode. Any test that would differentiate the two conditions would be of great value. Extein and colleagues found that 60% of manics, 26% of schizophrenics, and 0% of controls had a blunted ΔTSH. Although this was a relatively small study, the results are impressive. Using a ΔTSH cutoff of 7 μIU/ml, the sensitivity was 60%, specificity 84%, and diagnostic confidence 69%. Extein *et al.*[55] have postulated that increased noradrenergic or dopaminergic transmission in mania causes increased TRH release at the hypothalamic level. Pituitary TRH receptors then ''down-regulate'' in an attempt to maintain homeostasis. Therefore, the pituitary is less sensitive to the infused TRH, with resultant blunted TSH response. An alternate theory that is by no means incompatible with Extein's is that some manic patients are mildly hyperthyroid. Increased T_3 would make the pituitary thyrotrope cells less sensitive to infused TRH with the same result.

7. Thyroid Workup of the Depressed Patient

As has been reviewed in this chapter, hypothyroidism is common in ''depressed'' patients, and hyperthyroidism should also be considered in anxiety and manic disorders. The thyroid evaluation comprises history, physical examination, and laboratory testing.

7.1. History

The history elicited from a patient with thyroid disease will depend on both the severity of illness and the rigor with which thyroid-referable complaints are elicited. It is important to remember that hypothyroid patients may present with complaints only of depression or anergia, and hyperthyroid patients perhaps just with anxiety. A helpful tool is a standardized checklist of symptoms and signs of thyroid disease, such as the one presented in Fig. 5-1. Four or five positives on this list is highly suggestive of thyroid disease, especially if they point in the same direction, hyper or hypo. A patient with a positive family history for thyroid disease should always be evaluated.

SIGNS and SYMPTOMS of THYROID DYSFUNCTION

	Present	Absent
Goiter		
Thyroid Bruit		
Fine Tremor		
Weight Loss		
Increased Appetite		
Lid Lag		
Depressed Mood		
Sweating		
Heat Intolerance		
Positive Family History		
Lethargy/Anergia		
Weight Gain		
Hoarseness		
Dry Skin		
Nervousness		
Hair Loss		
Cold Intolerance		
Delayed Reflexes		
Constipation		
Exophthalmos		
Recent M. I.		
Coronary Artery Disease		
Arrhythmias		
Pulse>90/minute		
Hypertension		
TOTAL		

Patient with 5 or more signs/symptoms has high degree of suspicion of hypothalamic-pituitary-thyroid axis dysfunction.

Figure 5-1. Thyroid dysfunction checklist.

7.2. Physical Examination

Even a brief physical examination can give invaluable clues as to the patient's thyroid status. Vital signs will screen for altered blood pressure, tachycardia or bradycardia, and dysrhythmias. Inspection of the patient may reveal tremor, exophthalmos, diaphoresis, or loss of hair. The patient's clothing may reveal weight changes or heat or cold intolerance. Skin and hair changes may be palpable, and the thyroid should be checked for size, tenderness, and presence or absence of bruits. A neurological examination will pick up lid lag, tremor, and delayed or brisk ankle jerks.

7.3. Laboratory Testing

Presence of positive items on history or physical examination strongly increases the possibility of thyroid disease, and a laboratory workup is mandatory. We feel that all patients presenting with anergia or depression require at least T_4, T_3RIA, T_3RU, and TSH. This will pick up patients with grade 1 or grade 2 hypothyroidism.

7.4. Thyrotropin-Releasing Hormone Testing in Depressed Patients

The TRH infusion yields two pieces of information in depressed patients. First, it can be used in conjunction with the DST to confirm the presence of major depression or to tease apart diagnostic dilemmas. The indications are much the same as for the DST (see Chapter 4). Using the two tests together yielded a sensitivity of 84% in one study.[25] We realize, however, that the TRH requires a technical setup that is more complicated than the DST and that some clinicians may treat a patient empirically with antidepressants rather than refer for testing. The TRH is invaluable, however, if the diagnosis is uncertain and the patient is high risk. The TRH infusion is also a sensitive test for early hypothyroidism. We feel that all patients who are unresponsive to usual treatment for major depression should be tested with the TRH.

8. Thyroid Workup of Anxious or Manic Patients

Although the prevalence of hyperthyroidism in patients with generalized anxiety or mania is not fully known, it seems most prudent to screen all such patients with T_4, T_3RIA, T_3RU, and TSH. The TRH infusion is clearly of value in differentiating mania from acute schizophrenia, and a normal ΔTSH will help rule out hyperthyroidism. A blunted ΔTSH will not, however, differentiate "primary" mania from mania in which hyperthyroidism is etiologically responsible. Likewise, a normal TRH infusion test in a patient presenting with anxiety will rule out hyperthyroidism, but there is no definitive interpretation of a blunted TRH infusion test in such a patient.

Lithium-treated bipolar or recurrent unipolar patients present a unique problem. These patients are, by definition, predisposed to depressive episodes. In addition, they are at risk for lithium-induced hypothyroidism, which can cause or increase susceptibility to depression.[56] How should the psychiatrist work up the bipolar depressed patient who is taking lithium? A TRH infusion test can be of considerable help. Following a ΔTSH in the patient from before treatment to lithium maintenance is of considerable importance in the early identification of lithium-induced grade 3 disease. An increasing ΔTSH should raise the possibility of grade 2 or 3 hypothyroidism, and thyroid replacement should be considered before antidepressants are started.

9. Summary

The interactions between thyroid hormones and mental states are complex. Many questions remain unanswered concerning the interpretation of thyroid tests and subsequent treatment in borderline cases. Laboratory workup of depressed, manic, and anxious patients should include base-line T_4, T_3RU, T_3RIA, and TSH. The TRH infusion can be used to confirm the presence of major depression; it is often given in conjunction with the DST. An added bonus is that it picks up mild hypothyroidism masquerading as depression. Thus, it is especially indicated in treatment failures. The TRH test is also useful in differentiating mania from schizophrenia and in following patients on lithium who become depressed.

References

1. Demeester-Mirkine N, Dumont JE: The hypothalamo–pituitary–thyroid axis, in DeVisscher M (ed): *The Thyroid Gland.* New York, Raven Press, 1980, pp 145–152.
2. Martin JB, Reichlin S, Brown GM: *Clinical Neuroendocrinology.* Philadelphia, FA Davis, 1977.
3. Morley JE: Neuroendocrine control of thyrotropin secretion. *Endocrine Rev* 2:396–436, 1981.
4. Martin JB, Boshans R, Reichlin S: Feedback regulation of TSH secretion in rats with hypothalamic lesions. *Endocrinology* 87:1032–1040, 1970.
5. Wilber JF, Porter JC: Thyrotropin and growth hormone releasing activity in hypophysial portal blood. *Endocrinology* 87:807–811, 1970.
6. Jackson IMD: Thyrotropin-releasing hormone. *N Engl J Med* 306:145–153, 1982.
7. Hokfelt T, Fuxe K, Johansson O, et al: Distribution of thyrotropin-releasing hormone (TRH) in the central nervous system as revealed with immunochemistry. *Eur J Pharmacol* 34:389–392, 1975.
8. Hokfelt T, Johansson O, Ljungdahl A, et al: Neurotransmitters and neuropeptides: Distribution patterns and cellular localization as revealed by immunocytochemistry, in: *Nobel Symposium, 42nd, Stockholm 1978: Central Regulation of the Endocrine System.* New York, Plenum Press, 1979, pp 31–48.
9. Grimm Y, Reichlin S: Thyrotropin-releasing hormone (TRH): Neurotransmitter regulation of secretion by mouse hypothalamic tissue *in vitro. Endocrinology* 93:626–631, 1973.
10. Gold PW, Goodwin FK, Wehr T, et al: Pituitary thyrotropin response to thyrotropin-releasing hormone in affective illness: Relationship to spinal fluid amine metabolites. *Am J Psychiatry* 134:1028–1031, 1977.
11. Okuno A, Taguchi T, Nakayama K, et al: Kinetic analysis of plasma TSH dynamics after TRH stimulation. *Horm Metab Res* 11:293–295, 1979.
12. Vanhaelst L, Van Cauter E, Degaute JP, et al: Circadian variations of serum thyrotropin levels in man. *J Clin Endocrinol Metab* 35:479–482, 1972.
13. Grant G, Vale W, Guillemin R: Interaction of thyrotropin-releasing factor with membrane receptors of pituitary cells. *Biochem Biophys Res Commun* 46:28–34, 1972.
14. Larsen PR: Thyroid–pituitary interaction: Feedback regulation of thyrotropin secretion by thyroid hormones. *N Engl J Med* 306:23–32, 1982.
15. Sowers JR, Carlson HE, Brautbar N, et al: Effect of dexamethasone on prolactin and TSH responses to TRH and metoclopramide in man. *J Clin Endocrinol Metab* 44:237–241, 1977.

16. Re RN, Kourides IA, Ridgway EC, et al: The effect of glucocorticoid administration in human pituitary secretion of thyrotropin and prolactin. *J Clin Endocrinol Metab* 43:338–346, 1976.
17. Ingbar SH, Woeber KA: The thyroid gland, in Williams RH (ed): *Textbook of Endocrinology*. Philadelphia, WB Saunders, 1974, pp 95–232.
18. Blum M: Easier understanding of the new thyroid tests. *Resident Staff Physician* 27:72–90, 1981.
19. Warren DW, LoPresti JS, Nicoloff JT: A new method for measurement of the conversion ratio of thyroxine to triiodothyronine in euthyroid man. *J Clin Endocrinol Metab* 53:1218–1222, 1981.
20. Ormston BJ, Garry R, Cryer RJ, et al: Thyrotropin-releasing hormone as a thyroid-function test. *Lancet* 2:10–14, 1971.
21. Fink JN, Beall GN: Immunologic aspects of endocrine disease. *JAMA* 248:2696–2700, 1982.
22. Hawkins BR, Dawkins RL, Burger HG, et al: Diagnostic significance of thyroid microsomal antibodies in randomly selected population. *Lancet* 2:1057–1059, 1980.
23. Whybrow PC, Prange AJ, Treadway CR: Mental changes accompanying thyroid gland dysfunction: A reappraisal using objective psychological measurement. *Arch Gen Psychiatry* 20:48–63, 1969.
24. Haskett RF, Rose RM: Neuroendocrine disorders and psychopathology. *Psychiatr Clin North Am* 4:239–252, 1981.
25. Gold MS, Pottash ALC, Extein I, et al: Diagnosis of depression in the 1980s. *JAMA* 245:1562–1564, 1981.
26. American Psychiatric Association: *Diagnostic and Statistical Manual of Mental Disorders*, ed 3. Washington, American Psychiatric Association, 1980.
27. Spitzer RL, Endicott J, Robins E: *Research Diagnostic Criteria (RDC) for a Selected Group of Functional Disorders*. New York, New York State Psychiatric Institute, 1980.
28. Skodol AE, Spitzer RL: The development of reliable diagnostic criteria in psychiatry. *Annu Rev Med* 33:317–326, 1982.
29. Billewicz WZ, Chapman RS, Crooks J, et al: Statistical methods applied to the diagnosis of hypothyroidism. *Q J Med* 150:255–266, 1969.
30. Evered DC, Ormston BJ, Smith PA, et al: Grades of hypothyroidism. *Br Med J* 1:657–662, 1973.
31. Harvey RF: Grades of hypothyroidism. *Br Med J* 2:488–489, 1973.
32. Bastenie PA, Bonnyns M, Vanhaelst L: Grades of subclinical hypothyroidism in asymptomatic autoimmune thyroiditis revealed by the thyrotropin-releasing hormone test. *J Clin Endocrinol Metab* 51:163–166, 1980.
33. Wenzel KW, Meinhold H, Raffenberg M, et al: Classification of hypothyroidism in evaluating patients after radioiodine therapy by serum cholesterol, T_3-uptake, total T_4, FT_4-index, total T_3, basal TSH and TRH-test. *Eur J Clin Invest* 4:141–148, 1974.
34. Prange AJ, Lara PP, Wilson IC: Effects of thyrotropin-releasing hormone in depression. *Lancet* 2:999–1002, 1972.
35. Targum SD, Sullivan AC, Byrnes SM: Compensatory pituitary–thyroid mechanisms in major depressive disorder. *Psychiatry Res* 6:85–96, 1982.
36. Kirkegaard C, Bjorum N: TSH responses to TRH in endogenous depression. *Lancet* 1:152, 1980.
37. Prange AJ, Loosen PT: Some endocrine aspects of affective disorders. *J Clin Psychiatry* 41:29–34, 1980.
38. Gold MS, Pottash ALC, Extein I, et al: The TRH test in the diagnosis of major and minor depression. *Psychoneuroendocrinology* 6:159–169, 1981.
39. Ettigi PG, Brown GM: Psychoneuroendocrinology of affective disorder: An overview. *Am J Psychiatry* 134:493–501, 1977.
40. Sternbach H, Gerner RD, Gwirtsman HE: The thyrotropin-releasing hormone stimulation test: A review. *J Clin Psychiatry* 43:4–6, 1982.
41. Gold MS, Pottash ALC, Ryan N, et al: TRH-induced TSH response in unipolar, bipolar and secondary depressions: Possible utility in clinical assessment and differential diagnosis. *Psychoneuroendocrinology* 5:147–155, 1980.
42. Extein I, Pottash ALC, Gold MS, et al: The thyroid-stimulating hormone response to thyrotropin-releasing hormone in mania and bipolar depression. *Psychiatry Res* 2:199–204, 1980.
43. Linkowski P, Brauman H, Mendlewicz J: Thyrotropin response to thyrotropin-releasing hormone in unipolar and bipolar affective illness. *J Affective Disord* 3:9–16, 1981.

44. Gold MS, Pottash ALC, Extein I: Hypothyroidism and depression: Evidence from complete thyroid function evaluation. *JAMA* 245:1919–1922, 1981.
45. Sternbach HA, Gold MS, Pottash ALC, et al: Thyroid failure and protirelin (thyrotropin-releasing hormone) test abnormalities in depressed outpatients. *JAMA* 245:1618–1620, 1983.
46. Bonnyns M, Vanhaelst L, Bastenie PA: Asymptomatic atrophic thyroiditis. *Horm Res* 16:338–344, 1982.
47. Gold MS, Pottash ALC, Extein I: "Symptomless" autoimmune thyroiditis in depression. *Psychiatry Res* 6:261–269, 1982.
48. Bastenie PA, Vanhaelst L, Bonnyns M, et al: Preclinical hypothyroidism: A risk factor for coronary-heart disease. *Lancet* 1:203–204, 1971.
49. Ridgway EC, Cooper DS, Walker H, et al: Peripheral responses to thyroid hormone before and after L-thyroxine therapy in patients with subclinical hypothyroidism. *J Clin Endocrinol Metab* 53:1238–1242, 1981.
50. Hall RC, Gardner ER, Stickney SK, et al: Physical illness manifesting as psychiatric disease. II. Analysis of a state hospital inpatient population. *Arch Gen Psychiatry* 37:989–995, 1980.
51. Carney MWP, Macleod S, Sheffield BF: Thyroid function screening in psychiatric inpatients. *Br J Psychiatry* 138:154–156, 1981.
52. Josephson AM, MacKenzie TB: Thyroid-induced mania in hypothyroid patients. *Br J Psychiatry* 137:222–228, 1980.
53. Kronfol Z, Grenen JF, Condon M, et al: Application of biological markers in depression secondary to thyrotoxicosis. *Am J Psychiatry* 139:1319–1322, 1982.
54. Extein I, Pottash ALC, Gold MS, et al: Differentiating mania from schizophrenia by the TRH test. *Am J Psychiatry* 137:981–982, 1980.
55. Extein I, Pottash ALC, Gold MS, et al: Using the protirelin test to distinguish mania from schizophrenia. *Arch Gen Psychiatry* 39:77–81, 1982.
56. Reisberg B, Gershon S: Side effects associated with lithium therapy. *Arch Gen Psychiatry* 36:879–887, 1979.

Other Neuroendocrine Tests

H. Rowland Pearsall, M.D., and Mark S. Gold, M.D.

1. Introduction

The roles of the hypothalamic–pituitary–thyroid axis (HPT) and the hypothalamic–pituitary–adrenal axis (HPA) have been discussed in detail with regard to their role in psychiatric diagnosis. There are other neuroendocrine hormones that hold promise in helping to further our understanding of psychiatric illness and diagnosis. Growth hormone (GH), endorphins, prolactin, luteinizing hormone (LH), follicle-stimulating hormone (FSH), gonadal hormones, and melatonin are reviewed in this chapter both with regard to regulation and to their role in either theory or diagnosis of psychiatric illness.

2. Growth Hormone

Growth hormone is a single-chain polypeptide secreted from cells of the anterior pituitary. It circulates unbound in the plasma and has multiple effects throughout the body. These effects include regulation of cell growth, connective tissue growth, and the growth of a variety of viscera. The hormone is thought to exert these effects through a stimulating action on nucleic acid and protein synthesis. Growth hormone is also known to mobilize lipid stores in the body and is involved in glucose metabolism as well. It tends to increase blood glucose by impairing glucose metabolism in tissues such as muscle and fat. It is thought that some of the effects of growth hormone are mediated through a factor known as somatomedin, which circulates in the plasma and is believed to be secreted in the liver in response to growth hormone stimulation.

Secretion of growth hormone occurs in spontaneous bursts throughout the day with increased levels of secretion occurring during sleep. In this respect, it follows the patterns of other pituitary hormones. Secretion is also known to vary with age, with high levels noted at birth and during the growth period of adolescence.

H. Rowland Pearsall, M.D. • Stony Lodge Hospital, Ossining-on-Hudson, New York 10562. *Mark S. Gold, M.D.* • Research Facilities, Fair Oaks Hospital, Summit, New Jersey 07901, and Fair Oaks Hospital at Boca/Delray, Delray Beach, Florida 33445.

2.1. Regulation of Growth Hormone Secretion

Growth hormone secretion is a complex system influenced by multiple factors. Figure 6-1 outlines the currently understood central regulatory mechanism. The system operates primarily through influences of monoaminergic neurons acting on peptidergic neurons, which subsequently release a stimulating factor known as growth hormone-releasing factor (GHRH) or a growth hormone-inhibiting factor known as somatostatin to the anterior pituitary. In response to GHRH and somatostatin, cells of the anterior pituitary secrete growth hormone into the plasma. As indicated, a variety of mono-aminergic neurons have been implicated in the hypothalamic regulatory mechanism. Serotoninergic, α-adrenergic, and dopaminergic neurons have all been shown to have a stimulating effect on subsequent growth hormone release. β-Adrenergic input appears to be inhibitory. Following stimulation by the hypothalamic neurons, either GHRH or somatostatin is released to the anterior pituitary. Growth hormone-releasing hormone is a hormone mediator whose chemical nature is still not clearly identified. Somatostatin, on the other hand, is well characterized, and its inhibitory effects on growth hormone are well documented.

A variety of factors mentioned above can influence growth hormone secretion. Physiological, hormonal, pharmacological, and various pathological conditions have all been shown to have an impact on either stimulating or decreasing growth hormone secretion. As shown in Fig. 6-1, factors such as sleep, exercise, and stress can stimulate the hypothalamic pathways leading to a subsequent increase in serum growth hormone. Table 6-1 outlines some of the factors implicated in increasing and decreasing growth hormone secretion.

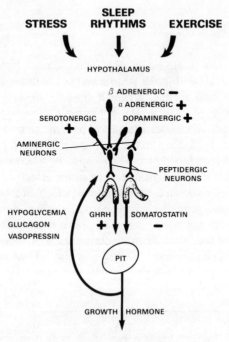

Figure 6-1. Regulation of growth hormone.

Table 6-1. Factors That Influence Growth Hormone Secretion

Physiological	Pharmacological	Pathological
Increase growth hormone		
1. Exercise	1. Insulin hypoglycemia	1. Acromegaly
2. Stress	2. Amino acid infusions	2. Renal failure
a. Physical	a. Arginine	3. Protein depletion
b. Psychological	b. Leucine	4. Fasting and starvation
3. Sleep	c. Lysine, etc.	5. Anorexia nervosa
4. Postprandial glucose decline	3. Small peptides	
	a. Vasopressin	
	b. ACTH	
	4. Monoaminergic stimuli	
	a. α-Adrenergic agonists	
	b. Dopamine agonists	
	c. Serotonin precursors	
	d. β-Adrenergic antagonists	
	5. Nonpeptide hormones	
	a. Estrogens	
	b. Diethylstilbestrol	
Decrease growth hormone		
1. Postprandial hyperglycemia	1. Somatostatin	1. Dwarfism
2. Elevated free fatty acids	2. Serotonin antagonists	2. Pituitary failure
3. Elevated GH levels	3. α-Adrenergic antagonists	3. Psychosocial deprivation
	4. Dopamine antagonists	
	5. β-Adrenergic agonists	

2.2. Growth Hormone in Psychiatric Disorders

Growth hormone has been studied in a variety of psychiatric disorders including affective disorders, alcoholism, stress, anorexia nervosa, and growth failure of infancy. Each of these areas is discussed briefly below.

2.2.1. Depression

Measurements of growth hormone in affective disorders have given conflicting results. Growth hormone secretion itself appears to be normal in depression. The responsiveness of growth hormone secretion to stimuli such as insulin hypoglycemia and TRH infusion has shown variation with changes in mood state. Part of the confusion about the significance of these changes arises from the variety of factors that can influence growth hormone.

Human growth hormone studies using the response of growth hormone secretion to insulin-induced hypoglycemia have in recent years suggested a significantly lower GH response in patients with depression.[1-3] Some studies have suggested that this is more severe in psychotic depressions and also that bipolar patients show more reduction in GH when depressed than even unipolar patients.[4]

Growth hormone response to stimulation with TRH infusions has been reported to be increased in depressed patients.[5] Normally only TSH and prolactin release are affected with TRH infusion. Reports indicated that 50% of unipolar and bipolar depressed patients show GH increases after TRH.

As mentioned above, α-adrenergic factors are thought to influence GH secretion at the hypothalamic level.[6] Clonidine stimulation has been used also to assess GH secretion. Depressed patients in some reports show blunted GH response to clonidine.[7]

These responses are of theoretical interest given the suspected adrenergic input to growth hormone response at the hypothalamic level. Assuming that some types of affective disorders represent either a real or functional deficiency of catecholamines in the central nervous system, it would be reasonable to expect a subsequent decrease in responsiveness of hormones controlled by similar systems. Given the serotonergic and adrenergic input involved in growth hormone regulation, variation in GH response and, in particular, response to α-adrenergic stimulating agents such as clonidine offer a hope for improved classification of depressions.

2.2.2. Stress

Human growth hormone release is increased by stress, although studies suggest that human growth hormone is not as sensitive to stress as is prolactin or ACTH.[8] It has also been suggested that growth hormone shows a fairly rapid adaptation to repeated encounters with the same stressful situation.

2.2.3. Anorexia Nervosa

Human growth hormone levels are elevated in anorexia nervosa in about one-third of the cases.[9] The GH response to insulin hypoglycemia and TRH stimulation are also frequently decreased. This is felt to be a function of poor caloric intake. Resumption of normal eating leads to rapid normalization of human growth hormone plasma levels as well as of human growth hormone response to various stimuli.

2.2.4. Maternal Deprivation

The syndrome of maternal deprivation with failure to thrive and poor growth is an example of a psychosocial situation interacting with a biological mechanism. In this syndrome there is a decreased growth hormone response to pharmacological stimuli such as insulin-induced hypoglycemia.[10] The mechanism for this syndrome is unclear; however, β-adrenergic activity is thought to be one possible mechanism. Generally, restoration of a supportive environment results in growth hormone response returning to normal over a period of time. One study has suggested that human growth hormone secretion in such cases of maternal deprivation can be restored with treatment by propranolol or another β blocker.[11]

2.3. Diagnostic Testing Using Growth Hormone

To date, the major utility of growth hormone as a diagnostic test has been its use in provocative testing with insulin-induced hypoglycemia. This has proven most helpful in confirming a diagnosis of depression. There do seem to be changes in GH response in depressed patients that change with a real improvement in the patient's mood. Given the neurotransmitter input for control of GH at the hypothalamic level, this axis has the potential to improve psychiatric diagnosis, perhaps in conjunction with other neuroendocrine or metabolic measures.

3. Endorphins

β-Endorphins are part of a group of substances called opioid peptides. These opioid peptides are defined as substances either endogenous or synthetic that have pharmacological activity similar to morphine. Endorphins themselves are molecules derived from β-lipotropin. They consist of 31 amino acids or some shorter segments of the β-lipotropin molecule. β-Endorphin was first isolated from pituitary in 1976, and subsequent studies revealed a relationship between the lipotropin molecule and corticotropin (ACTH). It appears that the β-lipotropin molecule is derived from a portion of the corticotropin amino acid sequence.

Current knowledge suggests the following relationships among opioid peptides (illustrated schematically in Fig. 6-2). Proopiomelanocortin or "big ACTH" is a precursor for the adrenocorticotropic hormone (ACTH). Within this larger molecule is contained a 91-amino-acid pituitary gland peptide, β-lipotropin. β-Lipotropin contains a 31-amino-acid sequence called β-endorphin, which has potent actions at opioid receptors. Smaller five-amino-acid groups, met-enkephalin (methionine enkephalin) and leu-enkephalin (leucine-enkephalin), are contained in the 31 amino acids of β-endorphin and have opioid activity. A final opioid peptide is dynorphin, which occurs in several forms, all of which incorporate leu-enkephalin in the amino acid sequence. The exact roles of all the opioid peptides remain to be worked out.

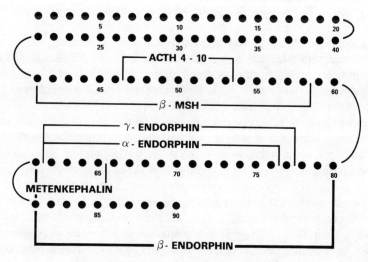

Figure 6-2. Schematic diagram of endorphins.

3.1. Roles and Distribution of β-Endorphins

β-Endorphins are located in high concentrations in two areas of the central nervous system. One is the ventral hypothalamus, which seems to contain endorphin cell bodies. There are also high concentrations in areas of projection of these cells, specifically the periaqueductal gray area. β-Endorphins are also found in the anterior pituitary in high concentration. Other areas of the body such as the pancreas and placenta have also been reported to have concentrations of β-endorphins.

The precise mechanism of action of opioid peptides is still unclear. Two possible roles in the central nervous system include functioning as neurotransmitters or functioning as neuromodulators. Neuromodulators are substances that do not have a detectable action on resting nerve cell membranes but do tend to modify actions of other known neurotransmitters. Although the exact mechanism of action of the β-endorphins is unclear, the general activation of opiate receptors leads to inhibition of neuronal firing. It has also been reported that opiate peptides tend to inhibit acetylcholine synthesis in the hippocampus and may effect dopamine, norepinephrine, and serotonin in other areas of the central nervous system.[12]

3.2. β-Endorphins and Psychiatric Disorders

The exact role of endorphins in psychiatric disorders is at present under exploration. The finding that there are high concentrations of opiate receptors in areas of the brain such as the limbic system and the theoretical suggestion of possible neuromodulator effects of the opiates in interaction with monoamine systems suggest possible roles in behavior. Areas of particular interest have been schizophrenic illness and affective disorders.

One research group[13] observed that animals given intraventricular or intracerebral doses of opioids developed a postural rigidity that seems suggestive of the catatonic posturing sometimes seen in schizophrenic illness. Subsequent attempts have been made to measure the activity of opioid substances in the cerebral spinal fluid of schizophrenic patients. Such tests have revealed increased levels of opioid activity in some schizophrenic patients[14] and suggested that at least in some patients who responded to treatment there was a decrease in such activity. Additional studies have yielded conflicting results, with some suggesting an overactivity of β-endorphins and others suggesting a relative deficiency. Research approaches using naloxone to block opiate receptors[15] as well as intravenous administration of β-endorphin, assuming a relative opiate deficiency, have yielded no conclusive results.

Given the positive effects of opiate substances on mood in many people, there has been interest in what role endogenous opioid systems might play in the pathogenesis of depression. Some studies have suggested that high doses of naloxone given to normal individuals can induce depressive symptomotology.[16] One recent study[17] looked at plasma cortisol levels of hospitalized patients meeting RDC criteria for major and nonmajor depression and attempted to correlate these with plasma β-endorphin immunoreactivity. Their findings suggest that patients with nonmajor depression tend to have lower levels of plasma β-endorphin immunoreactivity, whereas patients of both the major and nonmajor depression groups showed significantly elevated plasma cortisol compared to normals. The use of a ratio of plasma β-endorphin to cortisol immunoreactivity allowed separation of depressed patients from normal controls in most cases. Other groups looking at the relationship between plasma β-endorphin immunoreactivity and diagnosis have reported normal levels in unipolar depression.[18] Still other groups have suggested a higher plasma level of β-endorphin in patients with primary and secondary major depressions compared with normal subjects.[19]

At present, β-endorphin immunoreactivity levels and other measures of β-endorphin have been inconsistent in the various studies of affective disorders, and their potential utility remains to be fully understood.

4. Prolactin

Prolactin is a lactogenic hormone secreted from cells in the anterior pituitary. Prolactin in conjunction with estrogen and cortisol is directly responsible for normal growth of the nonlactating breast. Prolactin along with progesterone is essential for development of alveolar lobules and secretion of milk during and following pregnancy.

Prolactin secretion normally follows a sleep-related circadian pattern with peak values occurring approximately 1 hr after the onset of sleep. Prolactin levels are also increased by stress and certain medications.

4.1. Regulation of Prolactin Secretion

Control of prolactin secretion begins at the level of the hypothalamus (Fig. 6-3). In the hypothalamus, substances are secreted that move to the pituitary via the hypothalamic–pituitary portal vessels. These factors are grouped under the general heading of prolactin-inhibitory factors and prolactin-releasing factors. At the moment, the best-defined prolactin-inhibitory factor is dopamine, which is secreted from tuberohypophyseal nerve tracks of the hypothalamus and then appears to act directly on dopamine receptors of the pituitary prolactin-secreting cells. Its effect is to prohibit prolactin secretion. It is also possible that dopamine may act at the level of the hypothalamus to cause release of other, as yet undefined, prolactin-inhibitory factors.

It is thought that there are also specific factors that act from the hypothalamus to stimulate release of prolactin at the level of the pituitary. Thyrotropin-releasing hormone (TRH) has been shown to stimulate secretion of both prolactin and thryoid-stimulating hormone (TSH). Small doses of TRH have been shown to release both TSH and prolactin in humans. The fact that physiological stimuli of prolactin secretion such as suckling do not cause a concomitant increase in TSH secretion suggests that in addition to TRH there are other prolactin-releasing factors. The peptide hormone vasoactive intestinal polypeptide (VIP) has been shown to increase prolactin secretion in animals and has been shown to be present in the portal blood. At the level of the hypothalamus, serotonin pathways appear to stimulate prolactin secretion, and administration of serotonin precursors or serotonin agonists seems to increase prolactin secretion. Administration of drugs that block serotonin effects tends to cause a subsequent decrease in prolactin secretion. Prolactin secretion does not seem to be influenced significantly by adrenergic input, but cholinergic pathways do appear to exert an

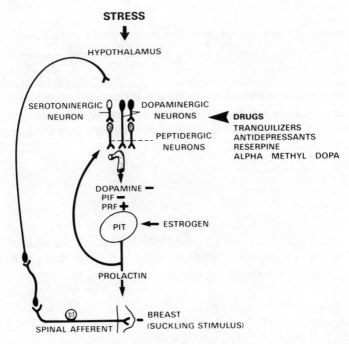

Figure 6-3. Regulation of prolactin.

inhibitory effect on prolactin release, possibly mediated via the dopaminergic pathways. There is also evidence that at least in animals the endogenous opiatelike peptides can influence prolactin secretion, possibly by interaction at the level of the hypothalamus with existing monoaminergic and peptidergic pathways.

Once prolactin is released from the anterior pituitary, it goes into the general circulation. The circulating level of prolactin in the plasma acts directly on the hypothalamus to inhibit further prolactin release and also acts on gonadotropin secretion, which may explain the anovulatory state observed in women who are nursing.

A variety of factors have been found to influence serum prolactin levels and include physiological, pharmacological, and certain pathological states. A limited number of factors have been found to decrease serum prolactin, and most important among these is administration of medication such as L-dopa, apomorphine, and bromocriptine. Table 6-2 reviews factors implicated in either increase or decrease of serum prolactin levels.

4.2. Utility of Prolactin in Psychiatric Disorders

Measurement of prolactin levels has been suggested to have several possible uses in psychiatric disorders, first with regard to assessing the effectiveness of certain antipsychotic medications that have effects on dopamine in the central nervous system and secondly as a possible neuroendocrine window into the function of the hypothalamic–pituitary axis. Each of these is discussed briefly below.

Table 6-2. Factors That Influence Serum Prolactin Levels

Physiological	Pathological	Pharmacological
Increase serum prolactin		
1. Pregnancy	1. Prolactin-secreting pituitary	1. TRH
2. Postpartum	tumors	2. Psychotropic drugs (e.g.,
a. Nonnursing mothers	2. Hypothalamic–pituitary disorders	phenothiazines, reserpine)
(days 1–7)	3. Pituitary stalk section or damage	3. Oral contraceptives
b. Nursing mothers after	4. Hypothyroidism	
suckling	5. Renal failure	
3. Nipple stimulation	6. Ectopic production by malignant	
4. Stress	tumors	
5. Exercise		
6. Sleep		
Decrease serum prolactin		
1. Water loading		1. L-Dopa
		2. Apomorphine
		3. Bromocriptine

4.2.1. Prolactin as a Measure of Antipsychotic Medication Effectiveness

Medications effective in the treatment of psychotic disorders, principally schizophrenia, share a common trait of being dopamine antagonists in the central nervous system. Dopamine exerts a strong inhibitory effect on prolactin secretion, and blocking dopamine in the CNS leads to increases in prolactin secretion. These changes in prolactin levels in response to antipsychotic medications offer a measure of the effectiveness of these medications in influencing central dopamine effects. This phenomenon has been widely used to screen drugs for possible antipsychotic activity.[20]

4.2.2. Prolactin as a Window to the Hypothalamus

Since prolactin secretion is influenced at the level of the hypothalamus by known neurotransmitters such as dopamine and serotonin, secretion of prolactin would seem to offer an opportunity to study illnesses that might potentially involve abnormalities in one or both of these neurotransmitters. In addition, endogenous opioid peptides have been implicated in the regulation of prolactin and may also be potentially studied by following variations in serum prolactin.

Prolactin levels in psychiatric disorders have not been well characterized to date. Some authors have suggested that base-line prolactin levels are elevated in depression,[5] whereas others have found the levels to be unchanged from normal controls.[21] There has been a suggestion that there might be an abnormal circadian secretion pattern for prolactin in depression.[22] Some authors have found that resting prolactin levels were significantly lower before treatment and increased after recovery from a major depression. Measurement of prolactin response to TRH hormone has given inconsistent results with reports of both increased and decreased levels in depressed patients. Linkowski suggested that prolactin responses to TRH were blunted in postmenopausal women with bipolar depression.[23]

Use of the opiate agonist morphine to stimulate prolactin release has suggested a deficient response in patients with major depression compared with normal controls. A study by Gold[24] using methadone to stimulate prolactin secretion found that depressed patients had lower mean basal prolactin levels than did other subjects and that their responses to methadone were decreased. Testing using prolactin either stimulated by TRH or by opiate agonists may eventually help to identify some types of depressive disorders.

In addition to the previously mentioned psychiatric uses, prolactin measurement is very useful in evaluating hypothalamic–pituitary dysfunctions, especially mass lesions of the stalk. This is because of the inhibitory effect of descending inputs, and with any interruption there is an increase in basal prolactin.

5. Luteinizing Hormone and Follicle-Stimulating Hormone

Luteinizing hormone (LH) and follicle-stimulating hormone (FSH) are part of the endocrine reproductive system. They have different effects in men and in women. In women, FSH brings about maturation of the ovarian follicle, and LH is involved in the process of ovulation as well as the development of the corpus luteum. Both LH and FSH are involved in influencing ovarian secretion of the steroid hormones estrogen and progesterone. In males, FSH is involved in maintenance of spermatogenesis, and LH stimulates secretion of testosterone by the testicular interstitial cells. A lack of LH and FSH leads to gonadal atrophy and impairment of the reproductive and steroid secretory patterns in the gonads.

5.1. Regulation of LH and FSH

Regulation of LH and FSH varies somewhat between the male and female systems. Figures 6-4 and 6-5 illustrate regulatory factors involved in the male and female, respectively. Both systems share some common response patterns to sensory and visual, or light-induced, changes as well as to stress. Control of LH and FSH secretion is complex and is influenced by positive and negative feedback at the level of the hypothalamus as well as the pituitary. Estrogen, progesterone, and testosterone all act at the level of the hypothalamus and pituitary as a direct feedback loop to FSH and LH secretion. In males, there is an additional feedback of FSH secretion via the testicular hormone inhibin. Positive control of LH and FSH secretion is exerted via gonadotropin-releasing hormone (GnRH), which is secreted from the basal hypothalamus and travels via the portal veins to the pituitary.

At the level of the hypothalamus, secretion of GnRH is influenced by neurotransmitter input. Most important seems to be α-adrenergic (norepinephrine) input. Administration of norepinephrine into the basal hypothalamus increases LH release in rats, and α-adrenergic blocking agents prevent an ovulatory response in some animals. It is also thought that cholinergic input is important for GnRH regulation. Atropine has been shown to block ovulation in animals. The cells of the hypothalamus that regulate GnRH output receive innervation from a variety of other sites in the central nervous system. It is through these stimulating and inhibitory influences that gonadal function

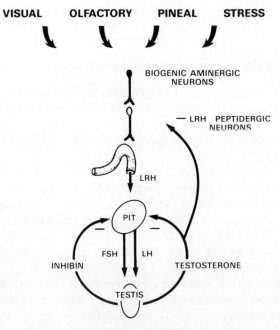

Figure 6-4. Regulation of LH and FSH in the male.

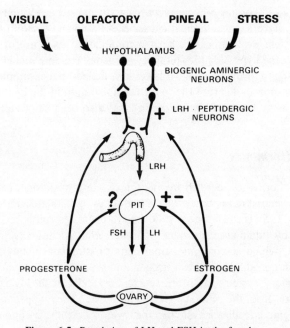

Figure 6-5. Regulation of LH and FSH in the female.

seems to respond to changes in the light–dark cycle, emotional stress, and sexual stimuli.

5.2. The Role of LH and FSH in Psychiatric Disorders

To date, the primary interest in LH and FSH has centered around changes in these hormones noted in anorexia nervosa. Studies of LH and FSH in other psychiatric diagnoses such as schizophrenia have revealed no consistent patterns, although these hormones are regulated by central aminergic pathways and therefore are of theoretical interest.

When LH patterns are measured over a 24-hr period at various times in the female life cycle, some consistent patterns emerge. In the period prior to puberty, LH concentration is generally low and shows no circadian pattern. In the beginning of puberty, LH shows pulsatile surges primarily during sleep. In late puberty, there is a pattern of pulsatile surges with a higher mean level of LH throughout the day. In the adult pattern, the higher mean level of LH persists with decreased surges but no change in the pattern of the sleep–wake cycle.

In anorexia nervosa, the presence of amenorrhea is a characteristic sign. Development of LH secretory patterns similar to those of prepuberty is characteristic of anorexia,[25] and reestablishment of a normal pattern is typical of clinical recovery. Gold[26] has suggested that LH patterns may remain abnormal despite restoration of ideal body weight and that this may be a biological marker of continued active anorexia nervosa.

One other use of measures of LH and FSH involves the evaluation of impotence. It has been suggested that despite the conventional wisdom that 90% of impotence is psychogenic in origin, subtle abnormalities of the hypothalamic–pituitary–gonadal axis may play an important role. In recent years it has been felt that 50% or more of impotence may have a physiological cause. Measurement of serum testosterone as a part of a complete evaluation has been recommended as a useful way to identify abnormalities in the hypothalamic–pituitary–gonadal axis in patients with impotence. Additional testing to further evaluate this system, including measurement of a base-line LH as well as response of serum LH to the administration of the hypothalamic peptide luteinizing-releasing hormone (gonadorelin), has also been suggested to be useful.

6. Gonadal Hormones

The major hormones secreted by the gonads are testosterone, estrogen, and progesterone. The general regulation of these hormones in the male and female is covered in Figs. 6-4 and 6-5. Testosterone is produced in the testes and is secreted in response to stimulation by luteinizing hormone. The secretion is indirectly regulated by the effects of FSH, which acts on interstitial cells to stimulate maturation and growth.

The female gonadal hormones estrogen and progesterone are involved in a more complex regulatory system. Both are secreted by cells in the ovary in response to central regulation from the pituitary via LH and FSH. There appears to be a complex positive and negative feedback system at the level of the pituitary and hypothalamus to ultimately regulate secretion and control the ovulatory cycle.

6.1. Testosterone

Interest in testosterone has centered around two major areas. The first has been the role of the hormone in the developing fetus with regard to central nervous system development and possible behavioral effects. The second is the potential influence of testosterone in sexual behavior of the adult.

In animal studies using testosterone administered to the mother during the course of pregnancy, some studies have suggested behavioral changes in the offspring.[27] Female offspring have been noted to show more malelike behaviors in terms of threatening, aggressiveness, and their sexual behavior compared with control animals. What role testosterone might play in development of the central nervous system with regard to promoting certain behavioral traits or brain organization typically characterized as being more male is yet to be determined. This is an area of interest and future research.

In adults, there has been a longstanding interest in whether serum testosterone levels could be connected with libido and sexual behavior.[28] Generally, studies trying to correlate sexual activity in normal males with plasma testosterone levels have been negative. Studies that have looked at frequency of intercourse in males have shown no higher levels of plasma testosterone in those who report frequent intercourse than in those who have less frequent sexual activity.[9] Grossly lower levels of serum testosterone caused either by castration or administration of antiandrogen medications[29] have shown some correlation with decreased libido and sexual activity. These changes in sexual behavior and interest do seem roughly to correlate with serum testosterone levels; however, the rates of change of sexual interest and lowering of serum testosterone are not highly correlated.

Impotence is a final area of interest with regard to serum testosterone. In males with normal serum testosterone and impotence, there is little benefit to administration of extra testosterone. Males who show decreased levels of testosterone with diminished libido often show a marked response with testosterone replacement. Measurement of LH and FSH in impotence can give useful information about whether the problem is primary gonadal failure or a problem at the level of the hypothalamus or pituitary.

6.2. Estrogen and Progesterone

Estrogen and progesterone play roles that are of interest in several areas. As noted with testosterone, there may be specific effects of estrogens and progesterone on the central nervous system of the developing fetus. These may take the form of behavioral variations or possibly organizational effects on the developing nervous system.

Estrogen and progesterone secretion has a major role in the normal menstrual cycle as well as in the menopause. Recent interest in these hormones has centered around their possible role in the premenstrual syndrome (PMS), which is being more commonly identified today.[30] Premenstrual syndrome is a symptom complex consisting of irritability, nervousness, crying spells, depressed mood, fatigue, water retention, headaches, changes in appetite, increased sweating, backache, and pelvic pain occurring during the 4 to 5 days prior to the menstrual period and ending some time after the onset of menses. There is no consensus at this time on the cause of premenstrual syndrome, and numerous etiologies have been suggested.[31] One hypothesis under investigation involves the relationship between estrogen and progesterone levels during the premenstrual phase. Some researchers have suggested that decreased progesterone is responsible for the symptoms noted in the premenstrual period. Follow-up studies with actual measurement of estrogen and progesterone levels have been inconclusive in providing an explanation for premenstrual syndrome, and active research is continuing.

7. Melatonin

Melatonin in the central nervous system is located in the pineal gland, where it is hypothesized that it serves to inhibit gonadotropin secretion. Since the pineal seems to be sensitive to light–dark cycles, it is thought that this may act as a mediator between the environment and the reproductive system. In addition, it is possible that melatonin may play a role in control of mood disorders that can also be sensitive to the light–dark cycle.

7.1. Regulation of Melatonin in the Central Nervous System

The hypothesized control of melatonin and the pineal gland is outlined in Fig. 6-6. It is hypothesized that light input enters through the retina and travels via the optic nerve to the suprachiasmatic nuclei. From there it travels through projections in the cervical spinal cord and via the sympathetic nervous system through the superior cervical ganglion to eventually reach the pineal gland. It is thought that the su-

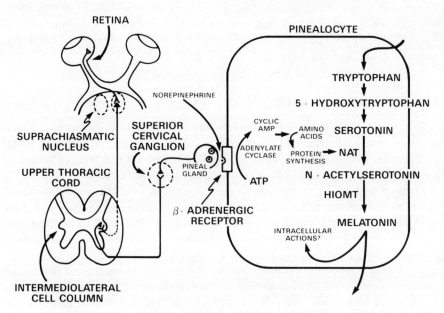

Figure 6-6. Regulation of melatonin.

prachiasmatic nucleus has an intrinsic circadian rhythm that determines both pineal and other circadian rhythms within the central nervous system. The melatonin itself is synthesized from tryptophan in the pinealocyte. It goes through a series of intermediate biosynthetic steps to become serotonin and then melatonin. This relationship between melatonin and serotonin offers intriguing possibilities regarding the relationship between melatonin and depression.

7.2. Seasonal Affective Disorder

One of the major interests in melatonin in the central nervous system is with regard to the possible mechanism of mood variation in response to light. This phenomenon has been under intensive study in recent years and has been defined as a syndrome called seasonal affective disorder (SAD).[32] Patients with SAD characteristically report changes in mood in response to the season or time of the year. Typically, they report feeling depressed in the late fall and winter and euthymic in the spring and summer. Their mood may also become depressed with changing latitude. The farther north, the higher is the incidence of depression.

Several areas of research have attempted to characterize more accurately the factors that might be involved in this phenomenon. Two active hypotheses at this point involve either the length of light exposure, which varies over the course of the year with the seasons, or the spectrum of light to which individuals are exposed. The first hypothesis suggests that the amount of light exposure is important in mood variation. During the winter months, especially at northern latitudes, the amount of daylight is considerably shortened. Studies investigating the length of light exposure have tried using light boxes in an effort to artificially increase the available amount of daylight during the winter season.[32,33] There are reports of patients having marked improvement in seasonal depressions in response to this therapy.

The second hypothesis suggests that it is not so much the amount of daylight but the spectrum or frequency of the light that is important. It is suggested that during the winter months there is a decrease in the red spectrum of the light we are exposed to. This decrease in red spectrum is hypothesized to lead to the depression of mood. Treatment has focused around attempts to increase the amount of red-spectrum light by artificially manipulating the environment. This has been most easily done by having patients wear glasses with a red tint, which increases red-spectrum light. Again, there seem to be some patients who report benefit with this particular type of treatment. Actual correlation of serum melatonin levels with seasonal affective disorder remains to be determined.

7.3. Serum Melatonin and Depression

A limited number of studies have attempted to measure serum melatonin directly and in some cases to correlate this with a variety of other neuroendocrine tests. Some studies have suggested that depressed patients with abnormal dexamethasone suppression tests also have lower melatonin levels than do patients with normal DSTs.[34] Other studies have suggested low melatonin levels in depressed patients but have not found the same correlation with the dexamethasone suppression test.[35] Since serum melatonin concentration in humans may reflect β-adrenergic activity at the level of the pineal (see Fig. 6-6), the decreased serum melatonin levels in depression may have implications for other central nervous system neurotransmitter activity. Some authors have also suggested low melatonin levels as a possible genetic trait marker for vulnerability to depression, but this is speculative at present. Further research and improvements in measurement techniques may eventually provide a more complete picture of the role of melatonin in mood disorders.

References

1. Gruen PH, Sachar EJ, Altman N, et al: Growth hormone responses to hypoglycemia in post-menopausal depressed women. *Arch Gen Psychiatry* 32:31–33, 1975.
2. Sachar EJ, Finckelstein J, Hellman L: Growth hormone responses in depressive illness, I. Response to insulin tolerance test. *Arch Gen Psychiatry* 25:263–269, 1971.
3. Carroll BJ, Mendels J: Neuroendocrine regulation in affective disorders, in Sachar EJ (ed): *Hormones, Behavior and Psychopathology*. New York, Raven Press, 1976, pp 193–224.
4. Mueller PS, Henninger GR, McDonald RK: Insulin tolerance test in depression. *Arch Gen Psychiatry* 21:587–594, 1969.
5. Maeda K, Kato Y, Ohgo S, et al: Growth hormone and prolactin release after injection of TRH in patients with depression. *J Clin Endocrinol Metab* 40:501–505, 1975.
6. Brown G, Reichlin S: Psychological and neural regulation of growth hormone secretion. *Psychosom Med* 34:45–61, 1972.
7. Checkley SA, Slade AP, Shaw E: Growth hormone and other response to clonidine in patients with endogenous depression. *Br J Psychiatry* 138:57–58, 1981.
8. Reichlin S: Regulation somatotrophic hormone secretion, in Greep RO, Astwood EB (eds): *Handbook of Physiology*, vol 4, part 2. Washington, American Physiological Society, 1974, pp 405–447.
9. Rose RM, Sachar E: Psychoendocrinology, in Williams RH (ed): *Textbook of Endocrinology*, ed 6. Philadelphia, W B Saunders, 1981, pp 646–671.
10. Powel GF, Brasel JA, Blizzard RM: Emotional deprivation and growth retardation simulating idiopathic hypopituitarism. I. Clinical evaluation of the syndrome. *N Engl J Med* 276:1271–1278, 1967.
11. Imwa H, Yoshimi T, Ikekuso K: Growth hormone secretion in a patient with deprivation dwarfism. *Endocrinol Jpn* 18:301–304, 1971.
12. Moroni F, Cheny DL, Costa E: Inhibition of acetylcholine turnover in the rat hippocampus by the intraseptal injections of beta endorphin and morphine. *Arch Pharmacol* 299:149, 1977.
13. Blum F, Segal D, Ling N, et al: Endorphins: Profound behavioral effects in rats suggest new etiological factors in mental illness. *Science* 194:630, 1976.
14. Teremius L, Wahlstrom A, Lindstrom L, et al: Increased CSF levels of endorphins in chronic psychosis. *Neurosci Lett* 3:157, 1976.
15. Pickar D, Cohen MR, Naber D, et al: Clinical studies of the endogenous opioid system. *Biol Psychiatry* 17:1243–1276, 1982.
16. Cohen MR, Cohen RM, Pickar D, et al: Behavioral effects after high dose naloxone administration to normal volunteers. *Lancet* 1:1110, 1981.
17. Cohen MR, Pickar D, Extein I, et al: Plasma cortisol and beta endorphin immunoreactivity in non-major and major depression. *Am J Psychiatry* 141:628–632, 1984.
18. Alexopoulos GS, Inturris CE, Lipman R, et al: Plasma immunoreactive beta-endorphin levels in depression. *Arch Gen Psychiatry* 40:181–183, 1983.
19. Brambilla F, Genazzani A, Facchinetti F, et al: Beta-endorphin and beta-lipotropin plasma levels in chronic schizophrenia, primary affective disorders, and secondary affective disorders. *Psychoneuroendocrinology* 6:321–330, 1981.
20. Langer G, Sacher EJ, Halpern FS, et al: The prolactin response to neuroleptic drugs, a test of dopaminergic blockade: Neuroendocrine studies in normal men. *J Clin Endocrinol Metab* 4:996–1002, 1977.

21. Gregoire E, Brauman H, DeBuch H, et al: Hormone release in depressed patients before and after recovery. *Psychoneuroendocrinology* 2:303–312, 1977.
22. Asnis GM, Nathan RS, Halbreich U, et al: Prolactin changes in major depressive disorders. *Am J Psychiatry* 137:1117–1118, 1980.
23. Linkowski P, Brauman H, Mendlewicz J: Prolactin secretion in women with unipolar and bipolar depression. *Psychiatry Res* 3:265–271, 1980.
24. Extein I, Pottash ALC, Gold MS, et al: Deficient prolactin response to morphine in depressed patients. *Am J Psychiatry* 137:845–846, 1980.
25. Katz JL, Boyer RM, Weiner H: Toward an elucidation of the psychoendocrinology of anorexia nervosa, in Sachar EJ (ed): *Hormones Behavior and Psychopathology*. New York, Raven Press, 1976, pp 263–284.
26. Gold MS, Pottash ALC, Sweeney DR, et al: Further evidence of hypothalamic–pituitary dysfunction in anorexia nervosa. *Am J Psychiatry* 137:101–102, 1980.
27. Ehrhardt AA, Meyer-Bahlburg HFL: Pre-natal sex hormones and the developing brain. Effects of psychosocial differentiation and cognitive function. *Annu Rev Med* 30:417, 1979.
28. Damassa DA, Smith ER: The relationship between circulating testosterone levels and sexual behavior. *Horm Behav* 8:275, 1977.
29. Lascattu L: Antiandrogens in the treatment of sexual deviation in men. *J Steroid Biochem* 6:821, 1975.
30. Rubinow DR, Roy-Byrne P: Premenstrual syndromes: Overview from methodologic perspective. *Am J Psychiatry* 141:163–172, 1984.
31. Reid RL, Yen SSC: Premenstral syndrome. *Am J Obstet Gynecol* 139:95–104, 1981.
32. Rosenthal NE, Sack DA, Gillin JC, et al: Seasonal affective disorder: A description of the syndrome in preliminary findings with light therapy. *Arch Gen Psychiatry* 41:72–80, 1984.
33. Lewy AJ, Sack RL, Fredrickson RH, et al: The use of bright light in the treatment of chronobiologic sleep and mood disorders: A phase response curve. *Psychopharmacol Bull* 19:523–525, 1983.
34. Steiner M, Brown GM: Melatonin/cortisol ratio: A biological marker? *Am Psychiatr Assoc Abstr New Res* abstract 53, 1984.
35. Kocsis JH, Brown RP, Frazer A, et al: Serum melatonin in melancholia. *Am Psychiatr Assoc Abstr New Res* abstract 54, 1984.

Norepinephrine and Serotonin Tests

Mark S. Gold, M.D., and Michael H. Kronig, M.D.

1. Introduction

In the field of affective disorders, research interests have focused on the neurotransmitters. The two that have been most extensively studied are the catecholamine norephinephrine (NE) and the indoleamine serotonin (5-HT). More recently, there has been work that also implicates dopamine (DA) and acetylcholine (ACh) in the pathogenesis of affective disorders, but tests with possible clinical utility center on NE and 5-HT.

The catecholamine hypothesis of affective disorders was advanced in the mid-1960s by investigators such as Schildkraut[1] and Bunney.[2] Briefly, the findings were that drugs such as reserpine[3] that deplete catecholamines can cause a condition remarkably similar to major depression. Drugs used to treat depression were found to be capable of increasing catecholamine neurotransmitters at the synaptic cleft.[4] Tricyclic antidepressants inhibit the reuptake of neurotransmitters into the synapse, and monoamine oxidase inhibitors (MAO-I) prevent the catabolism of the neurotransmitters. It was soon found that in these studies, both catecholamines and indoleamines were often affected, so that one could not with certainty differentiate between a norepinephrine effect and a serotonin effect. In any event, in its simplest form the catecholamine hypothesis read: (1) a NE deficiency results in depression; and (2) a NE excess causes mania. Treatment implications followed from there.

Clearly, the situation is much more complicated than that, and few researchers would consider the simplified scheme above the final word on affective disorders. Tricyclic antidepressants have numerous effects on neurotransmission. Given acutely they do increase neurotransmitter turnover, but after 2 to 3 weeks (considered the usual time course for clinical response), the situation is more complex.[5,6] Turnover may actually decrease, and there is also a down regulation of presynaptic adrenergic receptors.[7] The net effect in terms of actual neuronal firing is not known.

As reviewed in previous chapters, the neuroendocrine strategy is one way of assessing clinical conditions and can also shed light on neurotransmitter status. By

Mark S. Gold, M.D. • Research Facilities, Fair Oaks Hospital, Summit, New Jersey 07901, and Fair Oaks Hospital at Boca/Delray, Delray Beach, Florida 33445.   *Michael H. Kronig, M.D.* • Hillside Hospital, A Division of Long Island Jewish Medical Center, Glen Oaks, New York 11004.

working backwards, one can measure neuroendocrine abnormalities and then postulate changes in neurotransmission that may be responsible for such findings. In this chapter, we review other clinical and research strategies designed to look at the noradrenergic and serotonergic systems by other methods.

2. Norepinephrine Synthesis and Degradation

Norepinephrine is synthesized within specific neurons from the amino acid tyrosine. Tyrosine is converted to dihydroxyphenylalanine (dopa) by the enzyme tyrosine hydroxylase, which is normally saturated. This is the rate-limiting step. Dopa is decarboxylated by the enzyme dopa decarboxylase to become dopamine. Dopamine is then hydroxylated by the enzyme dopamine-β-hydroxylase to NE.

Norepinephrine is stored in granules in the presynaptic neuron. When a nerve impulse travels down the axon of a sympathetic nerve, NE is released into the cleft. Much is reabsorbed by the presynaptic neuron, where it is either stored or metabolized by MAO. There is also extracellular catabolism of NE by the enzyme catechol-O-methyltransferase (COMT). End products include 3-methoxy-4-hydroxymandelic acid (vanillymandelic acid, VMA), normetanephrine (NM), and 3-methoxy-4-hydroxy-phenylglycol (MHPG). From various studies it seems that measurements of NE, NM, and VMA principally reflect activity outside the central nervous system; MHPG is a major metabolite of central NE. Just how much of the MHPG measured in the blood or urine originates in the CNS is a controversial area.

Mannarino and associates[8] injected radioactive labeled NE into the lateral ventricle of cats. In the CNS, most was recovered as MHPG; in the urine, 50% of recovered radioactivity was in the form of MHPG or one of its conjugates. Isotope studies in other animals indicated that 25–60% of MHPG found in the urine was of central origin.[9,10] Stimulation of the brainstem nucleus locus coeruleus, the major center of NE neuron cell bodies, results in a significant increase in plasma MHPG.[11] These studies lead to three conclusions: (1) centrally, MHPG is a major metabolite of NE; (2) peripheral measures of MHPG include a significant amount of MHPG formed centrally; and (3) changes in central NE activity are reflected in peripheral MHPG levels.

A major problem is that the estimate of 25–60% stated above encompasses a large range. In the case of humans, there is one study indicating a significant peripheral conversion of MHPG to VMA, and the 25–60% range may be an overestimate.[12] Despite the uncertainties, the study of MHPG in patients with affective disturbances has yielded some interesting results.

3. MHPG in Patients with Affective Disorders

MHPG can be measured in CSF, blood, and plasma. A few research studies were done with CSF and yielded conflicting results.[13–16] One possible explanation is that lumbar MHPG may reflect local events in the spinal cord rather than brain events thought to be involved in psychiatric disorders.[17]

A number of investigators studied plasma MHPG, with one group finding increased levels in manics and decreased levels in unipolar and bipolar depressed patients.[18] There is a diurnal variation in plasma MHPG with an elevation in the morning and early afternoon compared with the night.[19] Plasma MHPG is difficult to measure. Mostly for technical reasons involving the determination of MHPG values, the majority of studies have looked at 24-hr urinary measures of MHPG.

4. Twenty-four-Hour Urinary MHPG

Many groups have studied MHPG output in the urine. Maas and colleagues[20] studied a heterogeneous group of severely depressed patients and found 24-hr urinary MHPG to be decreased compared with controls. There was overlap between depressives and controls, with no clear cutoff point to separate the two groups. Subsequent treatment studies by other groups [21-25] confirmed a wide variability in MHPG excretion in depressed patients, with an overall modest decrease compared with controls. Bipolar depressed patients have among the lowest values, and manic patients have elevated urinary MHPG.[26] There is no correlation between agitation/retardation and MHPG.[27,28] However, the first point is this: the 24-hr MHPG is not a diagnostic test for depression. Despite overall trends that are statistically significant, the overlap between depressives and normals is far too great to conclude anything about an individual test. Low MHPG appears to be a state marker that increases with successful treatment.[29]

4.1. MHPG as Predictor of Treatment Response

There has been great interest in the urinary MHPG as a predictor of treatment response. The theory is that decreased MHPG reflects decreased NE turnover. Therefore, drugs that increase central NE should be efficacious in treating these so-called "noradrenergic" depressions. Patients with high urinary MHPG presumably are deficient in 5-HT and have what are called "serotonergic" depressions. They should respond to 5-HT potentiation.[30] A preliminary study by Schildkraut[22] supported this idea. Patients with high pretreatment MHPG responded better to amitriptyline than did patients with low MHPG. Since the major effect of amitriptyline is to block serotonin reuptake (although its metabolite nortriptyline does block NE reuptake), this is consistent with expectations.

Fawcett et al. [31] administered dextroamphetamine and then imipramine or desipramine, both NE reuptake blockers, to depressed patients. Patients who responded to these drugs had significantly lower mean base-line MHPG excretion than nonresponders. This finding was confirmed by Beckman and Goodwin[23] in a study using imipramine and amitriptyline. Responders to imipramine had low pretreatment MHPG excretion, and responders to amitriptyline had high pretreatment MHPG, with no overlap. Nonresponders had the reverse, again with no overlap. These findings were extended by Cobbin et al.[25] to outpatient clinic practice. Although this was not double blind or tightly controlled, and some of the dosages are probably too low, there was an increase in improvement rate when drug treatment was tailored to MHPG excretion. Other studies have essentially confirmed this finding.

However, there is not total agreement on this issue. Coppen *et al.*[32] found MHPG not to predict response to amitriptyline. One possible explanation is that the dosage of amitripyline was 150 mg/day, which tended to be slightly less than the dosage used by other investigators. Schatzberg and colleagues[33] studied the MHPG predictor hypothesis using maprotiline, which is an essentially pure NE reuptake inhibitor. Neither the parent drug nor its active metabolites affect 5-HT reuptake. Patients with "low" MHPG ($\leq$ 1950 μg/24 hr) responded significantly better at both 2 and 4 weeks than patients with higher MHPG excretion. There was a suggestion of a "midrange" (1951 to 2500 μg/24 hr) group that was nonresponsive and a "high" (>2500 μg/24 hr) group that did respond but required higher doses, higher blood levels, and longer treatment than the "low" group. A recent study that was controlled for diet and activity found a trend toward increased response to imipramine or desipramine in low-MHPG patients, but this was not statistically significant.[34]

Overall, there is some, albeit controversial, evidence that urinary MHPG can help predict treatment response. Questions are also raised by blood level work of Glassman *et al.*[35] and Kragh-Sorensen *et al.*,[36] who adjusted dosages of imipramine and nortriptyline, respectively, to blood levels considered therapeutic and had higher response rates than would be predicted by a probable distribution of MHPG. A major problem with the treatment studies undertaken so far is the lack of specificity of the drugs used. With the exception of desipramine and maprotiline, which are quite specific for the NE reuptake pump, all the other drugs and/or their primary metabolites have significant effects on both NE and 5-HT. In addition, each group used somewhat different definitions of "high" and "low" MHPG, often picking the mean value of their group as an arbitrary cutoff. Another methodological question is whether all urine collections were complete.

4.2. Technical Consideration

Certain foods are known to contain measurable quantities of preformed catecholamines or to stimulate the release of endogenous catecholamines. This raises the question of how tightly one must control for diet when measuring MHPG. Reports on this are controversial. Muscettola *et al.*[37] found that depressed patients excrete significantly more urinary MHPG when encouraged to eat foods containing caffeine and catecholamines than when these foods are restricted. Normals, on the other hand, are unaffected by dietary changes. Sharpless[38] failed to confirm this, concluding that diet has no significant effect on urinary MHPG in depressives. The two studies differed methodologically. Muscettola's patients were on a restricted diet for 3 weeks compared with 2 days in the Sharpless study, and the patients in Sharpless' study were not encouraged to consume large quantities of previously restricted food. There may also have been differences in degree and/or type of depression. At this time it seems more prudent to have patients on a standardized diet.

Another variable is that of activity. Most investigators do not find that agitation or retardation *per se* correlate with base-line urinary MHPG excretion. In normals, exercise does not increase urinary MHPG[39]; another study did find an increase in plasma but not urinary MHPG in normals after exercise.[40] Depressed patients who were exercised beyond their base-line activity more than doubled urinary MHPG with exercise[41]; it is unclear whether this was a result of exercise itself or an unspecified "stress" factor.

Several investigators have found that males excrete more MHPG in the urine than do females when expressed as micrograms/24 hr. This apparent sex difference is eliminated by expressing MHPG excretion in terms of creatinine excretion: micrograms MHPG/24 hr per g creatinine.

The standard procedure is as follows. Patients are kept on a low-catecholamine diet for 2 days. On the third morning, the first urine is discarded. Urine is then collected for 24 hr including the first urine of the fourth morning. The urine is then refrigerated until the laboratory determination of MHPG is made. Absolute values of MHPG vary from laboratory to laboratory. Most define "high" versus "low" MHPG using a median split. The issue of "intermediate" MHPG is also arbitrarily defined.

The 24-hr MHPG has limitations, and we do not feel the final word is in. It may have some utility in the workup of the patient with major depression to guide the initial choice of antidepressants. If Schatzberg's work is replicated, it will become important to identify "high"-MHPG patients, who should remain on a given antidepressant at higher than usual blood levels and for longer than the standard 3 weeks before it is concluded that the patients are unresponsive.

5. Serotonin Biosynthesis and Degradation

The precursor of serotonin is the dietary amino acid tryptophan. Tryptophan is hydroxylated to 5-hydroxytryptophan (5-HTP) by the enzyme tryptophan-5-hydroxylase. This enzyme is not saturated, and the rate of synthesis depends on tryptophan concentration. The enzyme aromatic L-amino acid decarboxylase catalyzes the transformation of 5-HTP to serotonin (5-hydroxytryptamine, 5-HT). In man, 5-HT is metabolized by MAO and aldehyde dehydrogenase to 5-hydroxyindoleacetic acid (5-HIAA).

6. Serotonin Studies in Depressed Patients

Serotonin parameters in depressed patients have been studied by several teams of researchers. There are several lines of evidence implicating serotonin in the pathogenesis of depression. Some of the tests are obviously only for research, whereas others may prove to be of clinical value.

Postmortem research has shown that suicide victims have decreased concentrations of 5-HT and 5-HIAA in raphe nuclei,[42] which are major sites of serotonergic neurons. Similar decreases were found in depressed patients who died from other causes.[43]

Cerebrospinal fluid studies have been done by several groups. Asberg and colleagues[44] measured base-line 5-HIAA in the CSF and found a bimodal distribution; patients were indistinguishable in terms of symptoms. However, low CSF 5-HIAA correlated with later suicide attempts.[45] van Praag[46] studied patients with "vital depression" (similar to "endogenous" or major depression) both before and after probenecid loading. Probenecid inhibits the transport of 5-HIAA from the CSF to the bloodstream. The accumulation of 5-HIAA after probenecid loading is a rough indication of 5-HT turnover. In van Praag's work, about 40% of patients had decreased postprobenecid 5-HIAA: this correlated with a good response to serotonin precursors. Coppen and colleagues[47] found decreased CSF 5-HIAA in both manic and depressed patients as compared with controls. The decrease in 5-HIAA did not correlate with severity of illness. Importantly, low 5-HIAA persisted after clinical recovery. One theory is that low serotonin turnover may, in some patients, be a trait marker for vulnerability to affective illness, which then becomes manifest if other neurotransmitters are altered. If this is true, one could identify "at-risk" individuals and perhaps treat them prophylactically with serotonin precursors.

7. Platelet Serotonin Uptake

Most of the 5-HT in the blood is found within platelets. Platelets take up 5-HT both by an active transport mechanism and by passive diffusion. Although direct evidence is lacking, the possibility exists that platelet 5-HT uptake parallels the similar 5-HT uptake in the brain. Several groups have found a decreased maximum velocity (V_{max}) of 5-HT uptake in platelets of patients with major affective disease, both manic and depressed. Meltzer and colleagues[48] studied 72 patients and 20 normals. Compared with controls, bipolar depressed, unipolar depressed, and schizoaffective depressed patients had a decreased V_{max}. Except for bipolar depressed, however, the overlap with controls was fairly great. Coppen and colleagues[49] reported that this measure of serotonergic activity did not return to normal after recovery from depression.

Results with this test so far are intriguing but preliminary. The test has not yet been validated in large groups of patients, and for an individual it is hard to know how to interpret a "decreased" V_{max}. It may represent a "trait" marker for affective illness but clearly needs further study. In addition, the laboratory methods are complex.

8. Platelet Binding of Tritiated Imipramine

High-affinity binding sites for tritiated imipramine ([³H]imipramine) and other labeled tricyclics have been demonstrated in rat brain,[50] human platelets,[51] and human brain.[52] There is evidence that these binding sites are identical in platelet and brain. Moreover, these sites are associated with the uptake sites for 5-HT. Therefore, [³H]imipramine binding in platelets may be a model for studying 5-HT transport in the brain.

As with platelet 5-HT uptake, several groups have reported decreased [³H]imipramine binding in depressed patients. In a postmortem study, [³H]imipramine binding sites were found to be decreased in the frontal cortex of suicides.[53] Paul and colleagues[54] studied 14 patients with RDC major depressive disorder, endogenous subtype, and 28 age- and sex-matched controls. All subjects were medication-free for at least 2 weeks. Depressed patients had a significantly lower density of binding sites

(B_{max}) than controls. Additional data from this study supported a functional relationship between the [^{3}H]imipramine binding sites and the serotonin transport site. Thus, the [^{3}H]imipramine site may be the location where antidepressants inhibit 5-HT uptake. A small number of patients were studied after recovery and were found to have a low [^{3}H]imipramine binding, supporting the notion that it is a "trait" marker. Like the platelet serotonin uptake test, the [^{3}H]imipramine binding test awaits further validation in larger samples and in family members of depressed probands.

9. Tryptophan Levels and Competing Amino Acids

Tryptophan is the precursor of 5-HT. In animal studies, brain tryptophan, 5-HT, and 5-HIAA levels can be manipulated by changes in the dietary intake of tryptophan.[55] The only source of this precursor is dietary, as the body cannot synthesize tryptophan. Once tryptophan is absorbed, about 10–20% circulates free; the remainder is bound to albumin. Other large neutral amino acids compete with tryptophan for the same active transport system across the blood–brain barrier. The amount of tryptophan transported into the brain depends on the ratio of tryptophan (Trp) to five competing amino acids (phenylalanine, tyrosine, leucine, isoleucine, and valine). This ratio is noted as Trp/5aa.

DeMeyer and colleagues[56] studied plasma Trp/5aa ratios in patients who met Feighner criteria for depression. Patients were on a standard diet and medication-free. Depressed patients had lower Trp/5aa ratios than controls. As Hamilton depression scores improved, the Trp/5aa ratio increased significantly. Moller and colleagues[57] found that a decreased Trp/5aa predicted a good response to L-tryptophan. In a reanalysis of his data, Moller[58] concluded that the ratio of tryptophan to the three amino acids valine, leucine, and tyrosine was most predictive. As with the other peripheral 5-HT studies, more work is necessary before this test can be used as a routine clinical tool.

10. Summary

Most available antidepressants affect the NE and/or 5-HT systems. The best evidence to date indicates that the pathogenesis of depression includes alterations in these systems. Tests of NE and 5-HT could be important in pinpointing the biochemical abnormality(ies) in a given patient. Twenty-four-hour urinary MHPG has been advanced as predictive of response to specific antidepressants, with low-MHPG patients selectively responding to NE-potentiating drugs. Data for intermediate- and high-MHPG patients are less clear. Decreased CSF 5-HIAA is the most robust serotonin test, predicting suicide and violence. Peripheral tests of the 5-HT system are being studied as "trait" markers for depression. Decreased platelet serotonin uptake and decreased platelet [^{3}H]imipramine binding seem to correlate with susceptibility to major depression. The tryptophan/competing amino acid ratio may identify patients who respond to serotonin-precursor-loading strategies.

References

1. Schildkraut JJ: The catecholamine hypothesis of affective disorders: A review of supporting evidence. *Am J Psychiatry* 122:509–522, 1965.
2. Bunney, WE, Davis JM: Norepinephrine in depressive reactions: A review. *Arch Gen Psychiatry* 13:483–494, 1965.
3. Harris TH; Depression induced by rauwolfia compounds. *Am J Psychiatry* 113:950, 1957.
4. Schildkraut JJ, Dodge GA, Logue MA: Effects of tricyclic antidepressants on the uptake and metabolism of intracisternally administered norepinephrine-H^3 in rat brain. *J Psychiatr Res* 7:29–34, 1969.
5. Bunney WE, Post RM, Andersen AE: A neuronal receptor sensitivity mechanism in affective illness (a review of evidence). *Commun Psychopharmacol* 1:393–405, 1977.
6. Sulser F: New cellular mechanisms of antidepressant drugs, in Fielding S, Effland RC (eds): *New Frontiers in Psychotropic Drug Research.* Mt Kisco, NY, Futura, 1979, pp 29–50.
7. Crews FT, Smith CB: Presynaptic alpha-receptor subsensitivity after long-term antidepressant treatment. *Science* 202:322–324, 1978.
8. Mannarino E, Kirshner N, Nashold BS: The metabolism of (C^{14})noradrenaline by cat brain *in vivo. J. Neurochem* 10:373–379, 1963.
9. Maas, JW, Landis DH: *In vivo* studies of the metabolism of norepinephrine in the central nervous system. *J Pharmacol Exp Ther* 163:147–162, 1968.
10. Maas JW, Dekirmenjian H, Garver D, et al: Excretion of catecholamine metabolites following intraventricular injection of 6-hydroxydopamine in the *Macaca* speciosa. *Eur J Pharmacol* 23:121–130, 1973.
11. Crawley JN, Maas JW, Roth RH: Increase in plasma 3-methoxy-4-hydroxy-phenethyleneglycol following stimulation of the nucleus locus coeruleus. *Psychopharm Bull* 15:27–29, 1979.
12. Blombery PA, Kopin IJ, Gordon EK, et al: Conversion of MHPG to vanillylmandelic acid: Implications for the importance of urinary MHPG. *Arch Gen Psychiatry* 37:1095–1098, 1980.
13. Post RM, Gordon EK, Goodwin FK, et al: Central norepinephrine metabolism in affective illness: MHPG in the cerebrospinal fluid. *Science* 179:1002–1003, 1973.
14. Vestergaard P, Sorensen T, Rafaelsen OJ, et al: Biogenic amine metabolites in cerebrospinal fluid of patients with affective disorders. *Acta Psychiatr Scand* 58:88–96, 1978.
15. Berger PA, Faull KF, Kilkowski J, et al: CSF monoamine metabolites in depression and schizophrenia. *Am J Psychiatry* 137:174–180, 1980.
16. van Praag HM, Korf J, Schut D: Cerebral monoamines and depression: An investigation with the probenecid technique. *Arch Gen Psychiatry* 28:827–831, 1973.
17. Schildkraut JJ: Current status of the catecholamine hypothesis of affective disorders, in DiMascio A, Killam KF (eds): *Psychopharmacology: A Generation of Progress.* New York, Raven Press, 1978, pp 1223–1234.
18. Halaris AE, DeMet EM: Studies of norepinephrine metabolism in manic and depressive states, in Usdin E, Kopin IJ, Barchas J (eds): *Catecholamines: Basic and Clinical Frontiers.* New York, Pergamon Press, 1979, pp 1866–1868.
19. Markianos E, Beckman H: Diurnal changes in DBH, HVA, and MHPG in serum of man. *J Neural Transm* 39:79–93, 1976.
20. Maas JW, Fawcett J, Dekirmenjian H: 3-methoxy-4-hydroxy phenylglycol (MHPG) excretion in depressive states: A pilot study. *Arch Gen Psychiatry* 19:129–134, 1968.
21. Maas JW, Fawcett JA, Dekirmenjian H: Catecholamine metabolism, depressive illness, and drug response. *Arch Gen Psychiatry* 26:252–262, 1972.
22. Schildkraut JJ: Norepinephrine metabolites as biochemical criteria for classifying depressive disorders and predicting responses to treatment: Preliminary findings. *Am J Psychiatry* 130:695–699, 1973.
23. Beckman H, Goodwin FK: Antidepressant response to tricyclics and urinary MHPG in unipolar patients: Clinical response to imipramine or amitriptyline. *Arch Gen Psychiatry* 32:17–21, 1975.
24. Rosenbaum AH, Schatzberg AF, Maruta T, et al: MHPG as a predictor of antidepressant response to imipramine and maprotiline. *Am J Psychiatry* 137:1090–1092, 1980.
25. Cobbin DM, Requin-Blow B, Williams LR: Urinary MHPG levels and tricyclic antidepressant drug selection: A preliminary communication on improved drug selection in clinical practice. *Arch Gen Psychiatry* 36:1111–1115, 1979.

26. DeLeon-Jones F, Maas JW, Dekirmenjian H, et al: Diagnostic subgroups of affective disorders and their urinary excretion of catecholamine metabolites. *Am J Psychiatry* 132:1141–1148, 1975.

27. Taube SL, Kirstein LS, Sweeney DR, et al: Urinary 3-methoxy-4-hydroxyphenylglycol and psychiatric diagnosis. *Am J Psychiatry* 135:78–82, 1978.

28. Sweeney DR, Maas JW, Heninger GR: State anxiety, physical activity, and urinary 3-methoxy-4-hydroxyphenethyleneglycol excretion. *Arch Gen Psychiatry* 35:1418–1423, 1978.

29. Pickar D, Sweeney DR, Maas JW: Primary affective disorder, clinical state change, and MHPG excretion: A longitudinal study. *Arch Gen Psychiatry* 35:1378–1383, 1978.

30. van Praag HM: Significance of biochemical parameters in the diagnosis, treatment, and prevention of depressive disorders. *Biol Psychiatry* 12:101–131, 1977.

31. Fawcett J, Maas JW, Dekirmenjian H: Depression and MHPG excretion: Response to dextroamphetamine and tricyclic antidepressants. *Arch Gen Psychiatry* 26:246–251, 1972.

32. Coppen A, Rama Rao VA, Ruthven CRJ, et al: Urinary 4-hydroxy-3-methoxyphenylglycol is not a predictor for clinical response to amitriptyline in depressive illness. *Psychopharmacology* 64:95–97, 1979.

33. Schatzberg AF, Rosenbaum AH, Orsulak PJ, et al: Toward a biochemical classification of depressive disorders. III. Pretreatment Urinary MHPG levels as predictors of response to treatment with maprotiline. *Psychopharmacology* 75:34–38, 1981.

34. Muscettola G, Potter WZ, Pickar D, et al: Urinary 3-methoxy-4-hydroxyphenylglycol and major affective disorders: A replication and new findings. *Arch Gen Psychiatry* 41:337–342, 1984.

35. Glassman AH, Perel JM, Shostak M, et al: Clinical implications of imipramine plasma levels for depressive illness. *Arch Gen Psychiatry* 34:197–204, 1977.

36. Kragh-Sorensen P, Hansen CE, Baastrup PC: Relationship between antidepressant effect and plasma level of nortriptyline: Clinical studies. *Pharmakopsychiatr Neuropsychopharmakol* 9:27–32, 1976.

37. Muscettola G, Wehl T, Goodwin FK: Effect of diet on urinary MHPG excretion in depressed patients and normal controls. *Am J Psychiatry* 134:914–916, 1977.

38. Sharpless NS: Determination of 3-methoxy-4-hydroxyphenylglycol in urine and the effect of diet on its excretion. *Res Commun Chem Pathol Pharmacol* 18:257–273, 1977.

39. Goode DJ, Dekirmenjian H, Meltzer HY, et al: Relation of exercise to MHPG excretion in normal subjects. *Arch Gen Psychiatry* 29:391–396, 1973.

40. Tang SW, Stancer HC, Takahashi S, et al: Controlled exercise elevates plasma but not urinary MHPG and VMA. *Psychiatry Res* 4:13–20, 1981.

41. Ebert MH, Post RM, Goodwin FK: Effect of physical activity on urinary MHPG excretion in depressed patients. *Lancet* 2:766, 1972.

42. Lloyd KJ, Farley IJ, Deck JHN, et al: Serotonin and 5-hydroxyindoleacetic acid in discrete areas of the brainstem of suicide victims and control patients. *Adv Biochem Psychopharmacol* 11:387–397, 1974.

43. Birkmayer W, Riederer P: Biochemical post-mortem findings in depressed patients. *J Neural Transm* 37:95–109, 1975.

44. Asberg M, Thoren P, Traskman L, et al: "Serotonin depression": A biochemical subgroup within the affective disorders. *Science* 191:478–480, 1976.

45. Asberg M, Traskman L: Studies of CSF 5HIAA in depression and suicidal behavior. *Adv Exp Med Biol* 133:739–752, 1981.

46. van Praag HM: Central monoamine metabolism in depressions. I. Serotonin and related compounds. *Compr Psychiatry* 21:30–43, 1980.

47. Coppen A, Prange AJ, Whybrow PC, et al: Abnormalities of indoleamines in affective disorders. *Arch Gen Psychiatry* 26:474–478, 1972.

48. Meltzer HY, Arora RC, Baber R, et al: Serotonin uptake in blood platelets of psychiatric patients. *Arch Gen Psychiatry* 38:1322–1326, 1981.

49. Coppen A, Swade C, Wood K: Platelet 5-hydroxytryptamine accumulation in depressive illness. *Clin Chim Acta* 87:165–168, 1978.

50. Raisman R, Briley M, Langer SZ: Specific tricyclic antidepressant binding sites in rat brain. *Nature* 28:148–150, 1979.

51. Paul SM, Rehavi M, Skolnick P, et al: Demonstration of specific high affinity binding sites for ^{3}H imipramine on human platelets. *Life Sci* 26:953–959, 1980.

52. Rehavi M, Paul SM, Skolnick P, et al: Demonstration of specific high affinity binding sites for ^{3}H imipramine in human brain. *Life Sci* 26:2273–2279, 1980.

53. Stanley M, Virgilio J, Gershon S: Tritiated imipramine binding sites are decreased in the frontal cortex of suicides. *Science* 216:1337–1339, 1982.

54. Paul SM, Rehavi P, Skolnick P, et al: Depressed patients have decreased binding of tritiated imipramine to platelet serotonin "transporter." *Arch Gen Psychiatry* 38:1315–1317, 1981.

55. Biggio G, Fadda F, Fanni P, et al: Rapid depletion of serum tryptophan, brain tryptophan, serotonin and 5-hydroxyindoleacetic acid by a tryptophan-free diet. *Life Sci* 14:1321–1329, 1974.

56. DeMeyer MK, Shea PA, Hendrie HC, et al: Plasma tryptophan and five other amino acids in depressed and normal subjects. *Arch Gen Psychiatry* 38:642–646, 1981.

57. Moller SE, Kirk L, Honore P: Relationship between plasma ratio of tryptophan to competing amino acids and the response to L-tryptophan in endogenously depressed patients. *J Affect Dis* 1:47–59, 1980.

58. Moller SE: Evaluation of the relative potency of individual competing amino acids to tryptophan transport in endogenously depressed patients. *Psychiatry Res* 3:141–150, 1980.

Platelet and Trait Markers

Mark S. Gold, M.D., and H. Rowland Pearsall, M.D.

1. Introduction

The past decade has seen a tremendous expansion of the use of the laboratory both to understand and to diagnose psychiatric illness.[1-14] The use of 3-methoxy-4-hydroxyphenylglycol (MHPG) levels to predict antidepressant treatment response and the use of neuroendocrine tests such as the diurnal cortisol test (DCT), dexamethasone suppression test (DST), and thyrotropin-releasing hormone (TRH) test have become increasingly common in the assessment of patients with affective disorders. These tests are also being evaluated to assess their utility in patients with other psychiatric syndromes.[7-10,15-23] Research procedures that are being studied extensively and are approaching clinical usefulness can be divided into two main areas, state markers and trait markers.

State markers are those that assist in identifying particular conditions in patients. These tests confirm a primary psychiatric diagnosis, change with time, and may show change in response to treatment. State markers "mark" the presence of the active neurobiological disease state and may alert the clinician that the clinically improved patient still has active neurobiological disease and, therefore, high relapse potential. State markers such as the DCT, DST, and TRH test have already come into routine clinical use in the evaluation and treatment of patients with complaints of depression, anergia, mania, and other signs and symptoms. State markers can also assist clinicians in assessing spontaneous change of state over time. For example, mood swings from mania to euthymia to depression are preceded by state-dependent testing changes.

Trait markers identify patients with genetic or other life-long markers of risk or illness. On the biochemical and laboratory level, trait markers may identify specific traits that cut across psychiatric diagnostic groups. Patients may have a trait and either can express it or not. Many of the newest of the tests that may increasingly be used by psychiatrists fall into this trait category. The following discussion covers some of the tests that use platelets in psychiatric diagnosis and then some of the other potential trait marker tests.

Mark S. Gold, M.D. • Research Facilities, Fair Oaks Hospital, Summit, New Jersey 07901, and Fair Oaks Hospital at Boca/Delray, Delray Beach, Florida 33445. *H. Rowland Pearsall, M.D.* • Stony Lodge Hospital, Ossining-on-Hudson, New York 10562.

2. Platelets

Psychiatric research has attempted to improve diagnostic accuracy and at the same time add to an understanding of central nervous system processes in major psychiatric pathology. Although we do not have direct access to the central nervous system in the clinical setting, the more closely a biological system can mimic CNS processes, the closer to the presumed lesion one can get, and the more reliable a test is likely to be. Not having limbic or hypothalamic brain tissue available for routine examination, clinical researchers have focused on other approaches to potential information about central nervous system processes. Second only to tests of hypothalamic–pituitary function, blood platelets have proven to be one of the more accessible and reliable tissues for study. Platelets, with receptors and membrane phenomena that are very similar to CNS neurons, are ideal for use. They are relatively easy to process and readily available through vein puncture. Platelet research has focused psychiatric attention on combined trait/state markers and on pure trait markers that, with the improvement in measurement of platelet serotonin transport and levels of platelet monoamine oxidase, show strong correlations with depression, suicide, and stimulus seeking or need for psychiatric service.

2.1. Platelet Serotonin

There is considerable evidence that serotonin (5-HT) abnormalities may be present in a number of neuropsychiatric diseases.[24–27] In addition, disturbances of serotonin metabolism have been detected in numerous other human diseases. Perhaps the best known and understood serotonin disorder is the carcinoid syndrome, caused by the rapid synthesis of 5-HT by a carcinoid tumor originating from the enterochromaffin cells in the small intestine and characterized by blushing, angiomas, diarrhea, bronchial spasm, and mental changes. These symptoms result from excessive serotonin release. Other neuropsychiatric symptoms may result from abnormalities of serotonin in the CNS, and platelets can offer a vehicle to study these abnormalities.

Studies of serotonin in platelets have focused on two major biological measurements: (1) the number of serotonin receptor sites on the platelet and (2) the rate of serotonin transport or uptake by platelets. Platelets contain a high-affinity 5-HT uptake system similar to that in serotonergic neurons. The 5-HT uptake system in both platelets and brain contains specific binding sites for serotonin or [³H]imipramine, an antidepressant drug used as a ligand for neurochemical convenience since it blocks 5-HT uptake sites. Clinical investigations of the platelet 5-HT uptake system in neuropsychiatric disorders at the present time indicate possible abnormalities of neurotransmitter systems in the CNS.

2.1.1. Receptor Studies

Although this area of research is still considered controversial, numerous studies report a decrease in serotonin receptors in patients with major depression as well as a marked decrease in serotonin uptake in patients with major depression, unipolar type.[28,29] Studies in Europe and at NIMH[30,31] have examined the binding of

[^{3}H]imipramine to platelets from depressed patients and from age- and sex-matched controls. [^{3}H]Imipramine appears to bind to the receptor uptake site for serotonin in platelets and neuronal membranes. A highly significant decrease in the number of [^{3}H]imipramine binding sites was observed in platelets from depressed patients compared with controls.

These results, coupled with previous studies[32] showing a significant decrease in the maximum uptake of serotonin in platelets of depressed patients, suggest that an inherited or acquired deficiency of the serotonin transport mechanism(s) may be involved in the pathogenesis of depression. The discovery[33] of decreased serotonin uptake in platelets from depressed patients supports other evidence for a possible role of serotonin in the pathophysiology of some forms of depression. Furthermore, with postmortem brain tissue, it was shown[34,35] that imipramine binding was significantly reduced in the frontal cortex, hippocampus, and occipital cortex of suicides and depressed patients compared with normal controls.

2.1.2. Transport Studies

Receptor studies have focused on the number of apparent binding sites, whereas transport studies have attempted to look at the overall activity of the 5-HT uptake system. It has been reported that a decrease in serotonin turnover may be associated with an increased risk of suicide or violence; more recently, brain serotonin receptor transport has been found to be markedly reduced in the brains of human suicide patients. Low platelet serotonin transport has been reported in medication-free patients with unipolar depression, whereas increased transport has been observed in bipolar depressed patients.[36,37] Platelet serotonin has also been looked at in schizophrenic patients, with reports of increased platelet serotonin levels in some schizophrenic patients but of normal rates of platelet serotonin uptake.[38]

The group of patients with low platelet serotonin activity may reflect a subgroup of depressed individuals who are particularly responsive to serotonergic antidepressants and 5-HT precursors according to some studies.[28] Such a finding would be consistent with the concept of a serotonergic-deficient depression as one subtype of the unipolar spectrum. There have also been reports that platelet serotonin may be stable between episodes of affective illness and that there may perhaps be a subtype of depression characterized by platelet serotonin deficiency.[39]

Serotonin may provide data about more than the patient's state, however. For example, some studies have shown decreases in platelet serotonin activity in all involved first-degree relatives of affected individuals, indicating a possible trait marker function.[39]

2.2. Platelet Monoamine Oxidase

Like the central nervous system, platelets also contain monoamine oxidase, and assays have been developed to measure MAO activity in the platelet. Until recently, research has focused primarily on application of these activity measurements to diagnoses such as schizophrenia and affective disorders in the hope of improving the diagnostic process.[40-45] In addition, platelet MAO measurement has become routine in improving the treatment response to drugs such as the monoamine oxidase inhibitors. More recently, platelet MAO has been studied as a prognostic biological marker for personality, i.e., a possible trait marker function.[46-51]

Studies of some patients with schizophrenia have shown a decrease in platelet MAO activity. These studies have focused on patients with a chronic rather than acute form of schizophrenia, and low platelet MAO activity has been correlated with prognostic scales, indicating that such a finding is indicative of a poor prognosis. Low platelet MAO activity may also show the way to a possible genetic form of schizophrenia characterized by this state.

Platelet MAO has been reported to be low in bipolar depression; however, its application in unipolar depression has been more uncertain. The identification of a subset of unipolar depressed patients with symptoms of anxiety, agitation, somatic complaints, and with increased levels of pretreatment MAO activity may represent an MAOI-responsive group of patients.

Another application of platelet MAO activity levels already in widespread use is to improve the response rate to monoamine oxidase inhibitor-type drugs. Numerous studies have shown that patients achieving an MAO inhibition of greater than 80% from their own baseline have a much higher response rate for relief of depressive symptoms than patients achieving MAO inhibition below this level. One study reported a 50% increase in the response rate.[52] Response for those with inhibition greater than 80% was 68% compared with a 44% response for patients with less than 80% inhibition. These findings offer the potential for a useful clinical test for assessing the effectiveness of MAOI therapy in much the same way that one is increasingly able to monitor the blood levels of tricyclic antidepressants.

Platelet MAO levels have also been investigated as they relate to behavior. Recent studies have successfully correlated decreased MAO levels with personality traits and behavior such as sensation seeking or thrill seeking.[46-50] This use of MAO levels may eventually provide a useful trait marker. Studies looking at MAO levels in populations of "normals" have identified consistent correlations with personality traits and low MAO activity.[45-50] One study using college students found that those with low MAO activity reported more frequent psychological counseling and problems with the law and that their families had a higher incidence of suicide than a comparison group of students with high MAO activity.[48,49] Low-MAO males also had elevated scores on the hypochondria and hysteria scales of the MMPI. Other studies have correlated low MAO with sensation seeking, high ego strength, positive affect, and high leisure-time activity levels. Longitudinal studies of the nonsymptomatic population identified only by abnormal MAO activity levels may lead to the identification of a group at risk for development of personality disorder to major psychiatric illness. Low-MAO normals may not, in fact, be normal but may be a population "at risk" with a vulnerability that may or may not be expressed.

3. Other Potential Trait Markers

3.1. Cerebrospinal Fluid Metabolites

Attempts have been made to measure the metabolites of neurotransmitters such as serotonin, dopamine, and norepinephrine in the cerebrospinal fluid (CSF). To date, the most interesting finding has been a decreased amount of the serotonin breakdown product 5-hydroxyindoleacetic acid (5-HIAA) in the CSF of patients who have attempted suicide.[53] This lower level of 5-HIAA does not appear to be dependent on whether or not the patient has symptoms severe enough to be diagnosed as depression.

Swedish authors[54] described a bimodal distribution in the levels of the serotonin metabolite 5-HIAA in the CSF of 68 depressed patients. More of the patients who had attempted suicide, including two who eventually did commit suicide, were in the lower 5 HIAA group. In a more recent report, that same group[53] compared 30 patients who had attempted suicide with 45 normal persons. The suicide attempters, especially those who had made more violent attempts, had a significantly lower CSF 5-HIAA level than the controls. A follow-up study of these 30 and 89 earlier patients (depressed and/or suicidal) showed a 20% mortality by suicide within a year of the lumbar puncture in persons with a CSF 5-HIAA level below the median.

Brains of patients who have committed suicide have been studied with respect to serotonin measures. Low concentrations of serotonin,[55] 5-HTP,[56,57] and 5-HIAA[55,57] have been reported in suicide patients with postmortem studies. Consistent with these reports is the finding by Stanley of decreased imipramine binding sites in the frontal cortex of suicide patients.[34] Studies on living patients have confirmed this finding. Abbey found that low baseline CSF 5-HIAA measures correlated with the frequency of suicidal behavior in depressed patients[58] and that these patients employed more aggressive means, such as hanging, deep wrist slashing, and gas poisoning.[54] She found that 40% of low-CSF-5-HIAA patients had made a suicide attempt compared to 15% of patients without this finding.[54] The correlation between low CSF 5-HIAA accumulation and suicidality in depressed patients has also been reported by other investigators.[59,60] Traskman found that of 119 patients with low CSF 5-HIAA accumulation, 20% had killed themselves within a period of 1 year.[53] These patients were not exclusively depressed, suggesting that the serotonin abnormality correlates more with suicidality and violence than with depression.[53] Other investigators have found the correlation of low CSF 5-HIAA and suicidality in borderline patients,[61] mixed diagnostic groups,[62] psychotic illness,[63] and other nondepressed suicide victims.[64]

The relationship between suicidality and aggression has long been appreciated in clinical psychiatry. This relationship may have a biological basis. Brown studied 26 military men with histories of significant aggression and found low CSF 5-HIAA as well as high CSF MHPG concentrations after probenecid treatment.[65] This was consistent with reports of particularly violent suicide attempts in patients with low CSF serotonin metabolites.[53,58] Furthermore, criminals institutionalized for violence and aggression who also had 47,XYY syndrome were reported to show marked reductions in CSF 5-HIAA accumulation after probenecid.[66] Similarly, Agren found that unipolar and bipolar depressed patients with low CSF 5-HIAA levels scored particularly high on the anger-related items of the SADS interview.[67] Thus, as with suicidality, a predilection toward violence appears to correlate with this biological measure both with and without concomitant affective disease. It also suggests that serotonin may have a role as an inhibitor of aggressive behaviors.

Genetic loading has been described for both suicidality[68] and aggression.[69] Sedvall studied CSF 5-HIAA accumulation in a group of healthy volunteers.[70] He found that those with low values had significantly more affective illness in their families.[70] There has also been reported greater concordance in monozygotic than dizygotic twins for low CSF 5-HIAA accumulation.[71] Also consistent with genetic transmissibility of low CSF 5-HIAA accumulation is evidence that it represents a trait rather than state-related measure.[72,73] These findings suggest that this low serotonin measure is genetically determined and could indicate a genetic predisposition toward associated depression, suicidality, and aggressiveness.

Unfortunately, there is as yet no place in general clinical practice for determining CSF 5-HIAA levels as a possible predictor of suicidal behaviors. Rather than waiting for a homicide or suicide to occur, psychiatrists in the late 1980s may be able to do a spinal tap to compare 5-HIAA or other metabolic measurements with a known actuarial chart to assess risk more accurately. Low 5-HIAA has also been reported in other groups of patients such as violent patients, obsessive–compulsives, schizoaffective, and alcoholic patients, so this finding crosses diagnostic groups.[53]

3.2. Plasma/Urinary MHPG and Dexamethasone Suppression and TRH Tests

Although these three measurements have emerged during the past decade as useful diagnostic tests, their utility may be enhanced in the coming decade as their interrelationship is better understood. The diagnostic category of unipolar depression seems increasingly to contain a variety of subgroups that may be further classified biologically by findings in tests such as MHPG, DST, and TRH. Data already suggest that patients with low MHPG levels in plasma or urine are more likely to respond to treatments such as imipramine, desipramine, maprotiline, and nortriptyline antidepressant therapies.[15,16] These also correlate with the group of patients who show abnormalities in TRH testing.[1] A group of patients who have been found to have high and medium MHPG excretion may be more likely to have an abnormal DST. The medium-MHPG group appears to respond to serotonergic antidepressants, and the high-MHPG group appears to be responsive to noradrenergic treatment.

In the coming decade, the interrelationship among MHPG, DST, and TRH may provide useful insight into underlying mechanisms of affective disorder. Further, there may emerge some constant trait marker role for this interrelationship.

3.3. HLA Typing

Much interest has centered on trying to identify potential genetic or chromosomal markers that might specify or identify genetic defects leading to various kinds of psychiatric disorders.[74,75] The finding of increased frequency of affective disorders in certain families has focused attention on these disorders and the possible genetic implications. The HLA, or human leukocyte A system is a locus of genes that control antigens on the surface of cell membranes. These antigens probably consist of glycoproteins and can be tested for and typed in a similar way to the ABO blood group systems. There are four main antigens in the HLA system. Studies in this area have focused on the observation that HLA antigens appear with different frequencies than in the normal population in patients with primary affective disorders. Studies looking at families in which two siblings both have affective illness have detected an excess of

HLA similarities compared with families in which only one sibling has affective illness. Some authors feel that these findings imply a locus for primary affective disorder located somewhere near the HLA gene locus.[74] The nature of such a genetic defect, and, in fact, its existence, is still controversial; however, research of this type may eventually provide a technique for identifying patients at risk for affective or other psychiatric disorders.

3.4. Red Blood Cell Membrane Studies

Recently there has been considerable interest in the cell membrane as a possible experimental model for events taking place at the membrane level of neurons in the central nervous system. One of the most accessible sources of cell membranes is blood cells, in particular, the red blood cell. The red blood cell membrane in patients with a history of bipolar affective illness has been studied using a variety of techniques, and the results may some day provide us with a trait marker for these patients.

There are several sources of data about red blood cell membranes in affective disorders currently under active investigation[13,14,76–81]: (1) studies of lithium distribution, as reflected by the ratio of intracellular to extracellular lithium (lithium ratio); (2) changes in active transport of lithium across red cell membranes (lithium efflux); and (3) fluorescence spectroscopy of red blood cell membranes. Each of these approaches provides some interesting data with reference to predicting an affective disorder or separating clinically identical bipolar and unipolar depressives.

The lithium ratio involves the measurement of lithium concentrations both in and out of the red blood cells and is calculated by dividing the lithium concentration in the red blood cells by the lithium concentration in plasma or surrounding solution. Measurements of the ratio can be done both *in vivo* and *in vitro*. Generally, this ratio is considerably less than 1 and is indicative of some type of active transport process that allows lithium to be moved against a diffusion gradient out of red cells and into the surrounding plasma. When lithium ratios are measured in bipolar patients and in normal controls, there is a much higher lithium ratio in bipolar patients. This means that there is relatively more lithium in the red blood cells of the ill individuals, which may imply some defect in the active transport process that generally keeps lithium out. Some researchers have reported that lithium treatment responders tend to have higher lithium ratios than nonresponders.[76] Lithium ratio is the oldest of the red blood cell membrane tests and can be done "routinely" by some laboratories. The other membrane tests are newer and more complex and are not yet available outside of a few sophisticated laboratories.

Lithium efflux is a second technique used to evaluate red blood cell membranes. As mentioned, it is a technically more difficult test and involves the measurement of the rate of transport of lithium out of the red blood cells. Lithium kinetics across red blood cell membranes are complex but involve both influx and efflux with a presumed active transport process involved in the removal of lithium. Lithium efflux can be expressed as a rate constant K_O and reflects lithium accumulation in a Ringer solution after 1 hr divided by the mean concentration of lithium in the red blood cell during the incubation period. Data indicate that bipolar patients show a lower rate of lithium efflux than schizophrenic and unipolar patients as well as normal controls.[81] Generally, these patients also are lithium responders. Interestingly, giving lithium tends to bring about a change in lithium efflux and leads to an increase in the lithium ratio or a decrease in lithium efflux. This change seems to occur within 1 or 2 weeks after the beginning of lithium treatment and lasts for 1 to 2 weeks after lithium is discontinued. Although several explanations have been proposed for what causes this change in the lithium ratio or lithium efflux, the most likely seems to be the induction of some type of endogenous regulator that controls the rate of lithium movement across the cell membranes. Whether abnormalities in levels or activity of such an endogenous regulator have any clinical implications is unknown at present.

A third approach is fluorescence spectroscopy of red blood cell membranes. This involves the use of "probes" or substances with a known affinity for particular areas of the cell membrane. Fluorescamine binds to cell surface primary amines,[9,12] and anthroyl stearate binds to deep hydrocarbon regions of membranes. Red blood cell membranes labeled in this way and undergoing fluorescence spectroscopic analysis with measurement of emission spectrum show characteristic changes. Results show that hydrocarbon regions of membranes are altered in bipolar patients in a way that seems to be independent of their clinical symptoms and medications. Thus, this measurement may serve as a possible trait marker and also as a possible presymptomatic diagnostic test for bipolar disorders.

The results discussed above still vary among researchers, which may be a reflection of different populations of patients or different subgroups of bipolar illness.[14,76] It has been noted in some studies that schizophrenic patients or patients with other psychiatric diagnoses show abnormalities such as increased lithium ratio or decreased lithium efflux in a way similar to bipolar patients, suggesting that these patients could be potential lithium responders. This entire area is one of continued research and potential future usefulness, since separation of unipolar from bipolar depression and manic states from schizophrenia would greatly improve therapeutic response.

4. Endorphins

The endogenous opioid system in humans is increasingly being studied to determine its role in the regulation of mood and anxiety.[82,83] These studies may eventually elucidate some utility for the endorphin system as a trait marker. Several clinical research strategies have been used. Administration of high doses of the opiate antagonist naloxone to normal volunteers has shown dose-dependent increases in self-ratings of tension–anxiety and anger–hostility. These data support the hypothesis that modulation of human mood and feelings of well-being may be influenced by the endogenous opiate system. Studies measuring CSF opioid activity in psychiatric patients and normals using sensitive radioreceptor assays suggest that some schizophrenics have diminished endogenous opioid system activity.[82] Opioid activity may also be related to state changes in bipolar illness and anorexia nervosa.[82] In major depression, morning plasma concentrations of β-endorphin immunoreactivity are reported to be significantly higher than in age- and sex-matched normal controls or in psychiatric patients without affective disorders.[83] Schizoaffective disorders in the depressed phase show similar findings.[83]

It has been hypothesized that cholinergic mechanisms play a role in hypothalamic–pituitary release, and it has been found that giving physostigmine, a promoter of cholinergic activity, causes a significantly greater β-endorphin response in depressed patients than in normal controls.[83] This observation suggests a cholinergic supersensitivity in depression, and the cholinergically stimulated hypothalamic–pituitary β-endorphin release may some day be useful as a biological state or trait marker for some types of depression.

References

1. Davis KL, Hollister LE, Aleksander AM, et al: Neuroendocrine and neurochemical measurements in depression. *Am J Psychiatry* 138:1555–1562, 1981.
2. van Praag HM: Neuroendocrine disorders and depressions and their significance for the monoamine hypothesis of depression. *Acta Psychiatr Scand* 57:389–404, 1978.
3. Stahl SM: The human platelet: A diagnostic and research tool for the study of biogenic amines in psychiatric and neurologic disorders. *Arch Gen Psychiatry* 34:509–516, 1977.
4. van Praag HM: Neurotransmitters and CNS disease. *Lancet* 2:1259–1264, 1982.
5. Schildkraut JJ, Orsulak PJ, Schatzberg AF, et al: Toward a biochemical classification of depressive disorders. *Arch Gen Psychiatry* 35:1427–1433, 1978.
6. Leckman JF, Cohen DJ, Shaywitz BA, et al: CSF monoamine metabolites in child and adult psychiatric patients. *Arch Gen Psychiatry* 37:677–681, 1980.
7. Asnis GM, Sachar EF, Halbreich U, et al: Cortisol secretion and dexamethasone response in depression. *Am J Psychiatry* 138:1218–1221, 1981.
8. Sachar EJ, Hellman L, Roffwarg HP, et al: Disrupted 24 hour patterns of cortisol secretion in psychotic depression. *Arch Gen Psychiatry* 28:19–24, 1973.
9. Carroll BJ, Feinberg M, Greden JF, et al: A specific laboratory test for the diagnosis of melancholia. *Arch Gen Psychiatry* 38:15–22, 1981.
10. Carroll BJ: The dexamethasone suppression test for melancholia. *Br J Psychiatry* 140:292–304, 1982.
11. Loosen PT, Prange AJ: Serum thyrotropin response to thyrotropin releasing hormone in psychiatric patients: A review. *Am J Psychiatry* 139:405–416, 1982.
12. Sternbach H, Gerner RH, Gwirtsman AG: The thyrotropin releasing hormone stimulation test: A review. *J Clin Psychiatry* 43:4–6, 1982.
13. Pandey GN, Sarkadi B, Haas M, et al: Lithium transport pathways in human red blood cells. *J. Gen Physiol* 72:233–247, 1978.
14. Pettegrew JW, Nichols JS, Minshew NJ, et al: Membrane biophysical studies of lymphocytes and erythrocytes in manic depressive illness. *J Affect Dis* 4:237–247, 1982.
15. Schatzberg AF, Orsulak PJ, Rosenbaum AH, et al: Toward a biochemical classification of depressive disorders V: Heterogeneity of unipolar depressions. *Am J Psychiatry* 139:471–475, 1982.
16. Maas JW, Kocsis JH, Bowden CL, et al: Pre-treatment neurotransmitter metabolites and response to imipramine or amitriptyline treatment. *Psychol Med* 12:37–43, 1982.
17. Hollister LE, David KL, Berger PA: Subtypes of depression based on excretion of MHPG and response to nortriptyline. *Arch Gen Psychiatry* 37:1107–1110, 1980.
18. Sachar EJ, Hellman L, Fukushima D, et al: Cortisol production in depressive illness. *Arch Gen Psychiatry* 23:289–298, 1970.
19. Carroll BJ, Curtis GC, Mendels J: Neuroendocrine regulation in depression II: Discrimination of depressed from non-depressed patients. *Arch Gen Psychiatry* 33:1051–1058, 1976.
20. Brown WA, Johnston R, Mayfield D: The 24 hour dexamethasone suppression test in a clinical setting: Relationship to diagnosis, symptoms, and response to treatment. *Am J Psychiatry* 136:543–547, 1979.
21. Gold MS, Pottash ALC, Rein N, et al: TRH induced TSH response in unipolar, bipolar and secondary depressions: Possible utility and clinical assessment and differential diagnosis. *Psychoneuroendocrinology* 5:147–155, 1980.

22. Extein I, Pottash ALC, Gold MS, et al: Using the protirelin test to distinguish mania from schizophrenia. *Arch Gen Psychiatry* 39:77–81, 1982.
23. Extein I, Pottash ALC, Gold MS: Relationship of thyrotropin releasing hormone test and dexamethasone suppression test abnormalities in unipolar depression. *Psychiatry Res* 4:49–53, 1981.
24. Bowers MB, Heninger GR, Gerbode F: Cerebral spinal fluid in 5-hydroxy indoleacetic and homovanillic acid in psychiatric patients. *Int J Neuropharmacol* 8:255–262, 1969.
25. Apeschi R, McClure DJ: Homovanillic and 5-hydroxy indoleacetic acid in cerebral spinal fluid of depressed patients. *Arch Gen Psychiatry* 25:354–358, 1971.
26. Post RN, Ballenger JC, Goodwin FK: Cerebral spinal fluid studies of neurotransmitter function, in manic and depressive illness, in Wood JH (ed): *Neurobiology of CSF*. New York, Plenum Press, 1980, pp 685–717.
27. Cowdry RW, Goodwin FK: Amine neurotransmitter studies and psychiatric illness: Toward more meaningful diagnostic concepts, in Spitzer RL, Klein DF (eds): *Critical Issues in Psychiatric Diagnosis*. New York, Raven Press, 1978, pp 281–304.
28. Tuomisto J, Tukiainen E: Decreased uptake of 5-hydroxytryptamine in blood platelets from patients with endogenous depression. *Psychopharmacology* 65:141–147, 1979.
29. Briley MS, Langer SZ, Raisman R, et al: Tritiated imipramine binding sites are decreased in platelets of untreated depressed patients. *Science* 209:303–305, 1980.
30. Briley M, Raisman R, Langer S: Human platelets possess high affinity binding sites for [^{3}H]-imipramine. ᴱur J Pharmacol 58:347–348, 1979.
31. Paul SM, Rehavi M, Skolnick P, et al: Depressed patients have decreased binding of tritiated imipramine to platelet serotonin 'transporter.' *Arch Gen Psychiatry* 38:1315–1321, 1981.
32. Tuomisto J, Tukiainen E: Decreased uptake of 5-hydroxytryptamine in blood platelets from depressed patients. *Nature* 262:596–598, 1976.
33. Meltzer H, Arora RC, Baber R, et al: Serotonin uptake in blood platelets of psychiatric patients. *Arch Gen Psychiatry* 38:1322–1326, 1981.
34. Stanley M, Virgilio J, Gershon S: Tritiated imipramine binding sites are decreased in the frontal cortex of suicides. *Science* 216:1337–1339, 1982.
35. Perry E, Marshall E, Blessed G, et al: Decreased imipramine binding in the brains of patients with depressed illness. *Br J Psychiatry* 142:188–192, 1983.
36. Zemishlany Z, Munitz H, Rotman A, et al: Increased uptake of serotonin by blood platelets from patients with bipolar primary affective disorder bipolar type. *Psychopharmacology* 77:175–178, 1982.
37. Meltzer HY, Arora RC, Tricou BJ, et al: Serotonin uptake in blood platelets and the dexamethasone suppression test in depressed patients. *Psychiatry Res* 8:41–47, 1983.
38. Arora RC, Meltzer HY: Serotonin uptake by blood platelets of schizophrenic patients. *Psychiatry Res* 6:327–333, 1982.
39. Meltzer HY, Arora RC, Babe R, et al: Serotonin uptake in blood platelets as a biologic marker for major depression disorders, in Usdin E, Hanin I (eds): *Biological Markers in Psychiatry and Neurology*. Oxford, Pergamon Press, 1982, pp 39–48.
40. Davidson JRT, McLeod MN, Turnbull CD, et al: Platelet monoamine oxidase activity and the classification of depression. *Arch Gen Psychiatry* 37:771–773, 1980.
41. Fieve RR, Kumbaraci T, Kassir S, et al: Platelet monoamine oxidase activity in affective disorders. *Biol Psychiatry* 15:473–478, 1980.
42. Murphy DL, Weiss R: Reduced monoamine oxidase activity in blood platelets from bipolar depressed patients. *Am J Psychiatry* 128:1351–1357, 1972.
43. Gudeman JE, Schatzberg AF, Samson JA, et al: Toward a biochemical classification of depressive disorders VI: Platelet MAO activity and clinical symptoms in depressed patients. *Am J Psychiatry* 139:630–633, 1982.
44. Gruen R, Baron M, Levitt M, et al: Platelet MAO activity and schizophrenic prognosis. *Am J Psychiatry* 139:240–241, 1982.
45. Rosen AJ, Wirtshafer D, Pandey GN, et al: Platelet monoamine oxidase activity and behavioral response to pharmacotherapy in psychiatric patients. *Psychiatry Res* 6:49–59, 1982.
46. Schooler C, Zahm TP, Murphy DL, et al: Psychological correlates of monoamine oxidase activity in normals. *J Nerv Ment Dis* 166:177–186, 1978.

47. Buchsbaum MS, Coursey RD, Murphy DL: The biochemical high risk paradigm: Behavioral and familial correlates of low platelet monoamine oxidase activity. *Science* 194:339–341, 1976.
48. Buchsbaum MS, Murphy DL, Coursey RD, et al: Platelet monoamine oxidase, plasma dopamine-beta-hydroxylase, and attention in a biochemical high risk sample. *J Psychiatr Res* 14:215–224, 1978.
49. Coursey RD, Buchsbaum MS, Murphy DL: Two year follow-up of subjects and their families defined as at risk for psychopathology on the basis of platelet MAO activities. *Neuropsychobiology* 8:51–56, 1982.
50. Gattaz WF, Beckman H: Platelet MAO activity and personality characteristics. *Acta Psychiatr Scand* 63:479–485, 1981.
51. Demisch L, Georgi K, Patzke B, et al: Correlations of platelet MAO activity with introversion: A study on a German rural population. *Psychiatry Res* 6:303–311, 1982.
52. Georgotus A, Mann J, Friedman E: Platelet MAO inhibition as a potential indicator of favorable response to MAOI's in geriatric depressions. *Bio Psychol* 16:997–1001, 1981.
53. Traskman L, Asberg M, Bertilsson L, et al: Monoamine metabolites in CSF in suicidal behavior. *Arch Gen Psychiatry* 38:631–636, 1981.
54. Asberg M, Trasberg L, Thoren P: 5-HIAA in the cerebrospinal fluid. A biochemical suicide predictor. *Arch Gen Psychiatry* 338:1193–1197, 1976.
55. Lloyd KJ, Farley, IJ, Deck JHN, et al: Serotonin and 5-hydroxyindoleacetic acid in discrete areas of the brainstem of suicide victims and control patients. *Adv Biochem Psychopharmacol* 11:387–397, 1974.
56. Shaw DM, Camps FE, Eccleston EG: 5-Hydroxytryptamine in the hindbrain of depressive suicides. *Br J Psychiatry* 113:1407–1411, 1967.
57. Bourne HR, Bunney WE, Colburn RW, et al: Noradrenaline, 5-hydroxytryptamine, and 5-hydroxyindoleacetic acid in hindbrains of suicidal patients. *Lancet* 2:805–808, 1968.
58. Asberg M, Thoren P, Traskman L: Serotonin depression: A biochemical subgroup within the affective disorders? *Science* 191:478–480, 1976.
59. Agren H: Symptom patterns in unipolar and bipolar depression correlating with monoamine metabolites in the cerebrospinal fluid. I. General patterns. *Psychiatry Res* 3:211–222, 1980.
60. Banki CM, Molnar G, Vojnik M: Cerebrospinal fluid amine metabolites, tryptophan and clinical parameters in depression. II. Actual psychopathological symptoms. *J Affect Dis* 3:91–99, 1981.
61. Brown GL, Ebert MH, Goyer PF, et al: Aggression, suicide and serotonin: Relationships to CSF amine metabolites. *Am J Psychiatry* 139:741–746, 1982.
62. Oreland L, Wiberg A, Asberg M, et al: Platelet MAO activity and monoamine metabolites in cerebrospinal fluid in depressed and suicidal patients and in healthy controls. *Psychiatry Res* 4:21–29, 1981.
63. Leckman JF, Charney DS, Nelson CR: CSF tryptophan, 5-HIAA, and HVA in 132 psychiatric patients categorized by diagnosis and clinical state. *Recent Adv Neuropsychopharmacol* 31:289–297, 1981.
64. Barraclough B, Bunch J, Nelson B, et al: A hundred cases of suicide: Clinical aspects. *Br J Psychiatry* 125:355–373, 1974.
65. Brown GL, Goodwin FK, Ballenger JC, et al: Aggression in human correlates with cerebrospinal fluid amine metabolites. *Psychiatry Res* 1:131–139, 1979.
66. Bioulac B, Benezech M, Renaud B: Biogenic amines in 47,XYY syndrome. *Neuropsychobiology* 4:366–370, 1978.
67. Agren H: Symptom patterns in unipolar and bipolar depression correlating with monoamine metabolites in the cerebrospinal fluid, II: Suicide. *Psychiatry Res* 3:225–236, 1980.
68. Kety SS: Disorders of the human brain. *Sci Am* 241:202–214, 1979.
69. Hutchings B, Mednick SA: Registered criminality in the adoptive and biological parents of registered male criminal adoptees, in Fieve RR, Rosenthal D, Brill H (eds): *Genetic Research in Psychiatry*. Baltimore, Johns Hopkins University Press, 1975, pp 105–116.
70. Sedvall G, Fryo B, Bullberg B, et al: Relationships in healthy volunteers between concentration of monoamine metabolites in cerebrospinal fluid and family history of psychiatric morbidity. *Br J Psychiatry* 136:366–374, 1980.
71. Sedvall G, Nyback H, Oxenstierna G: Relationships between aberrant monoamine metabolite concentration in cerebrospinal fluid and family disposition for psychiatric disorders in healthy and schizophrenic subjects. *Coll Int Neuropsychopharmacol Abstr* 607, p 316, 1980.

72. Ashcroft GW, Crawford TBB, Eccleston D, et al: 5-Hydroxyindole compounds in the cerebrospinal fluid of patients with psychotic or neurological diseases. *Lancet* 2:1049–1052, 1966.

73. van Praag HM: Significance of biochemical parameters in the diagnosis, treatment, and prevention of depressive disorders. *Biol Psychiatry* 12:101–131, 1977.

74. Cazzullo CL, Smeraldi E: Genetic markers in psychiatry: Studies on HLA system, in Obiols J (ed): Developments in Psychiatry, Vol II: *Biological Psychiatry Today.* Amsterdam, North Holland Biomedical Press, 1979, pp 66–71.

75. Smeraldi E, Bellodi L: Possible linkage between primary affective disorders susceptibility locus and HLA haplotypes. *Am J Psychiatry* 138:1232–1234, 1981.

76. Flemenbaum A, Weddige R, Miller J: Lithium erythrocyte/plasma ratio as a predictor of response. *Am J Psychiatry* 135:336–338, 1978.

77. Rihmer Z, Arato M, Szentistvanyi I, et al: The red blood cells/plasma lithium ratio: Marker of biological heterogeneity within bipolar affective illness? *Psychiatry Res* 6:197–201, 1982.

78. Frazer A, Mendels J, Brunswick D, et al: Erythrocyte concentration of the lithium ion: Clinical correlates in mechanisms of action. *Am J Psychiatry* 135:1065–1069, 1978.

79. Meltzer HL, Kassir S, Dunner DL, et al: Factors effecting lithium efflux from human erythrocytes. *Psychopharmacol Bull* 14:19–21, 1978.

80. Goodnick PJ, Meltzer HL, Dunner DL, et al: Repression and reactivation of lithium efflux from erythrocytes. *Psychiatry Res* 1:147–152, 1979.

81. Pandey G: Lithium efflux from red cells in affective illness, in: *Continuing Medical Education: Syllabus and Proceedings in Summary Form,* vol 321. Washington, American Psychiatric Association, 1978, pp 104–105.

82. Pickar D, Cohen MR, Nase D, et al: Clinical studies of the endogenous opioid system. *Biol Psychiatry* 17:1243–1276, 1982.

83. Risch SC: Beta endorphin hypersecretion in depression. Possible cholinergic mechanisms. *Biol Psychiatry* 17:1071–1079, 1982.

Nutritional Deficiency Syndromes in Clinical Psychiatry

Frederick C. Goggans, M.D., and Mark S. Gold, M.D.

1. Introduction

The question of the role that vitamins, minerals, and other dietary substances play in normal and pathological mental functioning is one that has probably captured more popular than professional interest. Nevertheless, psychiatrists have become increasingly aware of the importance of a careful laboratory assessment of these substances in the modern diagnostic workup of their patients.[1] In the last decade, clinical nutrition has become a regular part of the undergraduate medical curriculum, and more recent basic science studies have extended our knowledge of the role that these substances play in those neurochemical processes that are relevant to the pathophysiology of the major psychiatric syndromes. For example, many vitamins and trace elements are cofactors or precursors in important metabolic pathways in the central nervous system, and it is becoming clearer that deficiencies of them are not limited to classical or obvious populations such as the skid-row alcoholic or the most unusual of ovolactovegetarians. If carefully examined, such individuals as the affluent cocaine abuser, the housebound agoraphobic, or the elderly depressive may show one or more deficiency states.

In some cases, these deficiencies may be considered as secondary phenomena that may or may not contribute to the morbidity imposed by the primary disorder. However, in other cases, vitamin deficiencies themselves may be reasonably considered as the primary causative factors in clinical illnesses. Most modern inpatient evaluation units have broadened their laboratory assessments to include screening for blood levels of such substances as tryptophan and tyrosine, zinc and magnesium, and vitamins C and B_6 in addition to such traditionally considered substances as folate, vitamin B_{12}, and thiamine.[2]

Frederick C. Goggans, M.D. • Neuropsychiatric Evaluation Unit, Psychiatric Institute of Fort Worth, Fort Worth, Texas 76104, and Department of Psychiatry, University of Texas Health Science Center, Dallas, Texas 75235.   *Mark S. Gold, M.D.* • Research Facilities, Fair Oaks Hospital, Summit, New Jersey 07901, and Fair Oaks Hospital at Boca/Delray, Delray Beach, Florida 33445.

2. Amino Acids

Tryptophan and tyrosine are among those required amino acids that cannot be manufactured by the body itself and are thus, by definition, vitamins. Both of these substances are precursors for the two most important neurotransmitters involved in mood regulation. Tyrosine becomes converted to norepinephrine, whereas tryptophan becomes serotonin. Although it is inherently obvious that availability of the substances in the diet and their presence in blood and brain would be important in the evaluation of mood states, appreciation of their roles and the clinical investigation of such issues as prevalence of amino acid deficiencies in major affective disorder patients and their role as therapeutic agents have only just begun. Recent case reports have shown that certain depressives may respond to tyrosine therapy alone.[3] Others have demonstrated at least an adjunctive role for these substances in potentiating the response to standard antidepressants.[4]

Both tyrosine hydroxylase and tryptophan hydroxylase are not fully saturated *in vivo*.[5] Therefore, administration of tyrosine or tryptophan may result in increased synthetic activity. It has also been shown that the ability of tyrosine administration to lead to an increase in catecholamine production is also dependent on the firing rate of the catechol-containing neurons.[5] This means that an indolent neuron system would be more responsive to the precursor-loading process than a well-functioning system would be. Also, there is evidence that tyrosine seems to increase norepinephrine synthesis more than dopamine synthesis and that administration of tyrosine and tryptophan themselves rather than more immediate precursors in the pathways may result in more specific increase in the desired neurotransmitters. Some depressed patients may have an inability to convert tryptophan to 5-hydroxytryptophan and may therefore require administration of this precursor instead of tryptophan itself.[6]

It remains to be seen whether persons who are most likely to benefit from the primary or supplemental administration of these substances have significantly decreased base-line levels of them. However, it is certainly reasonable to suspect that this may be so. Not only does the abovementioned evidence suggest that deficient patients would be more responsive to precursor loading in terms of amine synthesis, but the clinical responsiveness may be analogous to what we have recently learned about depressed patients with subclinical hypothyroidism. Targum and associates have recently demonstrated that patients with grade 2 and 3 hypothyroidism are those most likely to benefit from addition of thyroid hormone to their existing antidepressant program.[7]

There are certain populations of patients who may be most likely to be deficient in tryptophan or tyrosine. Cocaine and amphetamine abusers are likely to exhaust themselves of these precursors, especially tyrosine. It has been theorized that chronic stimulant usage results in depletion of the noradrenergic systems, and low 24-hr urinary MHPG is common in these patients (C. A. Dackis, personal communication, 1984). Therefore, tyrosine administration may be a useful technique in treating the poststimulant depression that is so common in these individuals. The other population that may be likely to show a precursor deficiency state is the elderly depressive group. Typically, these patients are socially isolated and do not get an adequate intake of high-quality protein foods, especially when they become depressed and are even more unable to fend for themselves.

The main question that remains is what is the best way to measure levels of tyrosine and tryptophan. Although blood levels can be assayed directly, some investigators feel that a better assessment is the ratio of these to other amino acids.[8]

3. Vitamins

Chronic malnutrition is often accompanied by psychiatric signs and symptoms such as apathy and depression, emotional lability and irritability, cognitive dysfunction, and even psychotic symptoms. Most frequently, members of the vitamin B family, such as thiamine, niacin, and B_{12}, have been closely associated with such disorders of mental functioning. Specific contributions of vitamins A, C, D, and E have not been so clearly related to mental symptoms. That this should be the case is not surprising since it has been known for many years that B vitamins play essential roles in brain metabolic pathways. For example, both thiamine and niacin are essential cofactors in brain metabolism of glucose, which is its main energy source.

One of the first vitamin deficiency syndromes to be associated with mental disorder was pellagra, the chief feature of which is niacin deficiency. The classical clinical triad included psychiatric disturbance, dermatitis, and gastrointestinal dysfunction. The most common psychiatric syndrome consisted of a mixture of mental depression and cognitive impairment. In the earlier part of this century, over 200,000 people were afflicted with pellagra, many of whom lived in the south. Although dietary deficiency is now rare, niacin-related disorders are still seen in drug addicts, alcoholics, and some patients with severe liver disease.[2] The early phase of illness presents with a strong sense of mental and physical sluggishness associated with irritability and depression. At a later stage of illness, frank dementia or psychosis may ensue. When the illness is detected early, the mental complications are quite readily reversible with niacin administration. The psychotic syndrome especially has been associated with rapid and dramatic recovery. Improvement of the dementia depends on the length of impairment. Probably, patients with acute psychosis as opposed to dementia are more likely to come to medical attention earlier in their clinical course, and this fact rather than the pattern of mental symptoms may underlie the differential prognosis.

The most commonly seen syndrome of thiamine deficiency is Wernicke's encephalopathy. This is a condition usually of relatively acute onset that is characterized by an apathetic acute confusional state, nystagmus and ocular gaze palsies, and ataxia of gait. Wernicke's encephalopathy is most frequently associated with chronic alcoholism, which is clearly the most frequent but not the sole cause of this disorder. Other illnesses that produce severe enough thiamine deficiency to cause this syndrome include primary carcinoma of the stomach, metastatic carcinoma, widespread tuberculosis, pregnancy, pernicious anemia, and severe, protacted gastrointestinal disease of any type.[9]

Wernicke's disease usually presents rapidly but occasionally evolves more slowly as an apathetic and fatigued state. The classical triad, if present, makes the diagnosis straightforward, but *formes frustes* do occur. The most common mental disturbance is a state of quiet rather than agitated global confusion and an especially severe derangement of memory. Although grossly agitated and severely delirious or psychotic behavior may be seen, that usually indicates superimposed delirium tremens (i.e., alcohol withdrawal state). Korsakoff's psychosis represents the amnestic syndrome that is the residual and sometimes permanent defect following the acute Wernicke disorder. In effect, these entities represent different aspects of the same pathological condition of thiamine deficiency.

Although the acute confusional state is almost always improved by parenteral thiamine replacement in those patients who survive their condition, as many as half of these patients may show a persistent memory defect of the Korsakoff type. Continued thiamine replacement, however, may lead to complete recovery in as many as 25% of the patients and at least partial recovery in 50%. Nonetheless, a substantial number of patients may have no recovery. In general, initial replacement should consist of at least 100 mg of parenteral thiamine and daily oral thiamine for at least 6 months, since delayed recovery is not uncommon. Whenever thiamine deficiency is suspected, a blood thiamine level should be quickly obtained and treatment not delayed. The laboratory report is then available as a reference that, if normal, may assist one in rethinking the diagnosis. Those unfortunate patients with the persistent amnestic dysfunction tend to be alert and responsive yet lacking in insight, neglectful of personal appearance and hygiene, and to tend toward idleness and apathy when not directly stimulated by their environment.

Deficiency of vitamin B_{12} has been associated with numerous psychiatric syndromes, and this condition is now considered as protean as neurosyphilis. The most common psychiatric syndromes associated with B_{12} deficiency are organic mental syndrome, violence, paranoia, and depression.[10] Recently, the full manic syndrome has been described as secondary to vitamin B_{12} deficiency.[11] Also, numerous reports have clearly shown that such syndromes as schizophreniform psychosis and mania, which are secondary to vitamin B_{12} deficiency, may occur in individuals who have not yet developed hematological or other neurological abnormalities at the time of clinical presentation.[12] These recent reports emphasize the value of vitamin B_{12} measurement in psychiatric syndromes other than dementia, especially in the older individual with no prior mental disorder.

It should also be known that radioisotope dilution methods may not always be accurate, and bioassays may need to be considered.[2] If there is very strong clinical suspicion of vitamin B_{12} deficiency, one should treat the patient anyway despite the blood level findings. All patients with vitamin B_{12} deficiency should have a Schilling test, which measures their capacity to absorb orally administered vitamin B_{12}. Pernicious anemia is an autoimmune disease that is associated with antibody production against gastric parietal cells and intrinsic factor. Decreased availability of intrinsic factor leads to impaired vitamin B_{12} absorption in the ileum. Patients with deficiency of vitamin B_{12} on an autoimmune basis will require continued parenteral therapy, usually at a dose of 1000 μg every 2 months. All patients who have pernicious anemia should also be screened for the coexistence of other vitamin deficiencies such as thiamine or folate deficiencies and for other autoimmune conditions such as thyroiditis, adrenal insufficiency, and diabetes. Those patients who have a normal Shilling test and absent antibodies may have a primary dietary deficiency or some other gastrointestinal illness that results in malabsorption, such as Crohn's disease. Such patients should have their cases reviewed by a gastrointestinal specialist to determine whether additional workup is indicated.

Folate deficiency may also result in considerable psychiatric morbidity, and the usual presentation is that of depression or dementia, although folate-related psychoses have been described. Folate deficiency may present as a macrocytic anemia similar to vitamin B_{12} deficiency. Patients must always be screened for low B_{12} as well, since folate replacement may allow continued neurological deterioration in the patient who also has that disorder.

Folate deficiency is often seen in alcoholics and other drug addicts but is not uncommon in very ill patients with poor nutrition. Folate deficiency is also seen in patients on certain medications such as anticonvulsants and oral contraceptives. In general, folate levels reflect the overall nutritional status of an individual. Differences in nutritional hygiene may underlie the finding that psychiatric patients as a whole have been noted to have decreased folate levels compared to normals. Other recent studies have suggested that at least 20% of nonanemic depressed inpatients may have abnormally low folate levels.[13] Nevertheless, it is not yet clear whether folate-related depression exists as a distinct entity or is rather a secondary process that then becomes a sustaining factor in clinical morbidity. Folate is a cofactor for tyrosine hydroxylase, which is the rate-limiting step in norepinephrine synthesis. The lack of folate, even if a secondary process, would then impair optimal biological recovery unless treated. Indeed, Sheffield *et al.* found that exogenous folate administration did decrease the hospital stays of patients with depression compared to those given standard treatments alone.[14] Usually, folate is given orally at a dose of at least 1 mg three times daily.

Very little research has been done on the role of pyridoxine (vitamin B_6) in psychiatric disorders. Its deficiency has been mentioned as a causative or aggravating factor in dementia, depression, premenstrual syndrome, and even autism. There are limited studies regarding its usefulness in these conditions, and no definite recommendations can be made. Megadose B_6 replacement has been associated with neurosensory dysfunction.[15] Pyridoxine levels are easily obtained, and replacement is indicated if the patient manifests a true deficiency. Replacement should not exceed 2 g daily because of the risk of toxicity.

4. Minerals

Hyponatremia does not always represent a sodium deficiency state. Although a low serum sodium is found in severe volume depletion, hyponatremia usually represents a relative excess of body water. The finding of hyponatremia requires an extensive clinical and laboratory investigation, which usually includes an assessment of volume status, serum and urinary osmolality, urinary sodium and electrolytes, and other studies. The workup of hyponatremia is beyond the scope of this chapter, and the reader should consult a standard medical textbook if necessary.[16]

Hyponatremia has been associated with numerous psychiatric conditions. To some extent, symptoms depend on the speed with which hyponatremia develops. For example, acute hyponatremia such as occurs with rapidly developing inappropriate ADH syndrome may result in an agitated delirium or psychosis. On the other hand, a chronic hyponatremia associated with gradual volume depletion may present with depression or dementia. Hyponatremia can also appear as a complication of antipsychotic or anticonvulsant treatment of psychiatric patients via the syndrome of inappropriate ADH secretion. This is an uncommon cause of hyponatremia, however, and hyponatremia in the psychiatric population most often arises from the usual medical causes, of which the most common is excessive diuretic therapy.

Certainly, the presence of hyponatremia may aggravate whatever psychiatric disorder is present previously. Psychogenic water drinking is seen occasionally. Typically, such patients can be distinguished from patients with diabetes insipidus by their lower plasma osmolality and by their better ability to concentrate their urine under conditions of fluid deprivation as well as their lack of response to exogenous vasopressin (ADH). Certain metabolic disorders can present with both hyponatremia and psychiatric disturbance and should always be remembered. These include porphyria, adrenal insufficiency, and hypothyroidism. Usually there are other clinical features of greater diagnostic import.

Potassium deficiency has been most commonly associated with depressive syndromes. This is most likely because potassium depletion usually results in a state of physical lethargy. Currently, the most common cause of potassium deficiency is diuretic therapy, although potassium deficiency is seen in certain special psychiatric populations such as the eating disorders. Patients with anorexia and bulimia often deplete themselves of potassium through self-induced vomiting, laxative abuse, and diuretic abuse. It is well known to be the most frequent cause of sudden death in these patients, usually because of a hypokalemia-induced cardiac dysrhythmia.

Recently, Strauss et al. emphasized the role that hypokalemia can play in the aggravation of chronic psychiatric conditions.[17] They reported a case in which an otherwise stabilized schizophrenic had two psychotic decompensations that were clearly related to severe thiazide-related hypokalemic states. They suggested that potassium levels be closely monitored in all psychiatric patients who are receiving coordinate therapy with medicines that may lower serum potassium levels.

There is little evidence to suggest that lithium plays a role in normal physiological processes even in trace amounts. The term "lithium deficiency" is usually encountered as a synonym for bipolar disorder in patients who have been poorly educated about this disorder by their physicians. Although lithium is an effective therapy for bipolar disorder, there is no evidence to suggest that this condition represents a deficiency of lithium. This would be tantamount to describing heart failure as digitalis deficiency.

Hypocalcemia can result from numerous medical conditions including renal failure, osteomalacia, vitamin D deficiency, hypoparathyroidism, and magnesium deficiency among others. Psychiatric syndromes may include weakness, anxiety, irritability and other manic symptoms, depression, and frank psychosis. Usually these conditions are associated with evidence of neuromuscular irritability, tremor, cramping, tetany, and even seizures. The diagnosis of hypocalcemia is based on the clinical picture as well as the serum calcium level. Attention to free calcium levels is important, as protein binding dynamics must be considered when a low calcium level is reported on automated profiles. The diagnostic workup should be addressed to the discovery of one of the numerous underlying causes, and therapy should be as specific as possible. It is most important to recognize that magnesium deficiency can be a frequent cause of hypocalcemia and that serum levels of magnesium must also be checked when hypocalcemia is detected. In the presence of hypomagnesemia, calcium replacement will not result in clinical improvement. When magnesium replacement is given, however, calcium levels will usually normalize.

Magnesium deficiency is rare since the element is abundantly present in most foods. Typically, significant hypomagnesemia most often results from chronic alcoholism, diuretic therapy, gastrointestinal illness, and inadequate replacement in patients on prolonged parenteral regimens. Conditions causing hypercalcemia may result in a secondary magnesium deficiency. The clinical signs and symptoms of magnesium deficiency are similar to those of hypocalcemia. The psychiatrist is most likely to encounter this condition associated with chronic alcoholism, but manic or schizophrenic patients who decompensate while on diuretic therapy should be checked for hypomagnesemia in addition to hypokalemia. Magnesium deficiency should be considered in all patients presenting with mania who are atypical or have no prior history of bipolar disorder.

The most common condition associated with copper deficiency is Wilson's disease or hepatolenticular degeneration. Actually, although serum copper is low, excess copper is deposited in various organs such as brain, liver, and the cornea. This condition is inherited as an autosomal recessive condition and is quite rare. The illness is most often associated with an inability to synthesize ceruloplasmin, which is the copper transport protein. Free copper deposits in those organ systems described above and their dysfunction account for the major clinical manifestations of the disorder. This condition usually presents early in life with psychiatric disturbance and basal ganglia dysfunction. Since the illness is treatable with penicillamine but fatal if missed, it is important that the diagnosis be considered in all first episodes of psychosis. Typically, one finds a low serum ceruloplasmin, low serum copper, and elevated urinary copper.

Zinc deficiency has been associated with numerous clinical signs and symptoms including poor appetite, depression, lethargy, and impaired sense of taste and smell. This latter condition may be quite dramatic as well as a good hint to the diagnosis. Low serum zinc levels have been associated with numerous medical illnesses but are most common in patients with chronic alcoholism. Zinc levels should also be considered in the alcoholic because zinc is a cofactor in the enzyme system involved in the metabolism of alcohol. Any psychiatric patient who reports impaired or bizarre sensations of taste or smell should have zinc levels checked in addition to the assessment of temporal lobe structure and function. In most cases, oral zinc replacement is rapidly effective.

5. Conclusion

Laboratory testing for deficiencies of amino acids, vitamins, and metals has become increasingly important and useful in the modern workup of the psychiatric patient. Assessment of these substances is particularly important in individuals who have no prior history of psychiatric disorder or who have an unexplained psychiatric relapse. In some cases, it is clearly established that deficiencies of these substances are directly causative of major clinical syndromes, whereas in other situations, such deficiencies may be secondary but sustain clinical morbidity. For example, the individual with folate deficiency that developed during an episode of major depression may not be able to respond to tricyclic antidepressant therapy until his vitamin lack is addressed. The psychiatrist should also realize that there is tremendous lay interest in the role that vitamins play in mental disorders. Although there is no evidence that the use of vitamins in the therapy of patients without true deficiencies is of value, absolute or relative deficiences will never be discovered if patients are not tested. A thorough assessment of vitamin and mineral status is always warranted in the treatment-refractory or especially unusual patient.

References

1. Gold MS, Lydiard RB, Carman JS: *Advances in Psychopharmacology.* Boca Raton, FL, CRC Press, 1984, pp 307–312.
2. Estroff TW, Gold MS: Psychiatric misdiagnosis, in Gold MS, Lydiard RB, Carman JS (eds): *Advances in Psychopharmacology.* Boca Raton, FL, CRC Press, 1984, pp 33–66.
3. Gelenberg AJ, Wojick JD, Growdon JH, et al: Tyrosine for the treatment of depression. *Am J Psychiatry* 137:622–623, 1980.
4. Walinder J, Carlsson A, Persson R: 5-HT reuptake blockers plus tryptophan in the treatment of endogenous depression. *Acta Psychiatr Scand [Suppl]* 290:179–180, 1981.
5. Gelenberg AJ, Gibson CJ, Wojick JD: Neurotransmitter precursors for the treatment of depression. *Psychopharmacol Bull* 18:7–18, 1982.
6. vanPraag HM, DeHaan S: Depression vulnerability and 5-hydroxytryptophan prophylaxis. *Psychiatry Res* 3:75–83, 1980.
7. Targum SD, Greenberg RD, Harmon RL, et al: Thyroid hormone and the TRH stimulation test in refractory depression. *J Clin Psychiatry* 45:345–346, 1984.
8. Moller SE, Kirk L, Honore P: Free and total plasma tryptophan in endogenous depression. *J Affect Dis* 1:69, 1979.
9. Lishman WA: *Organic Psychiatry.* Oxford, Blackwell, 1978, p. 677.
10. Zucker DK, Livingston RL, Nakra R, et al: B_{12} deficiency and psychiatric disorders: Case report and review of the literature. *Biol Psychiatry* 16:197–205, 1981.
11. Goggans FC: A case of mania secondary to vitamin B_{12} deficiency. *Am J Psychiatry* 141:300–301, 1984.
12. Evans DL, Edelsohn GA, Golden RN: Organic psychosis without anemia or spinal cord symptoms in patients with vitamin B_{12} deficiency. *Am J Psychiatry* 140:218–221, 1983.
13. Coppen A, Abou-Saleh MT: Plasma folate and affective morbidity. *Br J Psychiatry* 141:87, 1982.
14. Sheffield BF, Carney MWP: Associations of subnormal folate and B_{12} and effects of replacement therapy. *J Nerv Ment Dis* 150:404, 1970.
15. *Medical World News* Psychiatry ed. Oct 1983.
16. Schrier RW: *Renal and electrolyte disorders.* Boston, Little, Brown, 1976.
17. Hafez H, Strauss J, Aronson MD, et al: Hypokalemia-induced psychosis in a chronic psychiatric patient. *J Clin Psychiatry* 45:277–279, 1984.

Central Nervous System Neurodiagnostic Devices

William Hapworth, M.D.

1. Introduction

The field of psychiatry has suffered during the technological revolution from an inability to give biological definition to its various syndromes. Treatments for the most part have been discovered through serendipity and applied through empirical trial and error. At times, the field of psychiatry has appeared to fight progress to preserve the image of analytic purity. Nevertheless, the past 25 years has seen the emergence of psychiatry into a viable, healthy field of medicine. Perhaps, as in all transition, the pendulum of biological research has swung too far. This could only be explained by recognizing that psychiatry in the early 20th century devoted its exclusive attention to refining analytic technique. There can be no justification for either extreme. Psychiatry must ultimately incorporate itself into the modern technological revolution but should not do this at the expense or disregard of its analytic roots.

This chapter is an attempt to develop understanding of the latest technological advances in brain imaging, so that rational clinical applications can be developed. It is often the case that research findings regarding innovative advancements in psychiatry do not translate themselves into rational clinical applications. The rising cost of health care demands the need for succinct, definitive diagnostic and treatment strategies. This discussion attempts to highlight the history, theory, clinical findings, and future potentialities of CAT, PETT, and NMR scanning.

2. Nuclear Magnetic Resonance

The field of radiology underwent a revolution in imaging with the introduction of computed tomography in 1973.[1,2] The recent development of nuclear magnetic resonance (NMR) has excited the medical profession anew. The expectations of NMR

William Hapworth, M.D. • The Regent Hospital, New York, New York 10021.

imaging are only beginning to be realized with the research momentum that has developed in the past 3 years.

Nuclear magnetic resonance has been a physical phenomenon known since the 1940s[3,4] but was first applied to medicine in 1971. Damadian[5] showed that normal and malignant rat tissues differed in their proton nuclear magnetic resonance properties. Subsequently, in 1973, Lauterbur[6] was able to create images using phantoms with NMR. It was not until 1977 that Damadian[7] was able to make the first crude images of human volunteers. The clinical utility of NMR began to emerge in 1981 when investigators started to image the pathological states of brain,[8] thorax,[9] and abdomen.[10] Since that time, the technological and commercial investments in NMR have intensifed. At present, NMR provides a better anatomic, structural description of soft tissues than CAT scanning. It also offers, with recent developments in contrast media and topical magnetic resonance, the possibility for superior resolution capabilities as well as the capacity to generate *in vivo* metabolic data on specific human organs.

3. The Theory of NMR

The principles of NMR and the imaging processes involved are reviewed in several standard texts on the subject,[11,12] but a brief review of the principles that have made NMR a viable noninvasive diagnostic tool in modern medicine seems in order.

The theory of NMR revolves around the fact that most elements have at least one isotope in abundance whose nucleus is magnetic. Atomic nuclei consist of protons and neutrons. These nucleons rotate or spin about their axes and in most cases are paired in such a way that their spins cancel each other out. However, in the case of an upaired neutron or proton, the electric charge and net spin of the nucleus cause it to generate a magnetic field as it spins. In biological substances there are several such magnetic nuclei (^1H, ^{13}C, ^{23}Na, ^{31}P, ^{39}K). The most abundant by far of these nuclei is ^1H because of the high water content of nonbony tissues. The hydrogen nucleus or proton, when placed in an external magnetic field, acts like a small magnet and will either align with the external field or oppose the field.

Nuclear magnetic resonance imaging uses these physical properties of the hydrogen nucleus in the following manner. The body is immersed in a static magnetic field, which causes alignment or opposition of the nuclei to the field. In NMR scanning, a coil (see Fig 10-1) that surrounds the body produces an electromagnetic field that causes the nuclei of hydrogen to change their nuclear spins relative to their alignment in the static magnetic field. The coil produces the rapidly alternating magnetic field at an appropriate radio frequency, which will cause the nuclei to precess or change the orientation of their nuclear spins relative to the strong static magnetic field. The change in the nuclear spin causes the absorption of energy, which is released by the proton when the alternating field is turned off. This release of energy by the hydrogen proton returning to the equilibrated state of the static field is proportional to the frequency of the stimulating alternating field. This frequency is known as the resonance of Larmor frequency. The resonance frequency is unique for each species of nucleus and is the signal property that permits the hydrogen nuclei in the body to act as receivers and transmitters of radio-frequency energy. The transmissions from these nuclei are con-

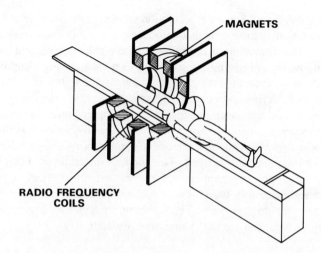

Figure 10-1. Depiction of NMR scanner showing the position of RF coils inside the main magnet. The RF coils surround the body part to be imaged.

verted by various techniques into spectra and/or images. The transmission of this specific nuclear resonance from hydrogen is the basis of NMR imaging.

Theoretically, by using relevant radio frequencies, one could tune into specific nuclei and record their reactions. Hydrogen is the logical nucleus because of its abundance and higher intrinsic NMR sensitivity. Nuclei such as ^{31}P, ^{39}K, and ^{23}Na are presently unable to be used in imaging because of their low concentrations; however, they are in high enough concentration to be measured spectroscopically.

The NMR signal, besides giving information on proton density, also gives two other measurable parameters that are relevant to biological investigations. Using the time variation of the NMR signal, one can measure T_1, which is the spin–lattice relaxation time, or T_2, which is the spin–spin relaxation time. T_1 can also be conceptualized as the longitudinal relaxation time and T_2 as the transverse relaxation time. These times are derived by measuring the time required for the hydrogen nucleus to return to the equilibrium of the applied static field after the radio frequency pulse is turned off. T_1 and T_2 are important because they are affected by the motion of the nuclei, the viscosity of the tissue, regional temperatures, and the magnetic effects of nearby nuclei. To this extent, T_1 and T_2 are tissue specific and can be used to delineate specific tissues in the body.

4. Strategies in NMR Imaging

Nuclear magnetic resonance imaging is presently restricted to the hydrogen proton. The usage of different radio-frequency pulse sequences to stimulate the proton has resulted in a number of different imaging techniques. The different methods produce slightly different images depending on whether they use pure proton density, pure T_1 or combinations of proton density, T_1, and T_2. The pulse sequences that are used in present NMR scanning are known as saturation recovery, inversion recovery, and spin echo. The saturation recovery method produces images that are related to proton density and T_1. The utilization of inversion recovery pulse sequencing adds enhancement to T_1 parameters of imaging, whereas spin-echo sequencing weights T_2 in terms of image production. Present research is focusing on the utility of using the various NMR parameters to define and characterize specific disease states.

Nuclear magnetic resonance imaging is also being enhanced by the utilization of surface coils to decrease signal-to-noise ratio as well as by the evaluation of scanners with higher field strengths. The potential development of contrast media for NMR is being researched aggressively as well. The contrast materials are comprised of two large groups, which are paramagnetic ion agents and nitroxide static-free radicals. These agents seek to modify tissue relaxation times and provide better enhancement and resolution of pathological states. These various strategies for expanding the role of NMR imaging in medicine are under intensive research.

5. Clinical Application of NMR

The central nervous system (CNS) offers the most practical starting point for evaluating the clinical applicability of NMR. The pulse sequencing that demonstrates lesions of the brain most clearly is the spin-echo technique. This weights the image production with T_2 relaxation times. Most lesions of the CNS have long T_1 and T_2 relaxation times, which provide an inherent contrast between normal and abnormal tissue. The imaging of cerebral infarctions, hemorrhages, tumors, and demyelinating plaques are all readily contrasted using spin-echo pulse sequencing. Several researchers using T_1-weighted images have shown that the lesions of infarctions, hemorrhages, cysts, tumors, and edema all have long T_1 values.[13,14] There is substantial overlap of these lesions with regard to T_1 values, and specific identification of and differentiation among these lesions are not possible at present.

The plaques of demyelinating disease are dramatically contrasted with NMR in a fashion never previously demonstrated[15]: NMR is particularly able to demonstrate multiple sclerosis plaques because of the absence of closely bound hydrogen to myelin (see Fig. 10-2).

Structures or lesions of the posterior fossa are markedly better imaged using NMR. The absence of bony artifact makes NMR very useful in identifying posterior fossa lesions.

Other researchers[16] have developed and demonstrated the ability to display intracranial lesions in a three-dimensional image. Another group[17,18] has developed the ability to collect contiguous simultaneous sections so as to shorten imaging time.

The application of NMR to psychiatric research has been explored by a few investigators. In a small group of chronic alcoholic patients, it was shown that the T_1 value of both gray and white matter decreased during alcohol intoxication and returned to normal during the withdrawal phase.[19] Another group produced results that attempted to show that the T_1 values in depressed bipolar affective disorder patients were higher than those of control patients.[20] They repeated the NMR scans after treatment with lithium and reported that the T_1 values in the patient with affective disorder

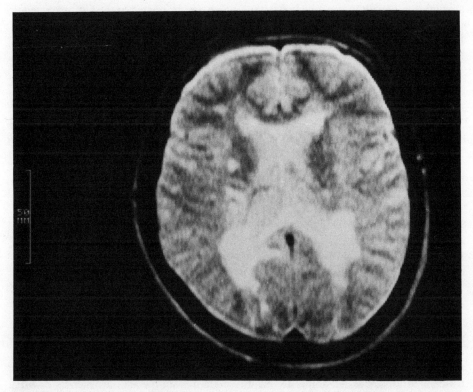

Figure 10-2. This transaxial magnetic resonance image was produced using the spin-echo pulse sequence with a long echo delay. This pulse sequence is used to examine parenchymal detail. There are numerous areas of increased signal intensity, as demonstrated by the white areas, in the region of the corpus callosum and the posterior portions of the centrum semiovale. These foci of abnormal increased signal intensity are most likely the result of a widespread demyelinating process. Courtesy of R. J. Mitnick, M.D., and J. S. Rosenthal, M.D.

returned to normal, whereas the lithium-treated normals had no change in T_1 values. The bulk of work that has applied NMR technology to the fields of neurological psychiatric research is still preliminary and speculative in nature. The need for carefully controlled studies is paramount for the development of a rational use of NMR's capabilities.

6. Safety of NMR

The major concern of the FDA in the licensing of NMR scanners is the permissible strength of magnetic fields in the scanning procedure. Their present position is that field strengths of 0.3T (3000 gauss) are safe. Anticipated future field strengths may be as high as 1.5 T. Clinical studies are under way to test the safety of these higher field strengths. Budinger and Lautebur[21] highlight in a review of NMR that higher field strengths will result in some body heating, which will be related to the radio-frequency pulse tuning, configuration of the radio-frequency probe, and ability of the body to lose heat. There are clearly no reported deleterious effects on human health in fields of up to 0.2 T. There are known hazards of NMR scanning on ferromagnetic objects such as surgical clips and joint replacements. Also, patients with pacemakers can have their pacemakers switched into a fixed-rate mode or reprogrammed. However, with these minor exceptions, NMR has proven to be exceedingly safe and produces images without subjecting the body to ionizing radiation.

7. Future of NMR in Psychiatry

The potential uses for NMR in medicine, especially in neurology, are great (see Figs. 10-3–10-5). The evolving ability for superior resolution and contrast will make NMR an imaging technique without rival. The potential for tissue-specific and lesion-specific T_1 and T_2 values would make pathological identification a noninvasive procedure. Additionally, the serial evaluation of tumors could demonstrate therapeutic efficacy by following the T_1 and T_2 relaxation values. These potentials are as yet unfulfilled but offer major advances over CAT scanning.

The potential for NMR in psychiatry is yet to be delineated. Several areas are of possible interest. The serial evaluations of T_1 or T_2 parameters during psychoactive treatments (e.g., medication treatment, electroconvulsive therapy) might define the mechanism of action of these modalities. The further development of *in vivo* spectroscopy will provide the ability to quantify certain brain metabolites such as cAMP, ATP, etc. These capabilities may prove valuable in studies of dementia, schizophrenia, and affective disorders. Nevertheless, whether the spectroscopic capabilities of NMR will prove useful in psychiatric research is still a matter of conjecture.

8. Positron Emission Transaxial Tomography

The emergence of positron emission transaxial tomography (PETT) as a major advance in neurodiagnostic procedures heralds a new frontier for neuropsychiatric research. Unlike the structural data generated by computerized tomography, PETT scanning permits the *in vivo* investigation of functional regional brain activity.

The development of PETT techniques has been based on the combination of technical advancements in several closely allied scientific fields. The collaboration among such fields as psychiatry, chemistry, physics, nuclear medicine, radiology, and engineering has contributed to the expensive development of PETT technology. Since 1979, an enormous number of man hours have been utilized as well as a major financial investment of research dollars by the National Institutes of Health (NIH) in an effort to develop and refine the PETT. To date, approximately a dozen centers have been funded by the NIH, creating a financial debt of approximately $20 million. The staggering cost of PETT development arises out of the complex technology and sophisticated manpower required to make PETT scanning a reality.

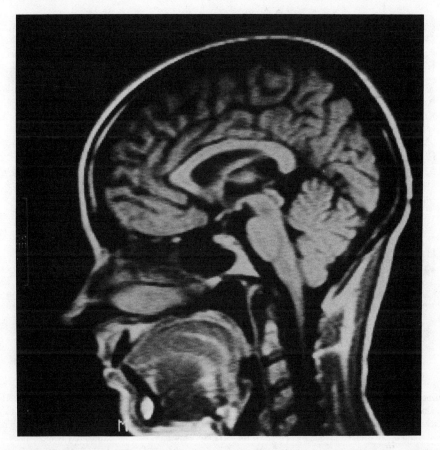

Figure 10-3. This sagittal image was produced using a spin-echo pulse sequence with a short echo delay. The image is taken in the right parasagittal location. The medial portions of the right cerebral and cerebellar hemispheres are demonstrated. The corpus callosum is clearly visualized. The normal brainstem and upper cervical spinal cord are visualized. Courtesy of R. J. Mitnick, M.D., and J. S. Rosenthal, M.D.

9. Historical Perspective of PETT

The fundamental theories of brain metabolism were postulated as early as 1890 by Roy and Sherrington.[22] They stated that enhanced brain activity in one part of the brain resulted in a regional hyperemia that paralleled neuronal activity as well as local metabolism. The pioneering work of Kety and Schmidt in 1948, with the introduction of the nitrous oxide technique for measurement of cerebral blood flow (CBF), provided the first data on the relationship between substrate delivery and its utilization in the human brain.[23] However, these methods lacked the ability to measure dynamic regional differences in both brain metabolism and circulation. It was not until 1966 that investigators developed methods to measure regional cerebral blood flow (RCBF) by the intracarotid injection of inert radioactive gases such as ^{133}Xe of ^{85}Kr.[24] These studies advanced our understanding of regional brain function, and these methods have

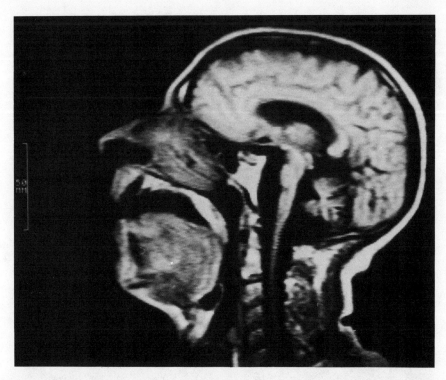

Figure 10-4. This midline sagittal magnetic resonance image was produced using a spin-echo pulse sequence with a short echo delay. There is atrophy of the cerebellum, brainstem, and cervical spinal cord. The findings are compatible with spinocerebellar degeneration, adult onset type. The visualized portions of the cerebral hemispheres are within normal limits. It should be noted that the brainstem and upper cervical spinal cord could not be well examined by computed tomography. However, they are exquisitely demonstrated by means of magnetic resonance imaging. Courtesy of R. J. Mitnick, M.D., and J. S. Rosenthal, M.D.

been refined to provide information on regional blood flow[25] as well as oxygen[26] and glucose[27] metabolism. Researchers have been able to map changes in regional brain activity under specific sensory stimuli or motoric tasks that yield landscapes of cortical functions.[28,29] However, these methods of measuring brain metabolism are not widely used because of the invasive nature of the procedure and inherent risks of intracarotid injection.

The need to develop safe, accurate, and noninvasive measures of regional brain metabolism was forwarded by several allied scientific advancements. In 1977, Sokoloff advanced the deoxyglucose (DG) method of measuring regional glucose uptake in the brain,[30] which is based on the principle that measurement of metabolic activity in the brain can be accomplished by deoxyglucose because it meets certain unique requirements of metabolism, transport, and excretion within the body. Metabolically, deoxyglucose acts as a substrate competitive with glucose, has a rapid turnover rate in cerebral tissue, and does not act as a substrate for further metabolism once it reaches the end-product stage of deoxyglucose-6-phosphate. The advantage of DG being only partially metabolized through the glucose cycle is the fact that it is

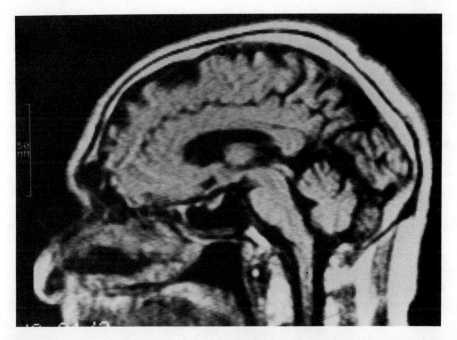

Figure 10-5. This sagittal image was produced using a spin-echo pulse sequence with a short delay time. The magnetic resonance image of this 71-year-old male displays diffuse prominence of the cortical sulci, indicating cortical atrophy. Courtesy of R. J. Mitnick, M.D., and J. S. Rosenthal, M.D.

trapped in the tissue as DG-6-phosphate. This entrapment allows the application of a quantitative autoradiographic technique that measures deoxyglucose in the tissue and relates it to glucose metabolism at a definable rate. It was the definition of this rate by the operational mathematical equation of Sokoloff that permitted the elucidation of regional glucose brain metabolic activity.

Two other areas contributed to the impetus of present-day PETT research: first, the appearance in the medical field of cyclotrons and linear accelerators for the bombardment of nuclei to produce radiopharmaceuticals suitable for metabolic investigations; and, second, the development of detection systems employing the concept of positron emission tomography. The historical background in these areas is too broad a topic for development in this chapter. There are several excellent reviews that encompass this subject and can be consulted.[31,32]

10. Radionuclides and Radiopharmaceuticals

Although operationally PETT is simply a matter of injecting a substance into the bloodstream and quantitatively measuring it as it functions in the body, the substances capable of being measured are limited in number, and the detection systems are extremely complex. Only a few radionuclides possess the chemical and physical properties that make them ideal for PETT technology. The primary positron-emitting radionuclides are ^{15}O, ^{13}N, ^{11}C, and ^{18}F.

Positrons are positively charged electrons that are emitted from the nuclei of these radionuclides because of the instability created by their neutron deficiency.

The positron travels a finite distance in space and comes to rest, where it interacts with an electron, and the two particles undergo annihilation. The annihilation of the two particles creates two photons, which travel at 180° from each other. This annihilation radiation can be detected by two radiation detectors placed outside of the field of interest but connected by a coincidence circuit (see Fig. 10-6). The annihilation is recorded only if the detectors simultaneously sense the emission of photons from the tissue at 180° from the event, hence the term annihilation coincidence detection, which forms the basis for detection systems used in PETT.

The potential uses of these radionuclides for investigation of metabolic processes can be gleaned by examining Table 10-1. The incorporation of these nuclides into the molecules that compose living matter make it possible to examine unlimited metabolic systems. As can be seen in Table 10-1, there is some limitation placed on research by the half-lives of these compounds. The need for an on-site cyclotron to rapidly process these radiopharmaceuticals has limited the number of centers capable of PETT imaging. However, the short half-lives of these compounds significantly reduce the dose of

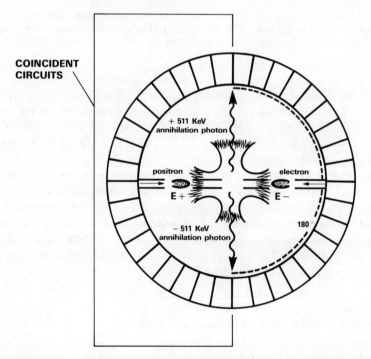

Figure 10-6. The decay of a radiopharmaceutical used in PETT causes the emission of a positron (E^+). This positron travels a finite distance in the tissue and encounters an electron (E^-) and undergoes annihilation. The subsequent release of two photons with 511 keV energy travelling 180° apart permits the detection of the event by the simultaneous arrival at two coincident circuits.

Table 10-1. Radionuclides, Their Investigative Functions, and Their Corresponding Half-Lives

Radionuclide	Investigative potential	Half-life
Oxygen-15	Transport and metabolism of oxygen	2.05 min
Carbon-11		
[^{11}C]Etorphine	Opiate receptors	20.34 min
[^{11}C]Flunitrazepam	Benzodiazepine receptors	
[^{11}C]Spiroperidol	Dopamine receptors	
Fluorine-18		
2-[^{18}F]2-Deoxy-D-glucose	Glucose metabolism	110 min
[^{18}F]Haloperidol	Dopamine receptors	
Nitrogen-13		
L-[^{13}N]Glutamate	Amino acid metabolism	9.96 min
-Alanine		
-Aspartate		
-Leucine		
-Valine		

radiation to the patient and permit possible repeating of studies because of the rapid elimination of these substances and the low radiation dose.

11. Principles of PETT Detection System

The properties of positron decay are well suited to the requirements of computed tomography. When a positron decays, the two photons released from the annihilation travel at 180° with an energy of 511 keV. This physical property of positron decay allows for annihilation coincidence detection (ACD)[33] by using an electronic form of photon collimation. Annihilation coincidence detection is crucial because it provides excellent spatial resolution, highly efficient detection, and simultaneous collection of linear and angular data from an imaged object.

Several types of detection systems have been developed for PETT,[34,35] but the basic principles are as follows (see Fig. 10-7). Multiple scintillation detectors are placed around the imaged object arranged in banks of either a circular or octagonal shape. The detectors are composed of either bismuth germanate or cesium fluoride. Each detector is operated in coincidence with multiple opposing detectors, creating a fan beam response through any given point of the imaged object. There are multiple banks of detectors, which are usually in motion around the image and provide three to seven tomographic planes for simultaneous collection of data, which helps to shorten the duration of the procedure. The image is reconstructed using a computed tomographic algorithm, which can be used to produce standard two-dimensional images through horizontal, coronal, or sagittal sections as well as to create three-dimensional images. The ability to color code as a means of quantifying radionuclide densities makes PETT images startling in their ability to convey information.

The resolution of a PETT image is theoretically limited to the distance that the positron travels in the brain prior to annihilation. This distance varies from 1 to 6 mm

SCINTILLATION DETECTORS

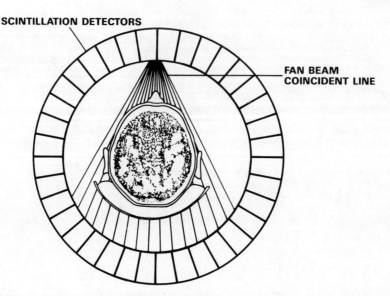

FAN BEAM
COINCIDENT LINE

Figure 10-7. The banks of multiple scintillation detectors are placed around the object to be imaged and are composed of either bismuth germanate or cesium fluoride. The fan beam of coincident lines permits maximum detector capabilities.

depending in part on the energy of a particular positron.[36] Some PETT images are already approaching this theoretical limit. Nonetheless, this level of resolution is capable of providing useful and valuable research information.

12. Clinical Applications of PETT Scanning in Psychiatry

Positron emission tomographic scanning has been controversial with regard to the significance of clinical findings. Recent controversy[37] has even challenged the deoxyglucose model as being a reductionistic view of how the brain utilizes glucose. Sokoloff and others contend that the model is sound but that there is some possible variation of the mathematical lumped constants. The resolution of this model is crucial to the continued viability of PETT. Virtually all of the research data accumulated to date utilizes Sokoloff's deoxyglucose model for computational purposes. If the model is unsound, than there will be a need to develop alternative techniques and tracers to monitor brain activity.

Nevertheless, a substantial body of research work has been done using PETT technology. At present there is no immediate clinical application for PETT scanning, but a review of the research data will illuminate potential future usages of the modality.

Much work has been done to define the anatomic and metabolic characteristics of the normal human brain by using PETT. This work has focused on the anatomic distributions of tracer activity as well as the variation in normal subjects under specific physiological tasks. The ultimate findings in each case depend on a number of parameters that must be controlled for as PETT data are collected.

These experimental parameters are discussed in various papers, but only a few will be mentioned here. One of the most important parameters is the ambient conditions under which a PETT scan is performed.[38,39] These researchers have shown how conditions of visual and auditory stimulation effect PETT images. They demonstrated that in normal right-handed subjects there is a left–right cerebral hemisphere symmetry when eyes are open but ears are occluded or *vice versa*. However, when both senses are deprived, there is a significant right-sided hypometabolism. The exact cause of this asymmetry is speculative, but it does highlight the need to specify ambient conditions and to interpret their effect on the images obtained. Other parameters such as the concentration in areas of interest relative to the surrounding areas effect the data obtainable from PETT images. Additionally, the signal-to-noise ratio, the size and shape of structures, as well as the final image resolution of the tomograph all affect the ultimate interpretations of information generated from PETT research. Finally, even the principle of superimposing structural computerized axial tomographic images on the same plane tomographs of PETT is subject to mechanical inaccuracy as well as other problems that relate to the principle that images of anatomic structure correspond to images of functional structure.

Nevertheless, despite the above difficulties with PETT technology, there have been many exciting studies that offer glimpses into future potentialities. The normal visual and auditory systems have been explored using PETT in several research groups. The utilization of clever paradigms has essentially shown that for the visual system the local cerebral metabolic rate for glucose (LCMRG) increased in proportion to the complexity of higher-order associative visual stimuli.[39,40] The auditory system has been researched in a study by Mazziotta *et al.*[41] They used a clever paradigm to investigate musically sophisticated and musically unsophisticated normals. They were able to show differences in the processing of tone sequences in these groups. The musically sophisticated normals used analytical strategies when listening to the tones and showed greater temporal asymmetries on the left as compared to the right, whereas the musically naive showed diffuse right-sided asymmetries when listening to the same tone sequences. These clever studies showed the capabilities of PETT to explore high-level mental processes and have impelled present-day researchers towards more sophisticated studies.

The neurological applications of PETT are extensively reviewed by Phelps *et al.*[31] and have evident advantages over the structural data generated by computed tomography. The metabolic definition of lesions of the CNS such as tumor, infarction, and seizure are dramatically shown by PETT technology. Generally, the metabolic image of such lesions is far more accurate and specific than the lesion that appears on structured CT scans. This applies particularly to seizure foci, which are rarely identified on CT scanning as structural defects. Further, PETT has superior ability to correlate abnormal EEG findings to their corresponding metabolic abnormality. This ability enhances the definition of epileptogenic foci and adds a dimension to our understanding of seizures never previously possible.

The field of dementia research has been greatly aided by PETT technology. The inability of CAT scanning to be able to accurately predict the degree of cognitive impairment has frustrated dementia research. Preliminary studies using PETT in evaluating dementia are very encouraging. Several investigators have looked at the effect of normal aging on the LCMRG. Kuhl *et al.* reported a mild but definite pattern towards a decrease in LCMRG from the second through seventh decades.[42] Yet others have shown less of a decrease in the utilization of oxygen with aging[43] and still others reported no significant change in LCMRG with normal aging.[44–46] Recently, Wong *et al.* published the first analysis of dopamine and serotonin receptors in normal aging.[47] They showed a significant decrease in these receptors from age 19 to 73 in the areas of the putamen, caudate nucleus, and frontal cerebral cortex. Males showed a slightly higher decrease than females. All the above findings need to be carefully replicated with close attention paid to methodological issues. The emergence of receptor studies offers new and better techniques to evaluate normal aging of the brain.

In the field of dementia, most investigators with PETT have concentrated on Alzheimer's disease. Alavi *et al.* reported a 20–30% decrease in glucose metabolic rate compared to normal age-matched controls.[48] Many investigators since have reported the marked decrease in metabolic usage of glucose in the brains of Alzheimer's patients.[49,50] The general percentages continue to range from 15% to 30% (see Fig. 10-8). The extensive analysis of regional areas of interest holds forth the hope of a better understanding of the role played by specific components of the central nervous system in Alzheimer's disease. The ability to compare CAT scan tomography to PETT scan tomography as described by de Leon *et al.*[50] may forward our understanding of this deadly disorder.

Investigations into schizophrenia with PETT began with Farkas, who demonstrated by using [18F]deoxyglucose that there was reduced frontal cortical metabolism (60% of normal), which increased (to 75% of normal) following drug treatment.[51] Another group used [11C]glucose and demonstrated decreased frontal-to-temporal cortical ratios.[52] Buchsbaum *et al.* reported similar findings of decreased frontal-to-posterior cortical ratios compared to age-matched controls.[53] This same group[54] extended their findings to include affective disorders. In a study of 11 depressed patients, the finding in common with schizophrenia was a decreased anterior–posterior gradient in glucose metabolism. In another study,[55] this group could show no specific clinical correlates to the decreased anteroposterior gradients in schizophrenic patients. Phelps *et al.*[56] have reported findings in depressed patients and their age-matched controls who were scanned before and after treatment with methylphenidate. Although the PETT scans showed no overall differences in metabolic activity between patients and controls, there were some findings in subgroups of patients. Bipolar depressed patients showed significantly lower hemispheric metabolic activity, and a subgroup of unipolar patients showed asymmetric metabolic gradients between frontal cortex and temporal cortex. Additionally, patients who showed an antidepressant response to methylphenidate showed a normalization of these asymmetries, whereas patients who became more depressed showed an increase in hemispheric asymmetries.

The above studies are preliminary findings that highlight the ability of PETT to accurately reflect brain metabolic activity. With the emergence of better resolution in the second-generation PETT scanners, we can hope for more specific findings of regional brain activity. The emergence of patterns in schizophrenia and affective disorders remains to be elucidated further. The synthesis[57,58] and utilization of labeled ligands such as [11C]ethrophine for opiate receptors, pimozide for dopamine receptors, flunitrazpam for benzodiazepine receptors, and spiroperidol for dopamine receptors[59]

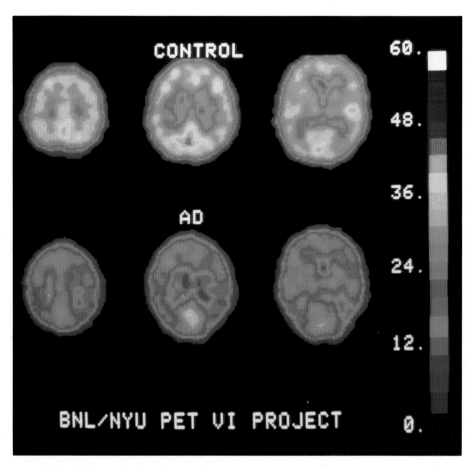

Figure 10-8. The images show representative PETT [¹¹C]deoxyglucose (CDG) scans from an elderly control (top row) and an age-matched Alzheimer (AD) patient (bottom row). From left to right, three levels of brain are depicted (centrum semiovale, ventricular bodies, and thalamic level). Using the color scale bar on the right, which color codes the metabolic rate for glucose (mg/min per 100 g), one sees the lower activity found in AD. On the average, AD patients show an about 15–20% decrease in glucose utilization compared with controls. The images are derived from the collaborative work of Drs. Mony J. de Leon, Steve H. Ferris, Ajax E. George (New York University Medical Center), and Alfred P. Wolf (Brookhaven National Laboratory) and are shown with their kind permission.

are all under evaluation and are undergoing feasibility studies, with appropriate tracer kinetic models being developed. Progress in this area is slow but offers the potential for enormous gains in the understanding of receptor physiology and the mechanism of action of many different medications.

13. Computerized Axial Tomography

Computerized axial tomography (CAT) was widely regarded when it was introduced into medical practice in 1973. It was heralded as a technological advancement in imaging that was equal to the invention of the X ray. Indeed, the invention of CAT by Hounsfield earned him the Nobel Prize in 1979. The implementation of CAT technology has greatly expanded our abilities to diagnose diseases of the central nervous system as well as refine the diagnostic expertise in the fields of neurology and psychiatry. The practical usage of CAT scanning in psychiatry is the major focus of this section.

14. Basic Principles of CAT

Computerized axial tomography technology has improved rapidly over the past 10 years but has now reached a plateau in its technical advancement. Equipment from different manufacturers is similar in design and is capable of high-resolution images, several-second computer reconstruction, and scanning times of less than 5 sec. All new models are multipurpose and provide images of both the head and body.

Computerized axial tomography functions on the principle that there are slight differences in the radiation absorption coefficients between various tissues. This fact permits the differentiation among bone, gray and white matter, cerebrospinal fluid, as well as pathological densities in the brain. Additionally, the intravenous injection of water-soluble contrast materials greatly enhances imaging of pathological lesions.

Computerized axial tomography utilizes detectors to pick up the radiation eminating from slices of tissue up to 1.3 cm thick. A total of 250,000 or more readings are obtained for each slice and are carried to a computer programmed with algorithms to solve huge numbers of simultaneous equations. The computer provides a digital printout of calculated density values for each slice. This is also transformed into a density image to be viewed on a brightness-modulated cathode ray tube. The operator is able to display selectively various density levels and alter contrast to improve vizualization. The final step produces photographs from an instant camera for a permanent viewing record.

15. Clinical Applications of CAT Scanning

Unlike the present status of clinical applications of NMR or PETT, usage of CAT scanning in the clinical practice of psychiatry is widespread. As is the case with all medical diagnostic procedures, CAT scanning is subject to abuse by inappropriate utilization.

A brief review of the clinical indications for ordering a CAT scan in psychiatry is warranted.

16. Clinical Indications

The increasing emphasis on ruling out organically based illnesses in patients presenting with psychiatric symptoms is a direct result of many studies documenting the high prevalence of undiagnosed medical illnesses in this population.[60,61] Clearly, if the CAT scan were not so expensive and did not involve X-ray exposure, it would make an ideal screening procedure for neurological illnesses. Often, the focal presentation of many neurological illnesses is preceded by disturbances of mood, perception, behavior, and thinking. Table 10-2 describes the psychiatric symptoms with which some neurological illnesses may present and lists the corresponding CAT findings. These patients often present to psychiatrists on referral from other specialists. The ruling out of organic illness should be the first priority.

Admittedly, it is rare that a structural neurological illness is diagnosed exclusively on the basis of psychiatric symptoms. The result is that psychiatrists often are not aggressive enough in working up patients with atypical presentations. Several clinical clues should point towards ordering a CAT scan. Any patient who presents with the recent onset of a dementia should be scanned. The appearance of a first-onset psychosis requires CAT evaluation. Patients who have undergone sudden severe personality transformations require a CAT. Additionally, a CAT evaluation is indicated in patients

Table 10-2. Partial List of Neurological Diseases Showing Their Psychiatric Symptoms and CAT Scan Findings

Neurological disease	Major psychiatric symptoms	CAT scan findings
Huntington's chorea	Psychosis, depression, movement disorder	Caudate atrophy
Wilson's disease	Psychosis, movement disorder	Atrophy: basal ganglia, cortex, cerebellum
Metachromatic leucodystrophy	Psychosis, dementia	Patchy decreased densities in subcortical white matter
Herpes simplex encephalitis	Psychosis	Decreased densities in temporal lobes
Lupus erythematosus	Psychosis, depression, movement disorder	Focal or generalized cerebral atrophy
Multiple sclerosis	Depression, movement disorder	Diffuse atrophy or focal hypodensities
Alzheimer's disease	Dementia	Diffuse cortical atrophy, ventricular enlargement
Fahr's disease	Psychosis, movement disorder	Calcifications of basal ganglia and cerebellum
Creutzfeldt–Jacob disease	Dementia	Cortical and subcortical atrophy

who present with the onset of psychiatric symptoms after the age of 40 years, patients with symptoms of anorexia, drug-abuse patients who are confused, patients with catatonia, and patients with involuntary movements. It is not enough to send a patient for consultation to a neurologist. Some neurological consultants are unfamiliar with the most subtle organic features of a mental status examination. They frequently fail to consider the psychiatric presentation as a possible prodromal phase of an organic mental syndrome.

The specific clinical indications for ordering a CAT scan ultimately rest with the psychiatrist's clinical intuition. There does not exist a randomly selected prospective study of psychiatric patients who were evaluated by CAT scan. As in all costly procedures, there needs to be a cost–benefit analysis to determine the rate of yield. It is impossible from existing studies[62–64] to determine the percentage yield on CAT scanning of randomly selected psychiatric patients. According to these studies, up to 10% of preselected hospitalized psychiatric patients have structural CNS lesions other than diffuse atrophy. This is an alarmingly high figure and painfully points out the need for research to develop rational guidelines for the ordering of CAT scans in psychiatric patients. The final point in this discussion is that the findings of a negative CAT scan are enormously reassuring to both clinician and patient. It provides the reassurance that the initiation of aggressive psychiatric treatment is not naively proceeding in the face of a structural CNS lesion.

17. Computerized Tomographic Findings in Schizophrenia

The proliferation of CAT scan research into defining structural abnormalities in the brains of schizophrenics began with the initial reports by Johnstone, who reported enlarged cerebral ventricles in schizophrenic patients.[64] Weinberger *et al.*, using ventricular brain ratios (VBR) as a measure of ventricular enlargement, reported that young chronic schizophrenics showed a statistically significant increase in VBR compared to controls.[65] These early reports have been replicated by several groups,[66,67] yet other groups have been unable to replicate the findings.[68,69]

Several explanations for this lack of consistent findings are possible. The first explanation is that there are differences among the patient populations between studies. Differences in previous medication treatment, duration and severity of illness, and diagnostic categories all potentially contribute to heterogeneous experimental populations. In addition, since there has not been a unified measure of ventricular enlargement, some groups have measured ventricular brain ratios,[68] whereas others have utilized linear measurements of ventricular size.[70] Another area of difficulty is the selection of controls for the experimental group. Clearly, no single fact accounts for the discrepent findings, but the discrepencies do not invalidate some very interesting speculation into the nature of ventricular enlargement in schizophrenia. The findings of Reveley and associates in the study of CAT scans obtained in monozygotic twins discordant for schizophrenia showed that the affected schizophrenic twins had significantly larger ventricles than the unaffected normal twins.[71] Additionally, there was a trend towards the nonschizophrenic twins having larger ventricles than those of the normal dizygotic twins. These findings are of interest when related to those of Weinberger, who compared the VBRs of unaffected siblings to their affected schizophrenic siblings.[72] He demonstrated significantly larger ventricles in the affected schizophrenics as well as a tendency for the nonschizophrenic siblings to have larger ventricles than control normals.

These studies are supportive of a genetic–environmental model of schizophrenia. The hypothesized emergence of schizophrenia occurs in a genetically disposed individual who suffers a brain insult such as a prenatal complication that breaks the threshold, causing the clinical appearance of schizophrenia.

Other arguments[73] seek to highlight the fact that the duration of illness should be considered as accountable for the degree of ventricular enlargement. These authors propose that the degree of ventricular enlargement is related to the progressive neuronal degeneration caused by an inherited progressive neurological syndrome. Their proposal needs to be validated by the follow-up of CAT scans in patients with schizophrenia.

Clinical correlates of enlarged ventricles have also been the subject of much recent research.[64,74,75] These studies have all found an association between enlarged ventricles and negative clinical features of schizophrenia. The symptoms of flat affect, retardation, and poverty of speech all correlated positively with enlarged ventricles. Another study[76] showed that chronic schizophrenic men with high VBR were at greater risk for suicide attempts. Additionally, the patients with increased VBR were less responsive to drug therapy.[65] Two other areas attempting to differentiate schizophrenic brain morphology from normals have been the subject of research. Brain asymmetry is a normal characteristic in humans. The normal pattern is a larger right frontal and left occipital brain region. Several studies have shown a reversal of this asymmetry,[77,78] but others have found no such reversal of brain asymmetry.[79,80] Another recent focus of CAT scan finding has been brain density measures in schizophrenia. Several studies have shown decreased brain densities, but this work needs replication.[81,82]

The variety of findings in schizophrenic patients with regard to CAT scan abnormalities is not surprising. Clearly, schizophrenia does not occur in a homogeneous group of patients. Nevertheless, it is clear that there exist on the basis of ventricular enlargement subgroupings among schizophrenic patients. There is much need for further research in correlating abnormal CAT scan findings to the longitudinal clinical pictures in these patients. It would be useful to follow the possible progression of ventricular enlargement as well as to define its clinical prognostic capability. Finally, agreement needs to be made on the standards of measurement with CAT scans, diagnostic selection of patients, and better definitions of neuropsychological exclusion criteria.

18. Computerized Tomographic Findings in Dementia and Affective Disorders

The usage of CAT scans in terms of correlating the mental decline in dementing processes has generally been accepted as having poor predictive capabilities.[83–85] These studies, however, are subject to methodological flaws in that they utilize absolute linear measurements in their analyses. Another problem in these studies was their reliance on measurements of cerebral sulci, which are subject to wide margins of error. Recent studies using ventricular brain ratios and gray matter/white matter discrimination have improved the CAT scan's ability as a predictive tool in assessing dementing processes.[86]

The most common dementing process by far is senile dementia of the Alzheimer's type (SDAT). Many studies attempting to correlate CAT scan abnormalities with the degree of cognitive decline in SDAT have found poor correlation. de Leon *et al.*,[87] in a study of different CAT scan evaluation strategies, found that the width of the third ventricle was the best linear ventricular correlate with the degree of cognitive impairment.

The essential issue with CAT evaluation in dementia is not whether it can accurately measure the degree of cognitive impairment but rather whether as a screening tool it can rule out treatable and reversible causes of dementia. It is clear that CAT has a superior ability to rule out brain tumors, hemorrhages, infarctions, subdural hematomas, hydrocephalus, and other potential causes for dementia. It remains to be seen whether, with the utilization of other measurement modalities, CAT can be better correlated to the degree of cognitive decline in SDAT.

The usage of CAT scan in examining the brains of affective disorder patients is poorly researched in the literature. One study found no significant differences between elderly patients with affective disorders and age-matched controls.[88] The investigators, however, examined a subgroup of patients with increased ventricular size, a later age of onset of their affective disorder, less anxiety, and more endogenous symptoms and reported that they had a poor outcome.[89] Two other groups published findings of combined groups of schizophrenic and affective-disorder patients and found them to have VBRs that were similar.[90,91] One of these studies reported that these two groups had VBRs that were significantly increased from their control group. A recent study has also shown that the lateral ventricular measurements of affective disorder, schizoaffective disorder, and schizophrenia were similar. Another study attempted to correlate the degree of cortisol hypersecretion in affective disorders to the increase in VBRs on CAT scan.[92] This group did not report repeating the scans after correction of the cortisol abnormality.

The fact that preliminary reports on affective disorders show increases in VBR similar to that seen in schizophrenia should not be surprising given their overlapping symptomatology and diagnostic blurring. More work needs to be done to define the relationship among extreme VBR values, genetic markers, and subgroups of affective disorders. The value of CAT in the area of prognostic outcome in affective disorders is a potential as yet unexplored.

19. Conclusion

The evidence that CAT, PETT, and NMR imaging will revolutionize medicine is irrefutable. The introduction of CAT technology 12 years ago has changed virtually every field of medicine. There are reports that CAT has been shown to reduce length of stay in hospitals as well as to eliminate certain surgical procedures.[93,94] It clearly has replaced less specific diagnostic procedures such as brain scans and pneumoen-cephalography. It has also decreased the use of other procedures such as abdominal arteriography, lymphangiography, and polytomography. In fact, wide availability and the general acceptance of CAT in diagnostic workups raise the fear of inappropriate utilization of a costly procedure. Several studies have shown that CAT scans when applied to the routine workup of headaches are not cost effective.[95,96] Additionally, as seen in this review, the development of rational guidelines for its usage in psychiatry are virtually nonexistent. It is of concern that a procedure that has been in wide use for over 10 years is still lacking such basic clinical indications for its usage.

The implementation of PETT and NMR into routine clinical practice should benefit from the mistakes in CAT implementation. Health care planning in the early 1970s sought to regionalize the usage of CAT. This created the paradox of patients being sent out of major medical centers to receive CAT scans in the private offices of doctors. The ensuing chaos was largely responsible for the demise of regional health care planning in some areas. The future of NMR in medicine undoubtedly will be bright regardless of the present lack of clear and specific indications for its usage.

Both PETT and NMR scanning require continued intensive research and develop-ment to avoid the stigma of escalating the cost of health care. Procedures such as PETT and NMR must undergo cost-effective studies before their usage can be widely accept-ed. These studies must demonstrate that the cost of this technology is outweighed by its diagnostic specificity. This can only be accomplished by developing their potentialities under carefully controlled research settings.

References

1. Hounsfield GN: Computerized transverse axial scanning (tomography). Part 1. Description of system. *Br J Radiol* 46:1016–1022, 1973.
2. Ambrose J: Computerized transverse axial scanning (tomography). Clinical application. *Br J Radiol* 46:1023–1047, 1973.
3. Block F: Nuclear induction. *Phys Rev* 70:460–474, 1946.
4. Purcell EM, Torvey HC, Pound RV: Resonance absorption by nuclear magnetic moment in a solid. *Phys Rev* 69:127, 1946.
5. Damadian R: Tumor detection by nuclear magnetic resonance. *Science* 117:1151–1153, 1971.
6. Lauterbur PC: Image formation by induced local interactions: Examples of employing nuclear magnetic resonance. *Nature* 242:190–191, 1973.
7. Damadian R, Goldsmith, M, Minkoff L: NMR in cancer. XV. Fonar image of the live human body. *Physiol Chem Phys* 9:97–108, 1977.
8. Doyle, FH, Gore, JC, Pennods JM, et al: Imaging of the brain by nuclear magnetic resonance. *Lancet* 2:53–57, 1981.
9. Smith, FW, Hutchison, JMS, Mallard, JR, et al: Esophageal carcinoma demonstrated by whole-body nuclear magnetic resonance imaging. *Br Med J* 282:510–512, 1981.
10. Smith FW, Mollard JR, Reid A, et al: Nuclear magnetic resonance tomographic imaging in liver disease. *Lancet* 1:963–966, 1981.
11. Abragam A: *Principles of Nuclear Magnetism*. London, Oxford University Press, 1983.
12. Mansfield P, Morris PG: *NMR Imaging in Biomedicine*. New York, Academic Press, 1982.
13. Bydder GM, Steiner RE, Young IR, et al: Clinical NMR imaging of the brain: 140 cases. *Am J Roentgenol* 139:215–236, 1982.
14. Buonanno FS, Pykett IL, Vielina J, et al: Protein NMR imagining of normal and abnormal brain.

Experimental and clinical observations, in Witcofski RL, Rarstaedt N, Partain CL (eds): *NMR Imaging*. Winston Salem, Bowman Gray School of Medicine Press, 1982, pp 147–157.

15. Young IR, Hall AS, Pallis CA, et al: Nuclear magnetic resonance imaging of the brain in multiple sclerosis. *Lancet* 2:1063–1066, 1981.

16. Alfidi RJ, Haaga JR, El Yousef SJ, et al: Preliminary experimental results in humans and animals with superconducting, whole body nuclear magnetic resonance scanner. *Radiology* 143:175–181, 1982.

17. Crooks LE, Mills CM, Brant-Zauadski M, et al: Visualization of cerebral and vascular abnormalities of NMR imaging. The effects of imaging parameters on contrast. *Radiology* 144:843–852, 1982.

18. Crooks, L, Aralsowa M, Hoenninger J, et al: Nuclear magnetic resonance whole-body images operating at 3.5 K Gauss. *Radiology* 143:169–174, 1982.

19. Bessor JAO, Glen AIM, Foreman EI, et al: Nuclear magnetic resonance observations in alcoholic cerebral disorder and the role of vasopressin. *Lancet* 2:923–924, 1981.

20. Rangel-Guerra RA, Perez Payan H, Minlsoff L, et al: Nuclear magnetic resonance in bipolar affective disorders. *AJNR* 4:229–231, 1983.

21. Budinger TJ, Lauterbur PC: Nuclear magnetic resonance technology for medical studies. *Science* 226:288–298, 1984.

22. Roy, CS, Sherrington CS: On the regulation of the blood supply of the brain. *J Physiol (Lon)* 11:85–108, 1890.

23. Kety SS, Schmidt CE: The nitrous oxide method for the quantitative determination of cerebral blood flow in man: Theory, procedure and normal values. *J Clin Invest* 27:476–483, 1948.

24. Hoedt-Rasmusser K, Sveinsdotter E, Lassen NA: Regional cerebral blood flow in man determined by intra arterial injection of radioactive inert gas. *Cir Res* 18:236–247, 1966.

25. Ter Pogossian MM, Eichling JO, Davis DO, et al: The determination of regional cerebral blood flow by means of water labeled with radioactive oxygen-15. *Radiology* 93:31–40, 1969.

26. Ter Pogossian MM, Eichling JO, Davis DO, et al: The measure *in vivo* of regional cerebral oxygen utilization by means of oxyhemoglobin labeled with radioactive oxygen-15. *J Clin Invest* 49:381–391, 1970.

27. Raichle ME, Larson KB, Phelps ME, et al: *In vivo* measurement of brain glucose transport and metabolism employing glucose-11C. *Am J Physiol* 228:1936–1948, 1975.

28. Olesen J: Contralateral focal increase in cerebral blood flow in man during arm work. *Brain* 94:635–646, 1971.

29. Lassen WA, Ingvar DH: Changes in the amount of blood flowing in areas of the human cerebral cortex reflecting changes in the activity of those areas are graphically revealed with the aid of radioactive isotope. *Sci Am* 239:62–71, 1971.

30. Sokoloff L, Reuvich M, Kennedy C, et al: The (^{14}C)deoxyglucose method for the measurement of local cerebral glucose utilization: Theory, procedure and normal values in the concious and anesthetized albino rat. *J Neurochem* 28:879–916, 1977.

31. Phelps ME, Mazziotta JC, Huang SC: Study of cerebral function with positron tomography. *J Cereb Blood Flow Metab* 2:113–162, 1982.

32. Sokoloff L: Localization of functional activity in the central nervous system by measurement of glucose utilization with radioactive deoxyglucose. *J Cereb Blood Flow Metab* 1:7–36, 1981.

33. Phelps ME, Hoffman EJ, Mullani NA, et al: Application of annihilation coincidence detection to transaxial reconstruction tomography. *J Nucl Med* 16:210–223, 1975.

34. Ter Pogossian MM, Mullani NA, Hood JT, et al: A multislice positron emission computed tomograph (PETTIV) yielding transverse and longitudinal images. *Radiology* 128:477–484, 1978.

35. Phelps ME, Hoffman EJ, Huang SC: ECAT: A new computerized tomographic imaging system for positron-emitting radiopharmaceuticals. *J Nucl Med* 16:210–224, 1978.

36. Phelps ME, Hoffman EJ, Huang SC, et al: Effect of positron range on spatial resolution. *J Nucl Med* 16:649–652, 1975.

37. Fox JL: Letter to the editor. *Science* 224:143–144, 1984.

38. Mazziotta JC, Phelps ME, Miller J, et al: Tomographic mapping of human cerebral metabolism: Normal unstimulated state. *Neurology (Minneap)* 31:503–516, 1981.

39. Phelps ME, Mazziotta JC, Kuhl DE, et al: Tomographic mapping of human cerebral metabolism: Visual stimulation and deprivation. *Neurology (Minneap)* 31:517–529, 1981.

40. Phelps ME, Kuhl DE, Mazziotta JC: Metabolic mapping of the brains response to visual stimulation: Studies in humans. *Science* 211:1445–1448, 1981.

41. Mazziotta JC, Phelps ME, Carson RE, et al: Tomographic mapping of human cerebral metabolism: Auditory stimulation. *Neurology (NY)* 32:921–937, 1982.

42. Kuhl DE, Metter EJ, Riege WH, et al: Effects of human aging on patterns of local cerebral glucose utilization determined by the (^{18}F)fluorodeoxyglucose method. *J Cereb Blood Flow Metab* 2:163–171, 1982.

43. Lammertsma AA, Frackowals RS, Lenzi GL, et al: Accuracy of the oxygen-15 steady state technique for measuring RCBF and $CMRO_2$: Tracer modeling statistics and spatial sampling. *J Cereb Blood Flow Metab* 1(Suppl 1):53–54, 1981.

44. de Leon MJ, George AE, Ferris SH, et al: Positron emission tomography and computed tomography assessments of the aging human brain. *J Comput Assist Tomogr* 8(1):88–94, 1984.

45. Rapaport SI, Duara R, London ED, et al: Glucose metabolism of the aging nervous system, in Samuels D, Algeri S, Gershon S, et al (eds): *Aging of the Brain,* vol 22. New York, Raven Press, 1983, pp 111–121.

46. Hawkins RA, Mazziotta JC, Phelps ME, et al: Cerebral glucose metabolism as a junction of age in man: Influence of the rate constants in the glucodeoxyglucose method. *J Cereb Blood Flow Metab* 3:250–253, 1983.

47. Wong DF, Wagner HN, Donnals RF, et al: Effects of age on dopamine and serotonin receptors measured by positron tomography in the living human brain. *Science* 226:1393–1396, 1984.

48. Alavi A, Ferris S, Wolf A, et al: Determination of cerebral metabolism in senile dementia using F-18-deoxyglucose and positron emission tomography. *J Nucl Med* 21:21, 1980.

49. Bensen DF: The use of positron emission scanning techniques in the diagnosis of Alzheimer's disease, in Arkin S, Davis KL, Growdan JH, et al (eds): *Aging,* vol 19: *Alzheimer's Disease: A Review of Progress in Research.* New York, Raven Press, 1982, 79–82.

50. de Leon M, George AE, Ferris SH, et al: Regional correlation of PET and CT in senile dementia of the Alzheimer's type. *Am J Neuroradiol* 4:553–556, 1983.

51. Farkias T, Wolf AP, Fowler J, et al: Regional brain glucose metabolism in schizophrenia. *J Cereb Blood Flow Metab* 1(Suppl 1):496, 1981.

52. Widen L, Bergstrom M, Blomgrist G, et al: Glucose metabolism in patients with schizophrenia: Emission computed tomography measurements with 11-C-glucose. *J Cereb Blood Flow Metab* 1(Suppl 1):455–456, 1981.

53. Buchsbaum MS, Kessler R, Bunney WE, et al: Simultaneous electroencephalography and cerebral glucography with positron emission tomography (PET) in normals and patients with schizophrenia. *J Cereb Blood Flow Metab* 1(Suppl 1):457–458, 1981.

54. Buchsbaum MS, DeLisi LE, Holcomb HH, et al: Anteroposterior gradients in cerebral glucose use in schizophrenia and affective disorders. *Arch Gen Psychiatry* 41:1159–1166, 1984.

55. DeLisi L, Buchsbaum M, Holcomb HH, et al: Clinical correlates of decreased anteroposterior metabolic gradients in positron emission tomography (PET) of schizophrenic patients. *Am J Psychiatry* 142:78–81, 1985.

56. Phelps MS, Mazziotta JC, Baxter L: Positron emission tomographic study of affective disorders: Problems and strategies. *Ann Neurol* 15(Suppl):S149–156, 1984.

57. Comor D, Berger G, Crouyel C, et al: Carbon-11 labelled radiopharmaceuticals for brain receptor studies. *J Label Compds Radiopharm* 18:3–4, 1981.

58. Marziere M, Berger B, Godot JM, et al: Etorphine "C": A new tool of the *in vivo* study of brain opiate receptors. *J Label Compds Radiopharm* 18:15–16, 1981.

59. Wolf AP, Fowler JS: Organic radiopharmaceuticals: Recent advances, in Sorenson JA (ed): *Radiopharmaceuticals II.* New York, Society of Medicine, 1979, p 73–93.

60. Larson EB, Mack LA, Watts B, et al: Computed tomography in patients with psychiatric illness: Advantage of a 'rule-in' approach. *Ann Intern Med* 95:260–364, 1981.

61. Hall RCW, Gardner ER, Stickney SK, et al: Physical illness manifesting as psychiatric disease. *Arch Gen Psychiatry* 37:989–995, 1980.

62. Owens DG, Johnston EC, Bydder GM, et al: Unsuspected organic disease in chronic schizophrenia demonstrated by computed tomography. *J Neurol Neurosurg Psychiatry* 43:1065–1069, 1980.

63. Evans NJR: Cranial computerized tomography in clinical psychiatry: 100 consecutive cases. *Compr Psychiatry* 23:445–450, 1982.

64. Johnstone EC, Crow TJ, Firth CD, et al: Cerebral ventricular size and cognitive impairment in chronic schizophrenia. *Lancet* 2:924–926, 1976.
65. Weinberger DR, Torrey EF, Neophytides AN, et al: Lateral cerebral ventricular enlargement in chronic schizophrenia. *Arch Gen Psychiatry* 36:735–739, 1979.
66. Golden CJ, Moses JA, Jr, Lelazowski R, et al: Cerebral ventricular size and neuropsychological impairment in young chronic schizophrenics. *Arch Gen Psychiatry* 37:619–623, 1980.
67. Andreasen NC, Smith MR, Jacoby CG, et al: Ventricular enlargement in schizophrenia: Definition and prevalence. *Am J Psychiatry* 139:292–296, 1982.
68. Jernigau TL, Zatz LM, Moses JA, et al: Computed tomography in schizophrenic and normal volunteers, I: Fluid volume. *Arch Gen Psychiatry* 39:765–770, 1982.
69. Benes F, Sunderland P, Jones BD, et al: Normal ventricles in young schizophrenics. *Br J Psychiatry* 141:90–93, 1982.
70. Tanaka Y, Hazama H, Kawshara R, et al: Computerized tomography of the brain in schizophrenic patients. *Acta Psychiatr Scand* 63:191–197, 1981.
71. Reveley AM, Clifford CA, Revelay MA, et al: Cerebral ventricular size in twins discordant for schizophrenia. *Lancet* 1:540–541, 1982.
72. Weinberger DR, DeLisi LE, Neophytides AN, et al: Familial aspects of CT abnormalities in chronic schizophrenic patients. *Psychiatry Res* 4:65–71, 1981.
73. Woods BT, Wolf J: A reconsideration of the relation of ventricular enlargement to duration of illness in schizophrenia. *Am J Psychiatry* 140(12):1564–1570, 1973.
74. Johnstone EC, Crow TJ, Firth DC, et al: The dementia of dementia pracox. *Acta Psychiatr Scand* 57:305–324, 1978.
75. Andreasen NC, Olsen SA, Dennert JW, et al: Ventricular enlargement in schizophrenia: Relationship to positive and negative symptoms. *Am J Psychiatry* 139:297–302, 1982.
76. Levy AB, Kurtz N, Kling AS: Association between cerebral ventricular enlargement and suicide attempts in chronic schizophrenia. *Am J Psychiatry* 141(3):438–439, 1984.
77. Luchins DJ, Weinberger DR, Wyatt RJ: Schizophrenia: Evidence for a subgroup with reversed asymmetry. *Arch Gen Psychiatry* 36:1309–1311, 1979.
78. Naeser MA, Levine HL, Benson DF, et al: Frontal leukotomy size and hemispheric asymmetrics on computerized tomographic scans of schizophrenics with variable recovery. *Arch Neurol* 38:30–37, 1981.
79. Jernigau TL, Zatz LM, Moses JA, et al: Computer tomography in schizophrenics and normal controls: II. Cranial asymmetry. *Arch Gen Psychiatry* 139:771–773, 1982.
80. Nyback H, Wiesel FA, Berggren BM, et al: Computed tomography of the brain in patients with acute psychosis and in healthy volunteers. *Acta Psychiatr Scand* 65:403–414, 1982.
81. DeMeyer MD, Gilmor R, Hendrie H, et al: Brain densities in treatment resistant schizophrenia and other psychiatric patients. *J Oper Psychiatry* 15:9–16, 1984.
82. Golden CJ, Graber B, Coffman J, et al: Structural brain deficits in schizophrenia. *Arch Gen Psychiatry* 38:1014–1017, 1981.
83. Roberts MA, Caird F: Computerized tomography and intellectual impairment in the elderly. *J Neurol Neurosurg Psychiatry* 39:986–989, 1976.
84. Earnest MP, Heaton RK, Wilkinson WE, et al: Cortical atrophy, ventricular enlargement and intellectual impairment in the aged. *Neurology (Minneap)* 29:1138–1143, 1979.
85. Ford CV, Winter J: Computerized axial tomograms and dementia in elderly patients. *J Gerontol* 36:164–169, 1981.
86. Damasia H, Eslinger P, Damasia AR, et al: Quantative computed tomographic analysis in the diagnosis of dementia. *Arch Neurol* 40:715–719, 1983.
87. de Leon MJ, Ferris SH, George AE, et al: Computed tomography evaluations of brain behavior relationships in senile dementia of the Alzheimer's type. *Neurobiol Aging* 1:69–79, 1980.
88. Jacoby RJ, Levy R: Computed tomography in the elderly: III Affective disorder. *Br J Psychiatry* 136:270–275, 1980.
89. Jacoby RJ, Levy R, Bird JM: Computed tomography and the outcome of affective disorder: A follow-up study of elderly patients. *Br J Psychiatry* 139:288–292, 1981.
90. Pearlson GD, Veroff AE: Computerized tomographic scan changes in manic depressive illness. *Lancet* 2:470, 1981.

91. Nasrallah HA, McCalley-Whitters M, Jacoby CG: Cerebral ventricular enlargement in young manic males. *J Affect Dis* 4:15–19, 1982.
92. Kellner C, Rubinow D, Gold P, et al: Relationship of cortisol hypersecretion to brain CT scan alterations in depressed patients. *Psychiatry Res* 8:191–197, 1983.
93. Bahr AL, Hodges FJ: Efficacy of computed tomography of the head in changing patient care and health costs: A retrospective study. *Am J Roentgenol* 131:45–49, 1978.
94. Wittenberg J, Fineberg HV, Ferrucci TJ Jr, et al: Clinical efficacy of computed body tomography II. *Am J Roentgenol* 134:1111–1120, 1980.
95. Larson EB, Omenn GS, Lewis H: Diagnostic evaluation of headache: Impact of computerized tomography and cost effectiveness. *JAMA* 243:359–362, 1980.
96. Kraus WA, Wagner DP, Davis DO: CT for headache: Cost/benefit for subarachnoid hemorrhage. *Am J Roentgenol* 136:537–542, 1981.

Therapeutic Drug Level Monitoring in Psychiatry

Sheldon H. Preskorn, M.D., Mark S. Gold, M.D., and Irl Extein, M.D.

1. The Significance of Drug Plasma Concentrations

Laboratory tests to monitor plasma levels of antidepressant drugs have enhanced the physician's ability to use these agents in a more rational manner. Although drug concentration is not the sole determinant of clinical response, it is an important refinement of the dose–response curve typical of classic pharmacological studies (see Fig. 11-1). Unlike the latter, which are performed in inbred laboratory animals, clinical pharmacology must contend with the substantial interindividual differences in metabolic rates observed in man. These differences can produce clinically important interindividual variability in the drug plasma concentrations that may be obtained with the same dose.

In most patients, we expect a normal or negative finding on most medical screening tests such as a screening electrocardiogram or chest X ray. In contrast, obtaining a drug plasma level of a well-studied medication always provides useful information. First, the test is directed to something that is expected to be there. Some concentration of drug in the blood should be detected and be quantifiable because the patient is presumably taking medication. If the drug is nondetectable, it suggests either insufficient dosage or a compliance problem. Second, a detectable level will be either appropriate or inappropriate. In the latter case, appropriate dosage adjustment would be indicated.

Drug plasma monitoring is becoming an integral part of medical practice. The goal of this chapter is to improve the understanding of such monitoring, specifically as it pertains to antidepressant agents. Comprehensive reviews are available elsewhere. [1–3] This chapter focuses on basic concepts and principles essential to understanding the relevance of therapeutic drug monitoring: (1) pharmacodynamics, (2) pharmacoki-

Sheldon H. Preskorn, M.D. • Departments of Psychiatry and Pharmacology, Washington University School of Medicine, St. Louis, Missouri 63110.   *Mark S. Gold, M.D.* • Research Facilities, Fair Oaks Hospital, Summit, New Jersey 07901, and Fair Oaks Hospital at Boca/Delray, Delray Beach, Florida 33445.   *Irl Extein, M.D.* • Fair Oaks Hospital at Boca/Delray, Delray Beach, Florida 33445.

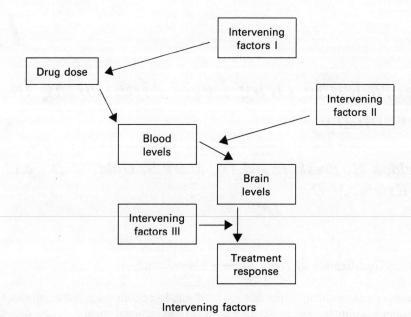

Intervening factors

Group I	Group II	Group III
Absorption	Bound : free ratio	Neurochemical variance
Distribution	Blood–brain barrier*	(e.g., receptor function,
Metabolism	Cerebral blood flow*	reuptake mechanisms,
Elimination		feedback systems)

Figure 11-1. The factors that lead to individual differences in human dose response. *Most critical under non-steady-state conditions.

netics, (3) methodological issues critical to routine monitoring and (4) concentration : response relationships.

2. Reasons for Drug Monitoring

There are essentially four major reasons to monitor:

1. To check compliance. This issue is important in regard to both initial and maintenance treatment response, especially in depressed patients whose concentration and motivation are impaired.
2. To maximize clinical response. Since a relationship between clinical response and drug plasma concentration has been established for certain antidepressant medications, plasma monitoring allows the physician to more rationally adjust drug dosage to enhance therapeutic effect.
3. To avoid toxicity. Since a relationship between drug plasma concentration and drug toxicity has also been demonstrated for some antidepressant agents, drug toxicity can also be minimized by rationally adjusting dosage based on plasma monitoring.

4. To protect the physician legally. This issue is particularly important in this era of malpractice suits, especially for physicians who give high doses of potent anticholinergic TCAs.

3. Pharmacodynamics

The elementary principle underlying drug monitoring is that pharmacodynamics is determined by drug concentration at some site in the body. From a clinical standpoint, pharmacodynamics can refer to either desired or undesired effects. Drugs such as the antidepressants (ADs) produce a multiplicity of concentration-dependent therapeutic, nuisance, and toxic effects. Tricyclic antidepressants (TCAs) may be annoyingly sedative for patients in remission even though this effect is desirable in other patients. Even toxicity is not unequivocal: TCAs can delay intracardiac conduction by inhibiting membrane excitability. At appropriate concentrations and in appropriate patients, these drugs can reduce specific cardiac arrhythmias. Yet, they can cause fatal arrhythmias at high concentrations.[4]

Regardless of their desirability, effects are mediated by the drug reaching an appropriate concentration at an effector site.[5,6] The interaction between drug and effector site (receptor or enzyme) may be either rapidly reversible or irreversible.[7] An example of a rapidly reversible interaction is TCA-induced delirium. This delirium results from excessive central acetylcholine receptor blockade and can be competitively overcome by increasing acetylcholine concentrations at the receptor.[8] An example of an irreversible drug : effector site interaction is monoamine oxidase inhibition by such drugs as phenelzine. The sustained effect of such monoamine oxidase inhibitors (MAOIs) results not from prolonged drug elimination but rather from the fact that new enzyme must be synthesized after drug discontinuation. Other examples of irreversible or slowly reversible drug action in psychopharmacology include withdrawal symptoms following discontinuation of neuroleptic drugs (i.e., tardive dyskinesia) or sedative–hypnotics (i.e., delirium tremens).

For most drugs exerting an irreversible or slowly reversible effect, it is difficult to demonstrate a relationship between effect and concentration. The reason is that the effect persists even after drug elimination. Yet the fact that it is technically difficult to establish a concentration : response relationship for irreversibly acting drugs does not mean that it does not exist. The antihypertensive effects of prazosin or clonidine are almost undoubtedly determined by the drug concentration reaching the effector site as well as by the number and functional state of the receptors and by factors such as integrity of feedback systems.[9] The same is probably true for MAOIs, with the components of response determination including drug concentration and basal MAO level. For these reasons, investigators studying the antidepressant and other effects of MAOIs have been correlating these actions to the degree of MAO inhibition achieved rather than to drug concentration.[10]

4. The Mechanism of Action of Tricyclic Antidepressants

The mechanism of action underlying antidepressant response to TCAs is less clear than those of other psychopharmaceuticals. For this reason, it would be speculative and arbitrary to pick one of these actions to monitor drug concentrations. Hence, most studies have either used multiple approaches or attempted to correlate response to actual drug concentration.

These drugs are complex medicines in terms of both their multiple mechanisms of action and their broad clinical effects.[5]

5. Receptor Effects

All TCAs have essentially comparable antidepressant effects but wide variation in side effects.[11-13] Important side effects include sedation, anticholinergic effects, conduction delays, and postural hypotension. These effects should be considered in making the initial choice for treatment and can often be tailored to a particular patient's requirements.

The degree to which sedation is produced by antidepressants corresponds to and is believed to result from H_1 histamine receptor blockade. Table 11-1 shows the relative potencies of the available antidepressants in blocking H_1 histamine receptors. As can be seen, many are more potent antihistamines than the standard antihistamine, diphenhydramine. Doxepin has the most potent antihistamine effects and is 800 times more potent than diphenhydramine. The rank order of these compounds correlates fairly well with their apparent sedative properties.

Desipramine is the least antihistaminic and least sedating of these compounds. For some patients, sedation may be a desirable side effect, particularly for those with extreme agitation and insomnia. Other patients are intolerant of these effects and may require a less sedating agent. Other clinically important effects that may be mediated via H_1 receptor blockade include weight gain, possibly hypotension, and potentiation of the CNS depressant effects of alcohol, other sedative hypnotics, and CNS depressants.

Table 11-1. Relative Antihistamine/Histamine H_1/Sedating Potencies of Antidepressants

Drug	Relative potency[a]
Doxepin (Adapin®, Sinequan®)	800
Trimipramine (Surmontil®)	250
Amitriptyline (Elavil®, Endep®)	190
Maprotiline (Ludiomil®)	25
Amoxapine (Asendin®)	4
Nortriptyline (Aventyl®, Pamelor®)	4
Imipramine (Janimine®, SK-Pramine®, Tofranil®)	2.5
Protriptyline (Vivactil®)	0.7
Trazodone (Desyrel®)	0.4
Desipramine (Norpramin®, Pertofrane®)	0.1
Diphenhydramine[b] (Benadryl®)	1

[a]Data modified from Richelson.[59]
[b]Not an antidepressant; given here for comparison.

Anticholinergic effects (dry mouth, constipation, urinary retention, blurred vision, increased heart rate) result from blockade of muscarinic acetylcholine receptors. As shown in Table 11-2, there is a substantial variation in the degree to which these effects are produced by TCAs. Amitriptyline, the most potent in this regard, is about one-tenth as potent as atropine in blocking muscarinic acetylcholine receptors and is 18,000 times more antimuscarinic than the newly released trazodone. Anticholinergic effects can be significant clinically and should be considered in choosing an antidepressant agent. For patients with a history of narrow-angle glaucoma, agents that are highly anticholinergic should be avoided. Elderly patients may be at risk for anticholinergic delirium, urinary retention (especially in males with enlarged prostates), or constipation. Patients with a cardiac history may experience an excessive increase in heart rate from highly anticholinergic agents.

Orthostatic hypotension is probably the most frequently encountered adverse effect resulting from α-adrenergic receptor blockade (Table 11-3). For patients who are sensitive to this effect, agents such as desipramine or protriptyline may be indicated, whereas highly anti-α-adrenergic agents such as doxepin, trimipramine, or amitriptyline should be avoided.

Amoxapine is a new antidepressant designated chemically as 2-chloro-11-(1-piperazinyl)dibenz[b,f](1,4)oxazepine. The antidepressant activity of amoxapine is related to the blockade of norepinephrine and serotonin uptake. There are two major metabolites, 7-OH-amoxapine and 8-OH-amoxapine. These metabolites may well be more responsible than the parent compound for pharmacological effects. 8-OH-Amoxapine is comparable to the parent compound in its norepinephrine reuptake-blocking properties; however, it is extremely potent on serotonin reuptake blockade. It has been demonstrated that 7-OH-amoxapine produces significant dopamine receptor blockade in laboratory animals, and its dopamine (DA)-blocking and neuroleptic activity in humans should be studied.

We have recent data in amoxapine-treated humans that demonstrated potent DA-

Table 11-2. Relative Anticholinergic Potencies
of Antidepressants

Drug	Relative potency[a]
Amitriptyline (Elavil®, Endep®)	11.0
Protriptyline (Vivactil®)	8.0
Trimipramine (Surmontil®)	3.4
Doxepin (Adapin®, Sinequan®)	2.6
Imipramine (SK-Pramine®, Tofranil®)	2.2
Nortriptyline (Aventyl®, Pamelor®)	1.4
Desipramine (Norpramin®, Pertofrane®)	1.0
Maprotiline (Ludiomil®)	0.4
Amoxapine (Asendin®)	0.2
Trazodone (Desyrel®)	0.0006
Atropine[b]	100

[a]Data modified from Richelson.[59]
[b]Not an antidepressant; given here for comparison.

Table 11-3. Relative Anti-α-Adrenergic/Hypotension-Producing
Potencies of Antidepressants

Drug	Relative potency[a]
Doxepin (Adapin®, Sinequan®)	5.0
Trimipramine (Surmontil®)	5.0
Amitriptyline (Elavil®, Endep®)	4.4
Trazodone (Desyrel®)	3.4
Amoxapine (Asendin®)	2.4
Nortriptyline (Aventyl®, Pamelor®)	1.9
Maprotiline (Ludiomil®)	1.3
Imipramine (SK-Pramine®, Tofranil®)	1.3
Protriptyline (Vivactil®)	0.9
Desipramine (Norpramin®, Pertofrane®)	0.9
Prazosin[b] (Minipress®)	2000

[a]Data modified from Richelson.[59]
[b]Not an antidepressant; given here for comparison.

blocking effects in some patients and negligible effects in others. Plasma samples were obtained on 30 patients maintained on amoxapine therapy for at least 3 weeks. Plasma was assayed for 8-OH-amoxapine by gas–liquid chromatography and for dopamine receptor-blocking activity by a neuroleptic radioreceptor assay (NRRA). Significant dopamine-blocking activity was noted by NRRA in samples independent of plasma 8-OH-amoxapine level. 7-OH-Amoxapine concentrations correlate with dopamine-blocking activity by NRRA. High concentrations of 7-OH-amoxapine and NRRA activity may be correlated with akathisia, extrapyramidal symptoms (EPS), galactorrhea, and antipsychotic efficacy. Occasional patients who are administered this compound on a chronic basis form high amounts of 7-OH-amoxapine and may be at risk for tardive dyskinesia.

As the preceding discussion of receptor effects indicates, pharmacological actions of TCAs may vary widely from patient to patient. The knowledge of these effects may help guide the initial choice and increase the likelihood of an adequate therapeutic trial with a minimum of unwanted effects (Table 11-4). For many patients, sedative, anticholinergic, or hypotensive effects can limit the ability to tolerate an adequate therapeutic trial with therapeutic blood levels. For this reason, we usually begin with a less sedating, less anticholinergic tricyclic such as nortriptyline or desipramine.[14]

6. Other Effects

A recent and important finding is that TCAs possess quinidinelike antiarrhythmic effects and actually suppress premature ventricular contraction.[13] Many patients with cardiac disease can be treated safely with TCAs if monitored closely.

Tricyclic antidepressants can be lethal in overdosage.[12] Although doxepin is alleged to be the safest in an overdose, this apparent safety is pharmacokinetically rather than pharmacodynamically mediated. Doxepin has the highest first-pass hepatic extraction of all TCAs. At equal concentration, doxepin is as cardioactive as amitrip-

Table 11-4. Clinical Significance of Receptor Activity

Property	Possible clinical consequence
1. Blockade of norepinephrine uptake at nerve endings	Antidepressive effects; blockade of the antihypertensive effects of guanethidine, clonidine, and α-methyldopa
2. Blockade of serotonin uptake at nerve endings	Antidepressive effects; ?postural hypotension
3. Blockade of histamine H_1 receptors	Potentiation of alcohol, tranquilizers, and other central depressant drugs, sedation, drowsiness; weight gain; hypotension
4. Blockade of muscarinic receptors	Blurred vision, urinary retention, dry mouth, constipation, sinus tachycardia
5. Blockade of α_1-adrenergic receptors	Potentiation of the antihypertensive effect of prazosin (Minipress®); postural hypotension, reflex tachycardia
6. Blockade of α_2-adrenergic receptors	Blockade of the antihypertensive effects of clonidine (Catapres®) and α-methyldopa (Aldomet®); ?antidepressive effects

tyline. Death can be from central nervous system or cardiorespiratory effects. Measurement of levels and EKG changes such as QRS widening are indicators of the severity of an overdose. The ratio of tertiary- to secondary-amine TCAs can also be used for this purpose. Because of the possibility of serious overdose in depressed patients, no more than a 1- to 2-week supply of a TCA should be prescribed at a time to outpatients.

Although some of the effects of TCAs are independent of each other, many impinge on different components of the same system or on related systems. Hence, these pharmacological mechanisms can be additive, synergistic, or even antagonistic. For example, the affinity for desipramine binding sites and the blockade of the neuronal reuptake pump for norepinephrine may be different aspects of the same action; that is, the desipramine binding sites may be the effector sites mediating pump inhibition.[15] The TCA-induced inhibition of neuronal reuptake of norepinephrine, blockade of α_1- and α_2-adrenergic receptors, and inhibition of MAO and COMT activity would be expected to interact in a complex manner to alter central actions of norepinephrine.[5] The establishment of well-defined concentration : response relationships could improve our understanding of the relative importance of these various actions in terms of mediating the response of interest (e.g., antidepressant response).

Given the multiplicity of TCA pharmacological mechanisms and their diverse nature, the fact that these drugs produce numerous desired and undesired responses is not surprising. With this background, the absurdity of attributing all their beneficial effects to antidepressant action is clear. This logical fallacy is even at times extended to using response to ADs to make a diagnosis. For example, if a patient with chronic pain or migraine headache responds to ADs, some will say that the patient must have had a "masked depression." Under this logic, perhaps excessive salivation is also a symptom of an affective disorder.

6.1. How Can Concentration : Response Studies Help?

What remains is a class of disorders (i.e., major affective syndromes) whose etiology is vague and uncertain and whose major treatment (i.e., TCAs) has a multiplicity of actions, each possibly being responsible for the antidepressant effects. It is with regard to this issue that well-defined concentration : response relationships can provide additional illumination.

6.2. Clinical Implications of Such Relationships

Beyond their impact on research, well-defined concentration : response relationships have clinical import in four ways. First, concentration monitoring is the only effective means of assessing patient compliance. Second, if a threshold exists for efficacy, then dosage can be adjusted rationally to increase response. Third, dosage can also be adjusted to avoid toxicity if an upper limit exists above which the risk of toxicity outweighs the probability of further therapeutic gain. Fourth, drug concentration monitoring can be useful from a medicolegal standpoint. For example, it can document the need for unusual doses, medication combinations in selected patients, or that a drug overdose did occur.

7. Antidepressant Levels

The use of standard dose regimens unrelated to drug plasma levels has been identified as a major source of antidepressant nonresponse. The reasons include pharmacokinetic, pharmacodynamic, and other factors. For example, hepatic microsomal enzymes that metabolize TCAs, including the conversion of tertiary-amine tricyclics to secondary amines, may show large intersubject variability (greater than 30-fold). Antidepressant absorption from the gastrointestinal tract can be variable among patients and within the same patient over time. Absorption may be affected by antacids, sodium bicarbonate, and vitamin C, to name a few variables. Drug interations may seriously affect plasma levels of antidepressants. Antipsychotic medications often increase antidepressant levels, whereas smoking and drug abuse will often lower levels. Physicians sometimes forget that poor compliance is a major factor in drug nonresponse even in the most motivated patients. All of these factors explain why measurement of antidepressant level is indicated for patients taking these medications, especially for inpatients, many of whom have just started treatment.

A significant number of patients who do not respond to antidepressants do not respond because of the use of routine dosages of "drug insert" treatment regimens. Increased response rate is seen when dosages are individually determined by TCA plasma levels.

Despite these facts, why have clinicians been slow to employ such tests as a routine part of their management of TCA-treated patients? We have encountered a number of factors to explain this hesitancy. Some early research showed mixed results with regard to correlation of response to medication level. However, methodology has improved both in the area of technical laboratory performance of the tests and clinical research with regard to precise diagnosis and evaluation of response. The results of new research show a clearer correlation between TCA plasma levels and both antidepressant response and side effects.

In addition, many clinicians have delayed use of TCA plasma levels because of suggestions in the past that all nonresponders merely require higher doses. It was once said that no antidepressant trial was complete without a period on high or very high doses for nonresponders. However, this practice is both incorrect and potentially dangerous. This approach would result in some nonresponders achieving toxic levels on high dosages. Instead, no antidepressant trial is complete until the patient has achieved therapeutic TCA plasma levels for at least 3–4 weeks. One factor contributing to this change in focus was the discovery that some TCAs have a therapeutic window, so that TCA plasma levels both below and above a specific range are correlated with poorer response to treatment.

8. Plasma Levels of Tricyclic Antidepressants

The four TCAs that have the best-defined and -studied concentration : response relationships are nortriptyline, imipramine, amitriptyline, and desipramine. In addition, with tertiary-amine TCAs, the levels of active metabolites, both demethylated and hydroxylated, are potentially as important as plasma levels of the parent drug.

Until drug plasma monitoring became available, the standard parameter used in determining the necessary dosage of these agents was clinical response. A patient was started on a relatively standard dose of the chosen TCA for a period of time to assess response. If response was inadequate, the dose was increased until the patient developed an optimum response, at which time the dose was maintained. If the patient developed intolerable side effects, the dose was decreased.

This approach works well only under the following conditions: (1) there is a fairly standard starting dose; (2) there is a short time between starting the drug and assessing the response; (3) response is objective; (4) there is a linear relationship between increasing the dose and achieving optimum clinical response; and (5) the side effects being monitored are related to excessive drug concentrations. Unfortunately, none of these conditions holds true for TCAs. First, the starting dose is not standard because of the substantial interindividual differences in drug metabolism. Second, the time between starting the drug and clinical response is on the order of weeks, so that rapid titration to optimize response is not possible. Third, the response is not nearly as objective as measuring, for example, blood pressure. Fourth, there is evidence that increasing the dose does not necessarily enhance the response. Fifth, the side effects that most physicians use as guides for titrating dosage are not related to excessive concentration but to anticholinergic effect, which may actually occur at concentrations well below those that are clinically therapeutic.

9. Pharmacokinetics of Tricyclic Antidepressants

In clinical psychopharmacology, we do not typically measure drug concentration at the effector sites. That is because the effector site is presumably located within the brain, a tissue remote from routine sampling. Instead, the concentration is measured in a readily obtainable but peripheral sample, usually plasma. An implicit but testable assumption in this approach is that the concentration in the peripheral sample reflects the concentration at the effector sites.[6] The plasma drug concentration achieved by a given individual on a specific dose is dependent on four pharmacokinetic variables: absorption, distribution, metabolism, and elimination.[16]

9.1. Absorption

Drug absorption, also termed bioavailability, refers to the fraction of the administered dose that reaches the general circulation and the rate at which it does so. Bioavailability is dependent on the route of administration: enteral, inhalation, or parenteral. The enteral route includes oral and rectal administration. Parenteral routes include intravenous, intramuscular, and subcutaneous injections. In contrast to the oral route, intravenous administration obviates absorption problems. Once injected, the drug reaches high concentrations rapidly. However, the oral route is used most often because of its convenience.

Efficiency of the oral route (i.e., completeness and speed of absorption) is determined by multiple factors: the nature of the drug, disease, and environmental factors. The speed and completeness of drug absorption can influence pharmacodynamics because they determine the magnitude of change in concentration in plasma and at the effector site mediating the action of interest. For example, sedative and membrane-stabilizing effects of TCAs have been related to the rate and magnitude of change from trough to peak levels.[17,18]

Besides the physiochemical characteristics of the drugs, the rate and completeness of absorption can be influenced by disease and environmental factors. Age-related changes in gastric pH, intestinal surface area, and gastrointenstinal motility can have important effects on absorption in the elderly and usually result in decreased bioavailability. Malabsorption syndromes of various etiologies can do the same. Environmental factors such as concomitant ingestion of agents that inhibit absorption (e.g., mineral oil) or slow gastric emptying (e.g., anticholinergics) can also reduce bioavailability and pharmacokinetically alter pharmacodynamics.

Absorption of tricyclic antidepressants is usually complete. However, TCA plasma levels in patients given the same dose can vary up to 30-fold. Such variation is probably related to first-pass metabolism through the intestine and liver. Genetic factors control the activity of hepatic microsomal enzymes that metabolize tricyclics and account for much of the intersubject variability in TCA plasma levels produced by standard dosages. There is up to tenfold individual variation in the rate of metabolism of the antidepressants.[2] It is important to monitor TCA plasma levels and not just dosage and clinical effects in a therapeutic TCA trial, especially in patients with idiosyncratic or poor response and patients with altered hepatic, cardiac, or renal function. A number of factors can affect hepatic metabolism in addition to liver disease. Many elderly patients metabolize antidepressant more slowly and hence achieve therapeutic plasma levels at markedly lower doses, as low as 25 to 50 mg daily, than younger individuals. Pharmacological factors such as cigarette smoking and use of concomitant medications can alter antidepressant levels in clinically significant ways. For example, neuroleptics slow the rate of metabolism such that when combined with a neuroleptic, the TCA dose may need to be reduced as much as 50% to achieve the same TCA plasma level.[19]

9.2. Distribution

Following absorption into plasma, TCAs are rapidly distributed to peripheral tissues such as brain. Uptake into brain tissue lags only briefly behind the rise in drug plasma concentration, which may be relevant to the observation that peak drug plasma concentrations may correlate better with sedative effects than do trough concentrations. This observation also suggests that sedative effects have a different mechanism of action than do effects that correlate with trough levels such as antidepressant response. Moreover, this observation and the fact that sedation with these drugs occurs acutely suggest that this effect is a direct and rapidly reversible one, perhaps mediated by changes in receptor occupancy status.

Drug plasma levels are also affected by the extent of the distribution in the body.[20] Most psychotherapeutic drugs are not distributed homogeneously. They are concentrated in tissue compartments such as brain, heart, liver, and adipose tissue as opposed to bodily fluids because of their lipophilic and protein-binding characteristics.[16] However, the relative volume of distribution (V_d) can vary from one individual to another even for a specific drug. V_d refers to the apparent volume of fluid into which the drug distributes with a concentration equal to that in the plasma. For example, female and elderly patients compared to young males have an increased amount of adipose tissues relative to lean body mass.[21] Consequently, lipid-soluble drugs such as amitriptyline may have a greater V_d in such patients.

The size of V_d can have clinical implications. A drug with a large V_d leaches slowly out of the tissue compartment following drug discontinuation and hence has a long duration of action. TCAs, like most psychoactive drugs, have a large V_d and hence persist longer in the body following drug discontinuation than do more water-soluble agents.

9.3. Metabolism

Following distribution, TCAs are metabolized mainly by hepatic microsomal enzymes.[16] The rate of metabolism and, consequently, concentration are influenced by the activity of these enzymes. Genetically determined differences in activity can lead to the large interindividual variability in drug plasma concentration previously described.[22]

However, other factors can also play a role in governing this activity. With liver and renal disease, larger variability can occur as a result of decreased rates of biotransformation and excretion. Impaired hepatic activity can lead to increased concentrations of the parent drug (e.g., amitriptyline, diazepam), whereas decreased renal excretion may lead to higher concentrations of more polar metabolites.[23,24] There has also been evidence that advancing age results in an increase in drug concentrations. Figure 11-2 illustrates the mean and standard deviation for total TCA levels of amitriptyline plus its active metabolite, nortriptyline, for each 5 years of life. Below age 40, no relationship was observed between drug concentration and age. After 40, a linear relationship between increasing years and higher drug concentrations became apparent. After 60, patients developed approximately twice the drug concentrations of those under 40, a finding that validates the clinical practice of reducing doses of tricyclics in

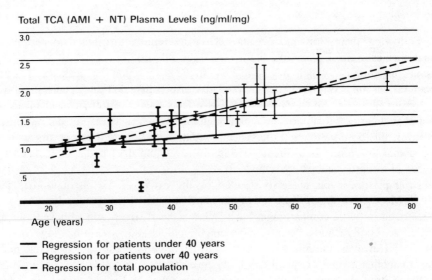

Total TCA (AMI + NT) Plasma Levels (ng/ml/mg)

Age (years)

—— Regression for patients under 40 years
—— Regression for patients over 40 years
– – Regression for total population

Figure 11-2. Age-related variability in total tricyclic (AMI and NT) levels for patients being treated with amitriptyline (AMI). NT, nortriptyline.

elderly patients. The use of TCA plasma concentrations, however, provides a more rational method for individual dose reduction than would a blanket halving of the dose for patients above 60 years of age. As is clearly seen in Fig. 11-2, there is still substantial variability in drug metabolism among the aged, with some achieving levels as low as some younger patients.

Interindividual variation may be pictured in a somewhat different way, as shown in Fig. 11-3. Figure 11-3 shows the percentage of patients on standard doses of amitriptyline with plasma levels of amitriptyline and its active metabolite, nortriptyline, for every 50-ng/ml interval starting with the interval 0 to 50 ng/ml. One can see that only approximately 30 to 50% of these patients fall within the optimally defined range of 150 to 250 ng/ml. This finding is especially interesting in that this percentage matches the response rates in early non-drug-concentration-adjusted clinical trials of amitriptyline.

One can also see in Fig. 11-3 the vast majority of patients who are not within optimum range have subtherapeutic concentrations, suggesting a generally conservative dosing approach. However, even with this conservative approach, around 5 to 7% of the patients developed concentrations in excess of 500 ng/ml, which puts them at risk both for failure to respond and for drug toxicity.

9.4. Concomitant Drug Administration

In clinical practice, situations frequently arise in which multiple-drug therapy is employed. If a patient on TCAs is started on an enzyme-stimulating drug such as a barbiturate, the TCA plasma level will decrease. Conversely, an enzyme-inhibiting drug will cause the TCA plasma level to increase. Examples of the latter include

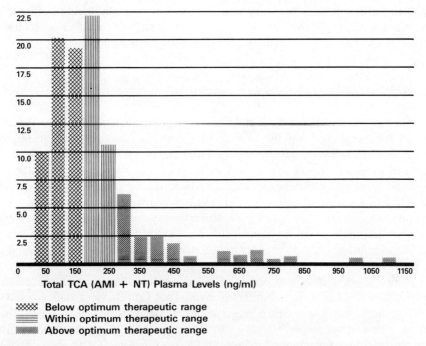

Figure 11-3. Percentage of patients (n = 330) achieving different steady-state plasma levels (ng/ml) of amitriptyline (AMI) and nortriptyline (NT) on routine doses of AMI. All patients were receiving AMI for treatment of depressive disorder, and in no case did the dose exceed 300 mg/day.

psychostimulants such as methylphenidate and most antipsychotic drugs.[25,26] The magnitude of such induction and inhibition can be clinically important. For example, standard doses of a neuroleptic drug can result in a 50–100% increase in the TCA plasma concentration.[27] Moreover, this effect can work both ways. If the neuroleptic drug is discontinued, a 50–100% fall in TCA plasma levels can occur following the loss in enzyme inhibition. Hence, the addition of a second drug may interact pharmacokinetically in addition to pharmacodynamically to determine response.

9.5. Elimination

Most psychotherapeutic drugs are metabolized from lipid-soluble substances to more polar compounds. Because of their more polar nature, they do not cross the blood–brain barrier as readily as do the parent drugs and hence may be less centrally active.

When a drug is ingested, it goes through all four phases: absorption, distribution, metabolism, and elimination. With regular, repeated ingestion, the concentration in the body rises until an equilibrium or steady-state condition occurs.[16] In this condition, the mean concentration remains constant from one interval to the next: the amount ingested equals the amount eliminated.

However, the brain adapts to the presence of drugs so that the number or functional state of the effector sites may change despite (or actually because of) a stable concentration of drug.[7] This latter phenomenon may be both time and concentration dependent and may alter the concentration : response relationship.

10. Major Affective Disorder in Children

A recently completed study of children aged 7 to 12 with DSM III major affective disorder has shown how the use of drug concentration measurements can improve clinical response and avoid adverse effects. These children were diagnosed at intake by structured diagnostic interviews as well as open clinical interviews. The structured diagnostic instrument used was the Diagnostic Interview for Children and Adolescents (DICA), which was developed at Washington University especially for use with children and adolescents. The severity of depressive symptomatology was measuring using: (1) a clinical global assessment, (2) a patient self-report scale, and (3) a researcher-administered test patterned after the Hamilton rating scale for depression but designed for use with children.

After a 2-week drug-free period of hospitalization during which the children received (1) individual, group, and family counseling, (2) behavioral therapy, and (3) school therapy, the severity of depressive symptomatology was reassessed. Those children who had not responded—the vast majority—were then treated with a fixed daily dose of 75 mg imipramine for 3 weeks. Plasma samples were drawn on days 10, 14, and 21 to determine the plasma concentration of imipramine and its demethylated and hydroxylated metabolites in each patient. At the end of the first 3-week trial, the clinician, unaware of the drug plasma monitoring results, was allowed to make one dosage adjustment based on clinical assessment only. The dose was then fixed, and treatment continued for an additional 3 weeks. Plasma samples for drug analysis were also obtained on days 10, 14, and 21 of this 3-week interval. At the end of this phase, response was again evaluated.

A sevenfold variation in the drug plasma concentrations was observed after 3 weeks on 75 mg imipramine. Approximately 60% of the response variance could be accounted for by the total TCA plasma concentration, with the principal determinant being the plasma concentration of the metabolite, desipramine (DMI) (Fig. 11-4). A linear concentration : response relationship was apparent up to a maximum of 225–250 ng/ml. However, a diminished response was observed in the few patients with levels above 250 ng/ml. Whether these patients were simply TCA nonresponders or whether this represents a curvilinear relationship with the drug having less efficacy at higher levels is not certain. What was found, however, was that if these high-level children had had their dose blindly adjusted downward at the end of the first 3-week study period, they clinically responded at the end of the second 3-week treatment period; whereas, those who were adjusted up failed to respond despite attaining even higher total TCA plasma concentrations.

Not surprisingly, after the first 3 weeks of drug therapy, drug dosage was advanced in most children who failed to respond. This approach mimics clinical practice and worked well in children who had low total TCA plasma concentrations. These children responded if their drug concentration was advanced to within a range of 115 to

Severity of depression (CDI residuals)

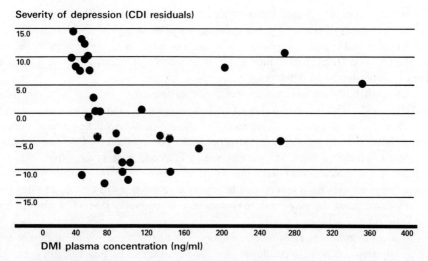

DMI plasma concentration (ng/ml)

Figure 11-4. Relationship between desipramine (DMI) plasma levels and antidepressant response in pre-pubertal depressed children being treated with imipramine (IMI). Although a relationship was observed between the total TCA (IMI and DMI) plasma level and antidepressant response, DMI, the active metabolite of IMI, was the principal determinant of that relationship.

250 ng/ml for imipramine plus DMI. There was a 90% remission rate at the end of 6 weeks of imipramine therapy for children with total TCA plasma concentrations within this range. In contrast, response rate was only 50% in children whose blood levels were either below or above this range.

11. How Is Concentration Quantitated?

Given the importance of concentration, the question then is how is it measured?

The most commonly used chemical assays include gas chromatography–mass spectrophotometry (GC–MS), gas chromatography (GC), and high-performance liquid chromatography (HPLC).[28] With these chromatographic techniques, parent drug and metabolites can be quantitated separately in the biological sample of interest. With optimum separation, attempts can be made to correlate the pharmacodynamic data with each of these concentrations separately.

This approach permits researchers to determine whether the parent drug and metabolites contribute equally to response or whether they have different potencies. In some instances, the concentration of parent drug may account for none of the response variance, suggesting that it is no more than a prodrug for the production of active metabolites.[29]

The first chromatographic technique used to measure plasma concentrations of TCAs was thin-layer chromatography (TLC).[30] This approach has now generally been replaced by GC or HPLC techniques because of inadequate sensitivity.[28] GC–MS is perhaps the single best technique for quantitating TCAs from the perspective of both sensitivity and specificity. Unfortunately, it is expensive and time consuming. Hence, it is mainly used to validate other methods. Both GC and HPLC are reasonably equivalent in terms of sensitivity and specificity and are adequate and reproducible for most research and clinical purposes. There are a number of different approaches with both the GC and HPLC techniques in terms of sample preparation, solvent systems, separation columns, and detectors.[31]

Although both sensitivity and specificity of these GC and HPLC methods are generally good, there is a possibility of cochromatography. This issue is important for research and clinical practice since many of the psychoactive drugs administered to patients have similar physiochemical properties. For example, TCAs are structural analogues of phenothiazines. If a patient is on a TCA and another drug that cochromatographs (e.g., thioridazine) with the TCA of interest and this problem goes undetected, erroneously high levels may be reported. Such a result can lead to improper dose adjustment, or the physician may conclude erroneously that TCA plasma level assays are not useful.

Radioimmunoassay, radioreceptor assay, and enzymatic assay are different techniques but share general advantages and disadvantages. In general, they are like biological assays in that they do not separately quantify parent drug and metabolites. In contrast to chemical assays, these approaches are less labor intensive, more reproducible, and have greater sensitivity. The radioimmunoassay requires an antibody that will react with the drug of interest.[32] This antibody may be sufficiently specific that it will only react with a single structure. Unfortunately, RIA usually shows variable cross-reactivity with active and inert metabolites and even with other structurally related compounds (e.g., phenothiazines). This can lead to erroneously high and clinically irrelevant levels.

12. Antidepressant Therapy

The physician may begin treatment with any TCA, since no clinical differences in response to various TCAs have been demonstrated conclusively. In general, in the absence of a positive personal or family history of past response to a specific TCA, we prefer to begin therapy with nortriptyline or desipramine and to monitor the plasma level closely to insure a trial at a therapeutic level for 21 days or longer after steady state is achieved. Under certain conditions (e.g., hospitalization), it may be advisable to begin therapy with a single "dose-prediction test."

The TCA dose-prediction test has been employed to ascertain in advance whether a patient is a rapid or slow metabolizer. With this information, the psychiatrist can determine the approximate dosage needed to achieve therapeutic levels.[33] This test consists of measurement of plasma level 24 hr after oral administration of a test dose of 50 or 100 mg of a specific TCA. A nomograms relating levels at 24 hr to anticipated daily dosages is needed.

One other practical application of pharmacokinetics is that the long half-lives (about 24 hr) of TCAs support the practice of giving medication in one dose at bedtime. This practice tends to minimize the impact of side effects, which peak, along with TCA plasma levels, 1 to 3 hr after oral administration. As almost all TCAs are sedating to some degree, single bedtime dosages concentrate the sedative effects when they are needed: at bedtime. Monoamine oxidase inhibitors are stimulating; therefore, they should be given in divided doses in the morning and early afternoon.

Therapeutic plasma level monitoring is useful in helping to define an adequate TCA trial (Table 11-5). In light of the high proportion of treated depressed patients who have inadequate pharmacological treatment,[34] criteria for adequacy are important. An adequate TCA trial consists of maintaining the patient at dosage adequate to achieve therapeutic TCA plasma levels for a minimum of 21 days with documented compliance.

If such monitoring is not available, begin therapy at a fairly low dosage and gradually increase it over a number of days to a therapeutically effective dose as defined in Table 11-6. Plasma levels of antidepressant should also be used as a check of compliance, since many patients do not take medication reliably. Medication given in an amount sufficient to maintain therapeutic plasma levels should, if effective, produce within 10 days some improvement in sleep, appetite, and even mood. However, the full effect does not appear until the end of the third week or occasionally even later. For an adequate trial, a minimum treatment duration of 21 days at a consistent therapeutic plasma antidepressant level is necessary. If improvement at this time is negligible or minimal, a change to another antidepressant is recommended.

Normally, once a clinical response is documented, antidepressant medication is continued for at least 6 months. During this time, the dosage may be altered as necessary to keep the plasma level in the therapeutic range. Plasma levels are usually monitored on an at least monthly basis or at any time that depressive signs and symptoms reemerge. The TCA may be given prophylactically following treatment of a recurrent depression. Unfortunately, the studies have not been conducted to determine whether the optimum concentration range for maintenance therapy is the same as or less than that needed for acute response.

13. Sources of Error

To derive the most benefit from the measurement of TCA plasma levels, their limitations and the sources of error must be recognized. A common one is inappropriate sampling time with regard to steady-state conditions and relative to dose interval. Most of the concentration : response data with TCAs are based on steady-state samples drawn 10–12 hr after the last dose.[35] Under steady-state conditions, an equilibrium

Table 11-5. Adequacy of a Tricyclic
Antidepressant Trial[a]

1. Dosage
2. Plasma levels
3. Duration
4. Compliance

[a]Minimal trial: 21 days at therapeutic plasma levels.

Table 11-6. Comparison of Antidepressants for Clinical Use[a]

Drug	Initial dose (mg)	Therapeutic plasma level (ng/ml)	Average daily maintenance dose (mg)
Imipramine (Tofranil®, Janimine®, SK-Pramine®)	100–300	With desipramine[b] >180	75–150
Amitriptyline (Elavil®, Endep®)	150–300	With nortriptyline[b] >120	75–150
Desipramine (Norpramine®, Pertofrane®)	100–300	>125	75–100
Nortriptyline (Pamelor®)	50–150	50–140	50–100
Doxepin (Adapin®, Sinequan®)	200–400	With desmethyldoxepin[b] >110	150–250
Protriptyline (Vivactil®)	30–60	90–170	20–40
Maprotiline (Ludiomil®)	75–150	n.a.[c]	75–125
Amoxapine (Asendin®)	200–1400	n.a.[c]	200–300
		n.a.[c]	
Trazodone (Desyrel®)	50–600	n.a.[c]	100–300

[a]In average adults (middle-aged, 150 to 200 lb, taking no other medication).
[b]Major active metabolite must be measured along with original tricyclic.
[c]n.a., not adequately studied.

exists between amount ingested and amount excreted per dosing interval and between various compartments such that concentration in the remote sample should reflect concentration at the effector site.[6] The attainment of steady-state conditions requires a stable dose regimen for a minimum of five times the drug half-life.[16] For most TCAs, 7 days on a stable dose is required to reach steady-state conditions. Samples should be drawn 10–12 hr after the last dose to insure being in the elimination phase rather than during absorption or distribution, since such samples tend to be more reproducible within a given patient. If samples are drawn at other times, both erratic and erroneous results may occur.

Another common source of error involves sample handling. Procedures as apparently innocuous as the use of certain types of vacuum tubes to obtain the sample can make a difference.[36–38] Most assays involve sample preparation in which percentage recovery of the drug and metabolites becomes critical. It must also be remembered that whole blood has several components: (1) plasma water, (2) plasma proteins, and (3) red blood cells (RBCs). The latter is a tissue compartment and has a higher TCA concentration than either plasma proteins or plasma water.[6,39,40] If the sample is hemolyzed prior to separation, RBC fragments containing drug may remain in the plasma sample. More than likely, drug on these fragments will be extracted with the plasma, yielding erratic and erroneously high values.

These examples of assay problems indicate that as laboratory tests become more useful, the psychiatrist will have to become more knowledgeable about potential sources of error. Moreover, these problems may be important factors in evaluating concentration : response studies because such errors can obscure such relationships (i.e., the type II error).

Noncompliance can occur with either inpatients or outpatients, although it is more of an issue in the latter case.[41] Although noncompliance often is associated with low concentration, it may also cause erroneous, high values. The latter results when the patient takes the drug shortly before returning for response evaluation and blood drawing. Approaches to detect noncompliance include (1) pill counts, (2) frequent intermittent blood sampling to look for excessive variance, and (3) use of single-dose prediction of steady-state.[42] In the latter case, the patient is given a single dose under observation, a sample is then obtained after a specified interval (e.g., 24 hr). The dose prediction test value obtained at this time can be used to predict the steady-state level that should occur on the fixed dose.[23,42] The values obtained under presumed steady-state conditions can then be compared to the predicted value as well as to each other.

14. Antiepileptic Medications

Neurologists have found antiepileptic drug monitoring helpful in determining patient compliance, preventing dose-related toxic effects, prescribing individual therapy, and achieving a "therapeutic range" of plasma drug levels for individual patients. The therapeutic range is a statistical concept representing the range of plasma drug concentrations that gives optimum clinical control without adverse effects in the majority of patients. Patients whose seizures are well controlled in spite of subtherapeutic plasma drug concentrations should not have their dosage increased: drug plasma monitoring is to aid treatment and is not a treatment endpoint. An unfortunate development with technical advancements in medicine is the tendency to treat the laboratory test result rather than the patient. In some patients, toxic effects may occur at low or even subtherapeutic drug concentrations because of individual differences in susceptibility to adverse effects. Table 11-7 gives the therapeutic ranges of the major and the minor antiepileptic drugs.

Table 11-7. Therapeutic Plasma Concentrations of the Antiepileptic Drugs

Nonproprietary name	U.S. trade name	Normal range (μg/ml)
Phenytoin	Dilantin	9–21
Phenobarbital	Luminal	20–50
Primidone	Mysoline	4–14
Ethosuximide	Zarontin	45–90
Carbamazepine	Tegretol	2–10
Clonazepam	Clonopin	0.04–0.1
Valproic acid	Depakene	40–100
Diazepam	Valium	0.2–0.5
Nitrazepam	Mogadon	0.04–0.09
Mephenytoin (measured as N-desmethylmephenytoin)	Mesantoin	12–25
Methsuximide (measured as N-desmethylmethsuximide)	Celontin	12–25
Mephobarbital (measured as phenobarbital)	Mebaral	20–50
Chlorazepate (measured as desmethyldiazepam)	Traxene	0.6–1.5
Trimethadione	Tridione	20–40
Dimethadione	Paradione	700–1400

Therapeutic plasma concentrations have been defined for most antiepileptic drugs, so that seizure control can be achieved with little risk or toxicity. The effective plasma level may vary from patient to patient because the severity of seizures may be different, which may explain why seizures in some patients are well controlled at subtherapeutic plasma drug levels.[43] The usefulness of antiepileptic drug monitoring in achieving optimum seizure control has been supported by many clinical studies.[44−49] We assume that these levels are useful in monitoring and titrating dose when these medications are used in psychiatry. It is important, however, that laboratories offering determinations of antiepileptic drugs participate in a quality control program to establish interlaboratory reproducibility[50] and report the method used to determine the blood level.

15. Lithium

When Cade first effectively treated mania with lithium, he stated "the original therapeutic dose decided on fortuitously proved to be the optimum." Once the patient responded, 2 months of further hospitalization was needed, in part because of "the necessity of determining a satisfactory maintenance dose."[51] This determination was achieved by trial and error, and it was not until many years later that blood level monitoring became a useful means of facilitating such dosage adjustment.

Although the toxicity of lithium had been recognized by the turn of the century, little heed was paid to appropriate monitoring when lithium chloride was used as a salt substitute in the late 1940s. Serious intoxications and deaths resulted.[52]

Although lithium concentrations were measured in both serum and urine in the early 1950s, a well-defined relationship between such levels and therapeutic effects, side effects, and toxicity could not be established.[53] Talbott[54] studied the use of lithium chloride as a salt substitute and concluded that adverse reactions occurred only in association with serum lithium levels greater than 1.0 mEq/liter (mM), although he also noted the absence of untoward effects in some patients with levels as high as 2.9 mEq/liter.

In 1959, Schou[55] advised that the serum lithium level be kept below 2.0 mEq/liter to prevent intoxication but otherwise suggested that maintenance dose be established by achieving a clinical balance between therapeutic and side effects. This approach was not unique, having its internal medicine counterpart in digitalis, another drug with a narrow therapeutic margin, whose effective use was and still is governed largely by clinical judgment.

Currently recommended therapeutic ranges vary depending on the information source but are generally similar. The package inserts used in the United States currently give 1.0–1.5 mEq/liter as an effective serum lithium level for acute mania and 0.6 to 1.2 mEq/liter as a desirable serum level for long-term control.

16. Methods for Lithium Measurement

Fortunately, the use of lithium blood levels in psychiatry has led to the development of inexpensive, commercially available, sensitive, and reliable techniques for quantitatively measuring lithium in the body.[56] Although qualitative spectroscopic techniques were available in the mid-1800s, the development and application of flame emission photometry and atomic absorption spectrophotometry in the last 30 years has made serum lithium determinations a routine clinical laboratory procedure.

17. Present Use of Antidepressant Drug Monitoring

The features that make plasma AD level monitoring helpful are summarized in Table 11-8. How often is plasma monitoring of TCA used in clinical practice? In the Kansas City area, about 45% of psychiatrists use plasma drug monitoring to adjust dosage, whereas only about 5% of internists or family physicians do.[57] Thus, most physicians treating patients with TCAs are not availing themselves of such tests to adjust drug dosage and should be educated about their value in making rational dosage decisions.

Physicians should also be educated in terms of how the test should be performed. Blood should be drawn when the patient is at steady state and at a postabsorptive, postdistributive time, which typically is 10 to 12 hr after the last dose. Physicians must also be aware of laboratory errors that can occur, such as (1) cochromatography of concomitantly administered drugs, particularly phenothiazine antipsychotics, (2) col-

Table 11-8. Features That Make Drug Plasma Monitoring Helpful

1. Well-defined relationship between concentration and beneficial response.
2. Well-defined relationship between concentration and toxicity.
3. A narrow range between beneficial and toxic concentration. Best example in psychiatry is lithium carbonate. For TCAs such as amitriptyline, beneficial response requires total AMI + NT levels in the 100–250 ng/ml range. Mild to moderate CNS toxicity is observed when the total AMI + NT levels exceed 500 ng/ml. Toxicity is routinely seen when levels exceed 1000 ng/ml. These figures mean that the therapeutic index is 2–4, whereas interindividual variability in metabolism is between 10- and 30-fold. The relationship between concentration and toxic effects under steady-state conditions (i.e., not overdose cases) has not been as well studied for TCAs other than AMI. However, the therapeutic index based on concentration is probably similar for all the tertiary-amine TCAs (i.e., doxepin, imipramine, and trimipramine) and somewhat broader for secondary-amine TCAs (e.g., nortriptyline, desipramine).
4. Sufficient interindividual variability in metabolism so that routine doses will produce subtherapeutic concentration in some patients, toxic concentrations in others, and therapeutic concentration in the remainder.
5. A sufficiently long delay in onset of beneficial response (e.g., antidepressant response) so that rapid titration based on clinical assessment of such response is not feasible.
6. A beneficial response (e.g., antidepressant response) that is clinically difficult to quantitate, so there is the possibility of substantial error in such assessment.
7. Toxic effects that are clinically difficult to detect or distinguish from worsening of the condition being treated (e.g., the distinction between TCA-induced confusional state and the confusional state observed in severe major depressive disorders).
8. The above conditions exist for TCAs such that clinical dose adjustment without the benefit of drug plasma monitoring can lead to prolonged illness in patients who develop suboptimum drug concentrations on routine doses and avoidable iatrogenic toxicity ranging from mild to potentially serious effects in patients who are slow metabolizers.

lection systems that influence plasma levels, and (3) specimens in which hemolysis has occurred.

In addition to the monitoring of steady-state TCA plasma concentrations, there is evidence that the use of single-dose predictions may permit rapid dosage adjustments to optimize drug concentration and accelerate clinical response. Data from one study[58] indicated that clinical response to amitriptyline was hastened in patients whose dosage was adjusted on the basis of single-dose predictions compared to those who were treated in the conventional way. If further research confirms the utility of this approach, it will assume even greater importance given the current pressures to reduce the length of hospitalizations.

18. Summary

Plasma drug monitoring of TCAs permits physicians to rationally adjust the dosage of drugs for which concentration : response relationships have been well characterized. Such monitoring of these medications can improve overall response rates, reduce the risk of drug toxicity, and perhaps also hasten clinical response by permitting more rapid dosage adjustments. This approach can also document noncompliance, which is a leading cause of both nonresponse and relapse.

References

1. Glassman AH, Perel JM: Tricyclic blood levels and clinical outcome: A review of the art, in Lipton MA, DiMascio A, Killiam KF (eds): *Psychopharmacology: A Generation of Progress*. New York, Raven Press, 1978, pp 917–922.
2. Amsterdam J, Brunswick D, Mendels J: The clinical application of tricyclic antidepressant pharmacokinetics and plasma levels. *Am J Psychiatry* 137:653–662, 1980.
3. Risch SC, Huey LY, Janowsky DS: Plasma levels of tricyclic antidepressants and clinical efficacy: Review of the literature—part II. *J Clin Psychiatry* 40:58–69, 1979.
4. Preskorn SH, Irwin H: Toxicity of tricyclic antidepressants—kinetics, mechanism, intervention: A review. *J Clin Psychiatry* 43(4):151–156, 1982.
5. Preskorn SH: Factors affecting the biphasic concentration : effect relationship of tricyclic antidepressants, in Dahl S, Gram L, Lingjaerde V, et al (eds): *Clinical Pharmacology in Psychiatry*. New York, Macmillan, 1981, pp 297–306.
6. Glotzbach R, Preskorn SH: Brain concentrations of tricyclic antidepressants: Single dose kinetics and relationship to plasma concentrations in chronically dosed rats. *Psychopharmacology* 78:25–27, 1982.
7. Creese, I, Sibley DR: Receptor adaptations to centrally acting drugs. *Annu Rev Pharmacol Toxicol* 21:357–359, 1981.
8. Preskorn SH, Kent T: Mechanisms and interventions in tricyclic antidepressant overdoses, in Stancer HC, Garfinkel P (eds): *International Symposium on Guidelines for the Use of Psychotropic Drugs*. Toronto, University of Toronto Press, 1984, pp 63–75.
9. Velasquez MT, Rho J, Maronde R, et al: Plasma clonidine levels in hypertension. *Clin Pharmacol Ther* 32:341–346, 1982.
10. Davidson J: MAO inhibitions: A clinical perspective, in Ayd F, Taylor I, Bruce T (eds): *Affective Disorders Reassessed*. Baltimore, Waverly Press, 1983, pp 41–55.
11. Klein DF, Gittelman R, Quitkin F, et al: *Diagnosis and Drug Treatment of Psychiatric Disorders*. Baltimore, Williams & Wilkins, 1980.
12. Baldessarini RJ: *Chemotherapy in Psychiatry*. Cambridge, Harvard University Press, 1977, p 1975.
13. Bigger JT, Giardina EGV, Perel JM, et al: Cardiac antiarrhythmic effect of imipramine hydrochloride. *N Engl J Med* 296:206, 1977.

14. Extein I, Gold MS, Pottash ALC: Psychopharmacologic treatment of depression. *Psychiatr Clin North Am* 7(3):503–517, 1984.
15. Raisman R, Sette M, Pimoule C, et al: High-affinity (^{3}H)DMI binding in the peripheral and central nervous system: A specific site associated with the neuronal uptake of noradrenaline. *Eur J Pharmacol* 78:345–351, 1982.
16. Friedel R: Pharmacokinetics in the geropsychiatric patient, in Lipton MA, DiMascio A, Killiam KF (eds): *Psychopharmacology: A Generation of Progress*. New York, Raven Press, 1978, pp 1499–1505.
17. Bianchetti G, Bonaccorsi A, Chiodawli A: Plasma concentrations and cardiotoxic effects of desipramine and protriptyline in the rat. *Br J Pharmacol* 60:11–19, 1977.
18. Elonen EL: Correlation of the cardiotoxicity of tricyclic antidepressants to their membrane effects. *Med Biol* 52:415–423, 1974.
19. Nelson JC, Jatlow PI: Neuroleptic effect on desipramine steady-state plasma concentrations. *Am J Psychiatry* 137:1232, 1980.
20. Sheiner LB, Tozer TN: The use of plasma concentrations of drugs, in Melmon KL, Morrelli HF (eds): *Clinical Pharmacology*. New York, Macmillan, 1978, pp 80–81.
21. Novak LP: Aging, total body potassium, fat-free mass, and cell mass in males and females between age 18 and 85 years. *J Gerontol* 27:438–443, 1972.
22. Alexanderson B: Prediction of steady state plasma levels of notriptyline from single oral dose kinetics: A study in twins. *Eur J Clin Pharmacol* 6:44–53, 1973.
23. Klotz U, Araut GR, Hoyumpa A, et al: The effects of age and liver disease on the disposition of diazepam in adult men. *J Clin Invest* 55:347–359, 1975.
24. Lieberman J, Cooper TB, Suckow RF, et al: Tricyclic antidepressant metabolite levels in depressed hemodialysis patients. *Clin Pharmacol Ther* 34:257, 1984.
25. Gram LF, Overo KF: Drug interaction: Inhibitory effect of neuroleptics on metabolism of tricyclic antidepressants in man. *Br Med J* 1:463–465, 1972.
26. Wharton RN, Perel JM, Dayton PA, et al: A potential clinical use of methylphenidate with tricyclic antidepressants. *Am J Psychiatry* 127:1619–1625, 1971.
27. Hirschowitz J, Bennett J, Zemlan F, et al: Thioridazine effect on desipramine plasma levels. *J Clin Psychopharmacol.* 4:376–378, 1984.
28. Vandermark GL, Adams RF, Schmidt GJ: Liquid chromatographic procedure for tricyclic drugs and their metabolites in plasma. *Clin Chem* 24:87–90, 1978.
29. Preskorn SH, Weller EB, Weller RA: Depression in children: Relationship between plasma imipramine levels and response. *J Clin Psychiatry* 43:450–453, 1982.
30. Nacy A, Treiber L: Quantitative determination of imipramine and desipramine in human blood plasma by direct densitometry of thin-layer chromatograms. *J Pharmacol* 25:599, 1973.
31. DeVane CL: Tricyclic antidepressants, in Evans WE, Schertag JJ, Jusko WJ (eds): *Applied Pharmacokinetics*. San Francisco, Applied Therapeutics, 1980, pp 574–576.
32. Maguire KP, Burrows GD, Normal TR, et al: A radioimmunoassay for nortriptyline (and other tricyclic antidepressants) in plasma. *Clin Chem* 24(4):549–554, 1978.
33. Cooper TB, Simpson GM: Prediction of individual dosage of nortriptyline. *Am J Psychiatry* 135:333–335, 1978.
34. Keller MB, Klevman GL, Lavori PW, et al: Treatment received by depressed patients. *JAMA* 248:1848–1855, 1982.
35. Risch SC, Huey LY, Janowsky DS: Plasma levels of tricyclic antidepressants and clinical efficacy: Review of the literature—part I. *J Clin Psychiatry* 40:6–21, 1979.
36. Brunswick DJ, Mendels J: Reduced levels of tricyclic antidepressants in plasma from vacutainers. *Commun Psychopharmacol* 1:131–134, 1977.
37. Cochran E, Carl J, Hanin I, et al: Effect of vacutainer stoppers on plasma tricyclic levels: A re-evaluation. *Commun Psychopharmacol* 2:495–503, 1978.
38. Veith RC, Raisys VA, Perera C: The clinical impact of blood collection methods of tricyclic antidepressants as measured by GC/MS-SIM. *Commun Psychopharmacol* 2:491–494, 1978.
39. Hammer W, Idelstrom CM, Sjoqvist F: Chemical control of antidepressant drug therapy, in Garattini S, Dukes NMG (eds): *Proceedings of the First International Symposium on Antidepressant Drug Therapy*. Amsterdam, Exerpta Medica, 1967, pp 301–310.

40. Linnoila M, Dorrity F, Jabson K: Plasma and erythrocyte levels of tricyclic antidepressants in depressed patients. *Am J Psychiatry* 133:5, 1978.
41. Ayd FJ: Once-a-day neuroleptic and tricyclic antidepressant therapy. *Int Drug Ther Newslett* 7:33–40, 1972.
42. Madakasira S, Preskorn SH, Weller R, et al: Single dose prediction of steady state plasma levels of amitriptyline. *J Clin Psychopharmacol* 2:136–139, 1982.
43. Feldman RG, Pippenger CE: The relation of anticonvulsant drug levels to complete seizure control. *J Clin Pharmacol* 16:51–59, 1976.
44. Kutt H, Penry JK: Usefulness of blood levels of antiepileptic drugs. *Arch Neurol* 31:283–288, 1974.
45. Lascelles PT, Kocen RS, Reynolds EH: The distribution of plasma phenytoin levels in epileptic patients. *J Neurol Neurosurg Psychiatry* 33:501–505, 1970.
46. Kutt H: Diphenylhydantoin. Relation of plasma concentration to seizure control, in Woodbury DM, Penry JK, Pippenger CE (eds): *Antiepileptic Drugs, ed 2. New York, Raven Press, 1982, pp 241–246.*
47. *Sherwin AL: Ethosuximide: Relation of plasma concentration to seizure control, in Woodbury DM, Penry JK, Pippenger CE (eds): Antiepileptic Drugs,* ed 2. New York, Raven Press, 1982, pp 637–646.
48. Cereghino JJ: Serum carbamazepine concentration and clinical control. *Adv Neurol* 11:309–330, 1975.
49. Eadie MJ: Plasma level monitoring of anticonvulsants. *Clin Pharmacokinet* 1:52–66, 1976.
50. Pippinger CE, Penry JK, White BG, et al: Interlaboratory variability in determination of plasma antiepileptic drug concentrations. *Arch Neurol* 33:351–355, 1976.
51. Cade JFJ: The story of lithium, in Ayd FJ, Blackwell B (eds): *Discoveries in Biological Psychiatry.* Philadelphia, JB Lippincott, 1978, pp 218–229.
52. Corcoran AC, Taylor RD, Page IH: Lithium poisoning from the use of salt substitutes. *JAMA* 139:685–688, 1949.
53. Amdisen A: Monitoring of lithium treatment through determination of lithium concentration. *Dan Med Bull* 22:277–291, 1975.
54. Talbott JH: Use of lithium salts as a substitute for sodium chloride. *Arch Intern Med* 85:1–10, 1950.
55. Schou M: Lithium in psychiatric therapy: Stock-taking after ten years. *Psychopharmacologia* 1:65–78, 1959.
56. Coombs HI, Coombs RRH, Mee UG: Methods of serum lithium estimation, in Johnson FN (ed): *Lithium Research and Therapy.* New York, Academic Press, 1975, pp 165–179.
57. Cono SV, Generaly JA, Letendre D, et al: Evaluation of amitriptyline use by internists and psychiatrists. *Hosp Forum* 19:1131–1155, 1984.
58. Madakasira S, Khazanie P: Reliability of amitriptyline dose prediction based on single-dose plasma levels. *Clin Pharmacol Ther* 37:145–149, 1985.
59. Richelson E: Pharmacology of the antidepressants in use in the United States *J Clin Psychiatry* 43:4, 1982.

Drug Abuse:
Interpretation of Laboratory Tests

Karl Verebey, Ph.D., David Martin, and Mark S. Gold, M.D.

1. Introduction

Knowledge of drug use or abuse by patients in psychiatric or drug abuse treatment is important to the attending physician. Depending on the specific drug used, symptoms of psychiatric illness may be mimicked by either the drug's presence or absence. This dichotomy of symptoms associated with drug presence or drug absence is best illustrated by the opioids. To the trained eye, it is obvious when the patient is under the influence of an opiate. Examination will demonstrate pupillary miosis, euphoric anxiolytic sedation, mental clouding, sweating, and constipation. Subjects dependent on opiates in the absence of the drug demonstrate various degrees of signs of withdrawal such as pupillary mydriasis, agitation, anxiety, panic, muscle aches, gooseflesh, and often diarrhea.

It is not unusual to find that behavior similar to a textbook description of psychosis identified as paranoid schizophrenia can be triggered in predisposed individuals by such drugs as phencyclidine (PCP), amphetamine,[1] or cannabis.[2] Drug-induced "model" psychosis can apparently be produced in anyone given the adequate dose by LSD, PCP, amphetamine, and cocaine.[3] Drug-induced psychoses have a different prognosis and must be treated differently than psychosis related to endogenous anatomic or neurochemical aberrations. Also, the treatment of drug abusers is extremely handicapped if drug abuse monitoring is not provided or not accurate. Therefore, comprehensive drug testing to distinguish the presence and/or absence of drugs, previously the province of the postmortem analysis, is now important for psychiatrists in making the precise evaluation and appropriate treatment of any patient.[4] For these and

Karl Verebey, Ph.D. • Department of Clinical Pharmacology, New York State Division of Substance Abuse Services, and Department of Psychiatry, SUNY Downstate Medical School, Brooklyn, New York 11217.   *David Martin* • Psychiatric Diagnostic Laboratories of America, Inc., Summit, New Jersey 07901.   *Mark S. Gold, M.D.* • Research Facilities, Fair Oaks Hospital, Summit, New Jersey 07901, and Fair Oaks Hospital at Boca/Delray, Delray Beach, Florida 33445.

other reasons,[5] psychiatrists have been interested in becoming more aware of laboratory testing of body fluids for drugs of abuse.

2. Drugs of Abuse

Illicit drug use should be in the differential diagnosis of almost every patient presenting to the psychiatrist. Although most physicians agree with this concept, few take a complete history from patient and family followed by comprehensive laboratory testing for drugs of abuse using a methodology sensitive to the low-dose use and abuse of illicit drugs.

Reported adverse psychiatric reactions to marijuana and THC include panic attacks and anxiety reactions usually lasting less than 24 hr,[6-8] depression severe enough to require psychiatric hospitalization,[8] and acute toxic psychoses with or without clouding of consciousness that clear within a few weeks.[8-10] Many of these reactions have a marked manic or schizoaffective manic quality.[8,10] The "marijuanaholic" diagnosis is made by observing behavioral change and Δ^9-THC levels in blood and/or urine.[11]

Chronic opiate administration is associated with high rates of major and minor depressions.[12-15] Three weeks after opiate detoxification,[15] there is 32% prevalence of RDC major depression and 10% minor depression. During opiate withdrawal, we have noted transient depressed moods, manic behavior, and, very rarely, emergence of a schizophreniform psychosis that cleared when opiates were again administered. Behavioral outbursts when they occur are carefully examined as possible signs of undetected withdrawal from another drug of abuse or alcohol.[16]

The acute effects of amphetamines are dose dependent and can range from increased alertness with decreased fatigue and need for sleep to severe anxiety and panic to euphoria and hypomanic behavior to acute psychoses that are limited to the presence of amphetamine in the body and can be indistinguishable from DSM III bipolar disorder—manic phase. Schizophrenic misdiagnosis and mistreatment are common.[7,17,18] There is also a characteristic "crash" or "discontinuation syndrome" characterized by hypersomic, psychomotoric retarded major depression.

As cocaine's abuse has skyrocketed, especially in middle- and upper-middle-class populations,[3] more attention is being paid to its acute toxic psychiatric effects, which often present as psychosis, mania, or extreme paranoia undistinguishable from classical DSM III psychiatric disorders.[10-21]

Phencyclidine (PCP) can cause an acute psychosis of several days' duration that clears rapidly. Yago *et al.*[1] have found a high prevalence of misdiagnosed PCP-induced manias, schizophrenias, and other "psychiatric disorders."

When psychiatric symptoms occur in association with LSD use, they may include a severe panic and anxiety reaction. Chronic psychoses of medium and prolonged term also are seen and can be indistinguishable from schizophrenia.[7] LSD abuse has also been associated with bipolar manic disorders, schizoaffective disorders, major depressions,[22,23] and successful suicide.[22,24] "Flashbacks" may also occur weeks to months after the last injection of LSD in which all the symptoms of an LSD trip may reoccur at unpredictable times.[25,26]

The best-studied group of volatile inhalers are persons who are exposed to these substances occupationally such as painters, refinery workers, and persons who work with or fuel airplanes. Less well studied are children and adolescents who intentionally abuse glue, toluene, gasoline, cleaning fluid (trichloroethane), and nitrous oxide in order to experience euphorigenic effects. Immediate effects include euphoria, hallucination in 50% of cases, and disordered behavior,[27] personality changes, irritability, anxiety, panic disorder symptoms, somatic complaints, fatigue, depression, and organic brain syndromes.[28,29]

3. Alcohol

Alcohol is rapidly absorbed from the GI tract, metabolized by the liver, and excreted unchanged in breath, urine, and sweat in small amounts. It can be given as an intravenous solution as well.[7,30] Blood levels of alcohol are useful at the time of an evaluation since they correlate with degree of acute intoxication.[30]

Alcohol idiosyncratic intoxication is a syndrome of extreme reactions to small amounts of alcohol and can include aggressive assaultive and destructive behavior. Partial complex seizures and concomitant barbiturate, sedative–hypnotic, or stimulant abuse must be ruled out. Unfortunately, rather than alcoholism being identified early in its course, it is usually identified prior to absolute dissolution of the family, loss of career, or severe alcohol-related physical disorder or substance-induced organic mental disorder. Alcohol withdrawal states occur after days to weeks of heavy alcohol ingestion. They may range from mild symptoms such as nausea and diarrhea, irritability, headaches, and mental sluggishness to delirium tremens. Delirium tremens is a life-threatening medical emergency occurring 2–4 days after the end of alcohol ingestion. It is characterized by delirium, hallucinations, agitation, tremens, tachycardia, and elevated blood pressure. Alcohol hallucinosis, auditory hallucinations in the presence of clear consciousness, often occurs during a period of decreased or no alcohol consumption. These states can be confused with anxiety disorders, mania, schizophrenia, and other forms of psychosis. Other substance(s), medical diseases, and vitamin and nutritional deficiencies must be identified and treated.

4. Polydrug Abuse

Drug-abusing individuals generally use more than one substance. Differential diagnosis of polydrug intoxication/withdrawal is difficult, as the patients' symptoms can range from those of alcohol intoxication to those of hallucinogens to naturally occurring psychiatric diseases. Diagnosis is only possible with sensitive antibody- or computer-assisted GC–MS comprehensive drug testing.

The great danger of polydrug abuse is that there will be a synergistic effect between drugs to produce a severe toxic, even lethal, result when two or more drugs are used together, whereas any one used alone would not have any significant effect.[30]

Irritability and attacks of anger,[31,32] depressed mood, and decreased social interaction may be seen in patients taking benzodiazepines or drinking. More severe and prolonged psychiatric reactions occur during the withdrawal phase of alcohol or sedative–hypnotic use. A syndrome indistinguishable from the delirium tremens (DTs) or schizophrenia can develop, with auditory and visual hallucinations, confusion, and even seizures, during withdrawal from any sedative–hypnotic including the barbiturates.[33,34] Gluthethimide (Doriden®) and ETH chlorvynal (Placydil®) are particularly notorious for the development of similar reactions.[16,35,36] To uncover a psychiatric disorder caused by or precipitated by a prescribed medication, illicit medication, or poison, the psychiatrist must, on the basis of the physical, neurological, and endocrinological examination and review of the history given by the patient and others, generate a formal differential diagnosis and exclude all viable competing diagnoses through testing or other active process of investigation.

Using the laboratory, as evidenced by the pathologist's or toxicologist's training, requires a working knowledge of laboratory methodology, pharmacology, and toxicology in order to utilize the proper body fluids for examination and to know the most favorable time of sample collection and the best testing methodology to order. The purpose of this chapter is to provide information to the practicing psychiatrist in analytical toxicology. After reading this chapter, the reader should have the information necessary for critical evaluation of negative and positive results and have the educated wisdom to interpret the overall reliability of tests.

5. Analytical Methodology

The choice of methods for the identification of drugs or their metabolites in body fluids depends on the patient's history, physical examination, past history, and available samples. Often there is some hint or knowledge about the type of substances used by the subject, which needs to be confirmed. These situations are the simplest for the analytical toxicologist because he/she can compare the suspected sample extracts with known standards. Also, the method of choice is determined by knowledge of the drug's biotransformation pathways and pharmacokinetic patterns.

Another common situation is that in which there is no specific idea what substance or substances were used by the subject whose body fluid is being analyzed. Such a patient sample is tested to rule out the now increasingly common but covert drug-induced or drug-related presenting symptoms. In this case, a broad screen is required and is generally called a "toxicological screen." However, there are various types of screens available, with markedly different sensitivity, specificity, and cost. Various methods will be described in detail along with specific examples showing a rationale for choosing appropriate methodology for specific needs.

5.1. Extraction

With the exception of some enzyme immunoassay (EIA) and radioimmunoassay (RIA) techniques, all methods require isolation of the drug. This is accomplished by extraction using appropriate organic solvents at the specific hydrogen ion concentration (or pH) at which the drug molecules favor movement from an aqueous biofluid into the organic solvent. Basic drugs such as morphine, methadone, and amphetamine are favorably extracted at alkaline pH, whereas acidic drugs such as the barbiturates and phenytoin are more soluble in organic solvents at acidic pH. Some neutral compounds are extractable at pH 7. Obviously, there is great advantage to the analytical chemist when the substance of interest is known or suspected; thus, the proper conditions can be selected for isolation. Unknowns are extracted at three different conditions in the hope of isolating the abused substances at one of the favorable conditions.

To provide the cleanest extract is of great importance so that interference by unrelated molecules is minimized. Biofluids providing clean extracts rank ordered from clean to dirty are saliva, spinal fluid (CSF), serum, urine, and whole blood (hemolyzed). In other words, the least interference is in salivary extracts and CSF, whereas the most interferences occur in urine and hemolyzed whole blood. Depending on the distribution of the drug in the body, which in turn is dependent on the drug's physicochemical properties, one or another biofluid is better suited for analysis. As a rule, urine has 100 to a 1000 times more drug in it than serum, but often it is more difficult to prepare a clean extract from urine, thereby making the theoretical advantages of urine testing disappear. Also, depending on the time after drug use, urine may be clean and serum dirty and *vice versa*. Thus, both biofluids have advantages and disadvantages, and one has to choose the best one suited for the clinical occasion. Following extraction and "clean up" of samples, the extracts are analyzed by various methods differing in sensitivity and specificity, which are discussed in the next sections.

5.2. Thin-Layer Chromatography

Thin-layer chromatography (TLC) is a technique that is utilized to separate different molecules that are present in a mixture. For those who are unfamiliar with analytical methods, Fig. 12-1 may be of some help to visualize the principles of this technique as it pertains to cocaine detection. The thin-layer plate is shown in the figure with several black dots on it, which represent different substances after development. A specific substance such as cocaine, given the same conditions, will always migrate to the same spot. Thus, if cocaine is in the mixture, a spot characterized by the cocaine standard will travel to that specific zone. Unfortunately, similar molecules and various drugs will travel to approximately the same zone. The spot location is identified by an R_f number, which is a ratio calculated from the distance traveled by cocaine divided by the distance traveled by the solvent front from the origin, where the mixture was originally spotted. As indicated in the figure, TLC is a qualitative method, and it is the least sensitive among the methods listed in the figure. Visualization of the spots on TLC is achieved in different ways. The plate can be illuminated by ultraviolet (UV) or fluorescence lights. Migration of molecules to specific R_f zones can be further identified or differentiated by color reactions of the spots after spraying with different chemical dyes. Identical molecules are expected to migrate to the same R_f zone and give identical color reactions.

Traditional "toxicology screen" by TLC was primarily designed to detect qualitatively very-high-dose recent drug abuse or toxic levels of drugs. It is the ideal test for an emergency room, where the drugs taken are unknown and quick determination of the toxic level(s) is the task. Psychiatrically relevant low-level substance abuse

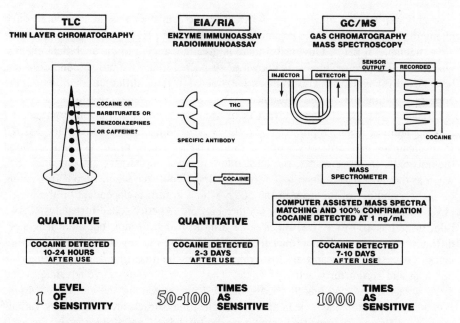

Figure 12-1. Major methodology used in quantitative and qualitative toxicology.

is not readily determined by traditional TLC. Thus, these toxicology screens are often not sufficiently sensitive for the differential diagnosis of drug-induced toxic psychosis mimicking depression, mania, or schizophrenia. Nor are they very well suited for diagnosis of chronic low-dose use of illicit drugs. Such TLC screens are generally not admissible as forensic-quality evidence. In addition to emergency rooms, TLC is also used in methadone programs as "routine drug screens" or "tox screens." Although TLC is the standard testing system, the programs themselves discount the reliability of positives. Patterns such as three consecutive morphine-positive urines rather than one positive test may be used to make a diagnosis. False negatives are the rule rather than the exception, thereby confusing the meaning of negative and positive drug screens by TLC. It must be understood that very often whether a sample is called positive instead of negative depends on the concentration of the drug in the sample or the sensitivity "cutoff" of the assay. With thin-layer chromatography for most drugs, sensitivity "cutoff" is the low-microgram range ($\approx 2 \mu g$); thus, a negative TLC urine may be positive by other methods such as RIA, EMIT, and/or GC–MS. Exception to low sensitivity is a new TLC method for marijuana detection which is sensitive to 20 ng/ml of THCA in urine.[37]

It should be emphasized that when a TLC is ordered, a positive should be confirmed by a second, more specific independent method. This is absolutely essential, since a TLC screen result is not reliable for confirmation of a psychiatric diagnosis by itself. Although the color specificity makes the assay reliable in the hands of experienced toxicologists, it is possible that some interfering substance migrates to the same spot. Furthermore, the boredom and labor-intensive nature of TLC makes experienced TLC master-level toxicologists hard to come by. Remember that negative results by TLC screen are not always negative by other analytical methods. The "negative"

Table 12-1. Sensitivity of TLC Methodology

Drug	Detection level (μg/ml urine)
Morphine	2.0
Codeine	2.0
Cocaine	2.0
Methadone	2.0
Barbiturates	2.0
Amphetamines	2.0
Propoxyphene	2.0
Quinine	0.5

result simply states that the level of sensitivity of the TLC was too low for the particular drug, and therefore none was seen. Table 12-1 shows some of the sensitivity ranges for commonly abused drugs detected by TLC. Most substances are detected only when the level of drug in the urine is above 2 μg/ml. This makes cocaine, for example, very very difficult to detect by routine TLC (see Fig. 12-1). Marijuana, PCP, LSD, and other important drugs are not identified at all in most TLC systems. For this reason, TLC should not be ordered for diagnostic purposes in children and adolescents and should be used with extreme caution in adults.

5.3. Gas Chromatography and Gas Chromatography–Mass Spectrometry

Gas chromatography (GC) is an analytical technique that separates molecules by similar principles as TLC except that the plate is replaced by glass or metal tubing (3 to 6 feet long) packed with materials of particular polarity (Fig. 12-1). The sample is vaporized at the injection port and carried through the column by a steady flow of gas. The column terminates at the detector, which registers the response, which can be recorded and quantitated. The response is proportional to the amount of substance present in the sample. Identical compounds travel through the column at the same speed since their interaction with the column packing is identical. The time from injection until a response at the recorder is observed is referred to as the retention time. Identical retention times of substances run on two different polarity columns is strong evidence that the substances are identical. Stronger evidence can be obtained by the use of GC–MS, which analyzes the substance by its fragmentation pattern. Since in various molecules not all bonds are of equal strength, the weak ones are more likely to break under stress. The exact mass of these fragments or breakage products is measured by a mass spectrometer. Gas chromatography–mass spectrometry is the most reliable, most definitive forensic quality procedure but is also the most expensive.

Information on the fragmentation pattern is compared to a computer library listing the mass of the parent compound and its most likely fragments. A perfect match is considered absolute confirmation of the compound. In fact, confirmation by GC–MS is referred to as the "fingerprinting" of molecules. The use of GC–MS has been out of the reach of most laboratories because of cost, technical expertise needed for operation, and complex sample preparation. However, recent advances in computerization, automated sample preparation, and analytical technology are now placing GC–MS capabilities within the reach of clinical analytical laboratories and clinicians. The sensitivity of GC for most drugs is in the nanogram range, but with special detectors for some compounds, picogram levels can be measured (Table 12-2). The GC–MS can also be used quantitatively, and its sensitivity ranges between nanograms and picograms depending on the drug measured. Although identification of compounds by GC–MS is absolute, this is only true when the instrument is operating in the fragmentation pattern mode. When the GC–MS is run in the search mode for the mass molecular ion only, some of the specificity of the technique is lost. Although the probability of interfering substances having the same mass molecular ion as the drug of interest in the sample is very low, it can occur in rare cases. The chances for error are much less if the instrument is monitoring the fragmentation pattern. Thus, testing should involve split samples and duplicate analysis.

Gas chromatography in most cases is about 100 to 1000 times more sensitive than TLC, and it is also more specific, especially when the two-column system is used. Commonly used and abused drugs are readily identified (e.g., marijuana, cocaine, heroin). The use of GC–MS is also 100–1000 times more sensitive than the TLC system, and when it is operated in the fragmentation pattern mode, identification of drugs is absolute in most cases. When a routine toxicological screen is ordered by the physician, it is usually performed by the cheapest technique (TLC). The physician is often not aware that he has options for more sensitive toxicological screens by either GC, GC/MS, or the more recently introduced and practical enzyme immunoassays (EIA) and radioimmunoassays (RIA).

5.4. Radioimmunoassay and Enzyme Immunoassay

The various immunoassays operate on the principle of antigen–antibody interactions. These techniques are commonly used to measure hormones, neurochemicals, and drugs. The drugs of interest are coupled to large molecules, then injected into rabbits or sheep to produce antibodies against the drug. The immunologic methods used for drug detection employ antibodies against the specific drug and competing drug molecules, which are tagged enzymatically or possess radioactivity. In a solution with the unknown sample, competition exists for available antibody binding sites between the tagged drug in the test and drug in the unknown sample. The binding ratio determines the presence or absence of specific drugs in the unknown sample.

Immunoassays depend on how specific and sensitive the antibodies are to a given

Table 12-2. Toxicology Common Units of Measure

1 g = gram (there are 28 g in 1 ounce)	1.0
1 mg = milligram (1/1000 of a gram)	0.001
1 μg = microgram (one-millionth of a gram)	0.000,001
1 ng = nanogram (one-billionth of a gram)	0.000,000,001
1 pg = picogram (one-trillionth of a gram)	0.000,000,000,001
1 liter = approximately 1 quart	
1 ml = milliliter (1/1000 of a liter)	

compound. Usually, they are extremely good; however, compounds architecturally similar to the drug of interest (often their metabolites) sometimes do cross react. Thus, specificity of the immunoassays is considered far less than that of GC and GC–MS. This can be an advantage in some cases, however, because interaction with drug plus metabolites in a sample by the immunoassay system increases sensitivity in "total" drug detection. In chromatography, a single molecular species is determined. The sensitivity, depending on the particular assay, ranges between micrograms and picograms. The EIA system is very popular and commonly used because no extraction or centrifugation is required, and the system lends itself to easy automation. Although an EIA screen is more costly than TLC, toxicological screens using EIA are much more sensitive for most drugs and are more likely to detect a lower level of drug use. However, EIA screens yielding one or many positives should be confirmed by GC–MS or other methods yielding lower sensitivity than EIA.

5.5. *Choice of Sample (Body Fluid) and Time of Collection*

The successful use of the toxicology laboratory by the physician is greatly dependent on the characteristics of the sample sent to the laboratory. The choices of body fluid and the estimated time after use depend on the suspected drug's pharmacokinetics. Some drugs are metabolized extensively and are very quickly excreted, wheras others stay in the body for an extended period of time. Thus, success of detection depends not only on the time factor but also on whether the analysis is performed for the drug itself or for its metabolites.

The following questions should be asked: (1) How long does the drug stay in the body? (2) How extensively is the drug biotransformed? Should one look for the parent compound or its metabolites? (3) Which body fluid should be analyzed? The importance of asking these questions is illustrated by two drugs, cocaine and methaqualone (Quaalude®), which are biotransformed significantly differently by the body.

Cocaine has a half-life of about 1 hr in the plasma.[38] It is rapidly biotransformed into inactive metabolites; the major metabolite is benzoylecgonine. Less than 5% of the unchanged cocaine is excreted into the urine. What does all this suggest to the clinician who wants to know whether his patient is taking cocaine? The short half-life indicates that unless use is suspected within hours or the patient is suspected of being under the influence cocaine itself, the parent compound is not likely to be found in detectable concentration in either the blood or the urine. However, a blood test that includes cocaine and the cocaine metabolite may be reliable for many hours after use. Plasma enzymes continue to metabolize cocaine even after the blood is taken from the subject. Blood samples should be collected into sodium fluoride, which inactivates these enzymes.[39] It is clear that detection is best accomplished by collecting blood or urine samples and having them analyzed for benzoylecgonine. Since benzoylecgonine is the major metabolite of cocaine, it is excreted in urine at levels of approximately 45% of the dose. It has been observed that of those subjects who had enough benzoylecgonine in their urine to be detected, only 2% had enough cocaine present (urine) for detection. Thus, 98% of the subjects who were tested would have been found negative if the physician had ordered specific testing for cocaine instead of benzoylecgonine in urine. For this reason, we automatically test for both the parent and metabolite.

The other example is methaqualone. This substance is extremely lipid soluble and has a long half-life. It is not biotransformed rapidly; thus, either blood or urine tests are effective for detection of the parent compound. In our studies, we were able to detect methaqualone for 21 days in the urine after a single 300-mg oral dose, and in blood for 7 days.[40]

Which biofluid is choice for drug detection analysis? As a rule, urine has about 1000 times more drug present than plasma. On the other hand, it is often much easier to prepare clean extracts from serum than from urine. A cleaner extract greatly reduces background interference, reduces the chances for false positives, and makes it easier for the chromatographer to interpret and confirm the results.

Many physicians prefer blood for drug screen rather than urine because they believe that it is stronger evidence of recent use and is clearly related to brain levels and drug-related behavior change. Blood levels, for example, are directly related to the emergence and persistance of amphetamine and other model psychoses. Urine is an ultrafiltrate of plasma; thus, it is normally sufficiently accurate for drug and metabolite determination. However, the collection of urine specimens must be supervised in order to insure that the person in question is the source of the sample and to guarantee the integrity of the specimen. It is not unusual to receive someone else's or a highly diluted sample when collection of samples is not supervised. For these and other reasons (e.g., many psychiatrists can draw blood, and few have office bathrooms; few psychiatrists have staff members of both sexes to supervise urines), supervised first morning urine samples where specific gravity is measured are preferred, as they are more concentrated and drugs are more readily detected. The decision for using blood or urine should be based on information on the specific drug suspected. Utilization of pharmacokinetic and excretion data of the drug is valuable. As a rule, urine drug levels are higher and should be the choice biofluid for drug and metabolite detection.

6. The Meaning of Positive and Negative Reports

When one receives reports on drug analysis, whether positive or negative, there are certain questions about the absolute truth of the results. The following questions should be asked: (1) What method was used? (If the lab does not tell you on the report, call and ask.) (2) Did the assay analyze for the drug, metabolite, or both? What is the "cutoff" value for the assay? (Again, call and ask.) (3) Was the sample time close enough to the suspected drug exposure?

First let us examine positive results. Some scrutiny is needed to determine whether or not a false-positive result is a possibility. Knowledge of the method of determination is helpful. Thin-layer chromatography, although not very sensitive, is reasonably specific for drugs that have both the parent and metabolite identified as present on the TLC plate. Also, some specific color reactions[5] help to eliminate false positives for certain drugs. However if GLC or GC–MS was the analytical technique, the positive result is acceptable by itself in most cases. Use of RIA or EMIT is considered rather sensitive, but chemically similar compounds may cross react, registering false positives. This possibility depends on the specificity of the antibody used for the particular test. Some antibodies are more specific and more accurate than others. Therefore, each test should be individually evaluated for specificity. Because individual tests can result in false positives, to be legally acceptable or used for diagnosis, the test should be confirmed by two independent methods. Usually, an immunoassay can be confirmed by a chromatographic procedure (GC/MS).

False-negative results can result perhaps even more easily than false positives, mainly because of the insensitivity of commonly used screening procedures such as the TLC (for most drugs ≥2 µg/ml). Thus, a negative report based on TLC alone may have missed the detection of drugs because the TLC "cutoff" between positives and negatives is too high. Another possibility for false negatives is that the sample was taken too long after the exposure, or the wrong biofluid was collected and analyzed for the wrong substance, or the sample was too diluted for TLC.

Whatever the case may be, if the suspicion of drug use is strong, inquire at the laboratory for more sensitive screening procedure such as immunoassays, GC, and ultimately GC–MS and acquire information on the best biofluid and time of collection for the optimum detection of the suspected drug. Collect a first-void urine, supervise it, measure the specific gravity, and draw a blood sample to hold if the urine is negative and clinical suspicion remains high.

In general, analytical toxicology methods have significantly improved in the past decade, and the trend is for further improvement. Even if everything that goes on in the laboratory is foreign, you can use Table 12-3 if you know which drug intoxication or withdrawal states must be ruled out. As technology continues to improve, more drugs and chemicals will be analyzed in the future in biofluids at the nanogram and picogram level. Advancement, however, does not mean that modern methodologies are infallible, nor do they replace the psychiatric clinician. A solid laboratory with the full spectrum of drug abuse tests enables the well-trained clinician to make diagnoses that are not otherwise possible. Theoretically and practically, technical or human error can influence all testing results. Thus, with some knowledge of the available analytical systems, one can scrutinize the results and be more confident about their validity.

Table 12-3. Tests to Confirm Suspected Drug Use by Class of Drugs

Suspected problem		Test
Opioids	Intoxication	Blood or urine levels of opioids
	Withdrawal	Urine test for opioids or quinine, which may be present for 24 to 84 hr after the last dose
Depressants	Intoxication	Blood or urine levels of depressant; EEG nonspecific depressant effect
	Withdrawal	EEG showing bursts of spiked high-amplitude slow waves in nonepileptics
Stimulants	Intoxication	Blood or urine levels of amphetamine or cocaine
	Withdrawal	Abnormal sleep EEGs; urine screen for amphetamine or cocaine metabolites; depression scales
Hallucinogens	Intoxication	None widely available; some laboratories can assay urine and blood levels
	Withdrawal	
Phencyclidine	Intoxication	Blood or urine levels of phencyclidine; either EIA or GC apparatus with a nitrogen detector or GC–MS is required for detection in the low-nanogram range; otherwise, a false negative may confuse the diagnosis
	Withdrawal	The test may be positive up to 7 days after the last dose

References

1. Yago KB, Pitts FN Jr, Burgoyne RW, et al: The urban epidemic of phencyclidine (PCP) use: Clinical and laboratory evidence from a public psychiatric hospital emergency service. *J Clin Psychiatry* 42:193–196, 1981.

2. Thacore VR, Shukla SRP: Cannabis psychosis and paranoid schizophrenia. *Arch Gen Psychiatry* 33:383–386, 1976.

3. Gold MS: *800-COCAINE.* New York, Bantam, 1984.

4. Pottash ALC, Gold MS, Extein I: The use of the clinical laboratory, in Sederer LI (ed): *Inpatient Psychiatry: Diagnosis and Treatment.* Baltimore, Williams & Wilkins, 1982, pp 205–221.

5. Gold MS, Pottash ALC, Estroff TW, et al: Laboratory evaluation in treatment planning, in Karasu TB (ed): *Part I: Psychiatric Therapies, The Somatic Therapies.* Washington, American Psychiatric Association, 1984, pp 31–50.

6. Smith DE: Acute and chronic toxicity of marijuana. *J Psychedel Drugs* 2:37–47, 1968.

7. Jefferson JW, Marshall JR: *Neuropsychiatric Features of Medical Disorders.* New York, Plenum Press, 1981.

8. Knight F: Role of cannabis in psychiatric disturbance. *Ann NY Acad Sci* 282:64–71, 1976.

9. Tennant FS, Groesbeck CI: Psychiatric effects of hashish. *Arch Gen Psychiatry* 27:133–136, 1972.

10. Rottanburg D, Robins AH, Ben-Arie O, et al: Cannabis associated psychosis with hypomanic features. *Lancet* 2:1364–1366, 1982.

11. Bloodworth RC: Medical aspects of marijuana abuse. *Psychiatry Lett* 1(2), 1983.

12. Weissman MM, Pottenger M, Kleber H, et al: Symptom patterns in primary and secondary depression. A comparison of primary depressives with depressed opiate addicts, alcoholics, and schizophrenics. *Arch Gen Psychiatry* 34:854–862, 1977.

13. Croughan JL, Miller JP, Wagelin D, et al: Psychiatric illness in male and female narcotic addicts. *J Clin Psychiatry* 43:225–228, 1982.

14. Rounsaville BJ, Weissman MM, Crits-Christoph K, et al: Diagnosis and symptoms of depression in opiate addicts: Course and relationship to treatment outcome. *Arch Gen Psychiatry* 39:151–156, 1982.

15. Dackis CA, Gold MS: Opiate addiction and depression—cause or effects. *Drug Alcohol Depend* 11:105–109, 1983.

16. Gold MS, Estroff TW: The comprehensive evaluation of cocaine and opiate abusers, in Hall RC, Beresford TP (eds): *Handbook of Psychiatric Diagnostic Procedures.* New York, Spectrum, 2:213–230, 1984.

17. Beamish P, Kiloh LG: Psychoses due to amphetamine consumption. *J Ment Sci* 106: 337–343, 1960.

18. Snyder SH: Amphetamine psychosis: A "model" schizophrenia mediated by catecholamines. *Am J Psychiatry* 130:61–67, 1973.

19. Estroff TW, Gold MS: Medical and psychiatric complications of cocaine abuse and possible points of pharmacologic intervention. *Adv Alcohol Subst Abuse* in press.

20. Post RM, Kopanda RT: Cocaine kindling and psychosis. *Am J Psychiatry* 133:627–634, 1976.

21. Gawin FH, Kleber HD: Cocaine abuse treatment. *Yale Psychiatr Q* 6:4–15, 1983.

22. Bowers MB: Psychoses precipitated by psychomimetic drugs a follow-up study. *Arch Gen Psychiatry* 34:832–835, 1977.

23. Vardy MM, Kay SR: LSD psychosis or LSD-induced schizophrenia? A multimethod inquiry. *Arch Gen Psychiatry* 40:877–883, 1983.

24. Hensala JD, Epstein LJ, Blacker KH: LSD and psychiatric inpatients. *Arch Gen Psychiatry* 16:554–558, 1967.

25. Dimijian GG: in Goth A (ed): *Contemporary Drug Abuse in Medical Pharmacology,* 7th ed. St. Louis, Missouri, C.V. Mosby, 1974, p 316.

26. Schick JFE, Smith DE: Analysis of the flashback. *J Psychedel Drugs* 3:13–19, 1970.

27. Wyse DG: Deliberate inhalation of volatile hypocarbons: A review. *Can Med Assoc J* 108:71–74, 1973.

28. Struwe G, Knave B, Mindus P: Neuropsychiatric symptoms in workers exposed to jet fuel—a combined epidemiological and causistic study. *Acta Psychiatr Scand* 67:55–67, 1983.

29. Struwe G, Wennberg A: Psychiatric and neurological symptoms in workers occupationally exposed to organic solvents—results of a differential epidemiological study. *Acta Psychiatr Scand* 67:68–80, 1983.

30. Schuckit MA: *Drug and Alcohol Abuse: A Clinical Guide to Diagnosis and Treatment.* New York, Plenum Press, 1979.

31. Ayd F: A critical appraisal of chlordiazepoxide. *J Neuropsychiatry* 3:177–180, 1962.
32. Griffiths RR, Bigelow GE, Liebson I: Differential effects of diazepam and pentobarbital on mood and behavior. *Arch Gen Psychiatry* 40:865–873, 1983.
33. *Medical Letter:* Drugs that cause psychiatric symptoms. *Med Lett* 23:9–12, 1981.
34. Preskorn SH, Denner LJ: Benzodiazepines and withdrawal psychosis. *JAMA* 237:36–38, 1977.
35. Flemenbaum A, Gunby B: Ethchlorvynol (Placidyl) abuse and withdrawal (review of clinical picture and report of 2 cases). *Dis Nerv Syst* 32:188–192, 1971.
36. Heston LL, Hastings D: Psychosis with withdrawal from ethchlorvynol. *Am J Psychiatry* 137:249–250, 1980.
37. Kogan MJ, Newman E, Willson NJ: Detection of marijuana metabolite 11-nor-9-tetrahydrocannabinol-9-carboxylic acid in human urine by bonded-phase absorption and thin-layer chromatography. *J Chromatog* 306:441–443, 1984.
38. Ritchie JM, Cohen PJ: Cocaine, procaine and other synthetic local anesthetics, in Goodman LS, Gilman A (eds): *The Pharmacological Basis of Therapeutics.* New York, Macmillan, 1980, p 308.
39. Kogan MJ, Verebey KG, DePace AC, et al: Quantitative determination of benzoylecgonine and cocaine in human biofluids by gas–liquid chromatography. *Anal Chem* 49(13):1965–1969, 1977.
40. Kogan MJ, Jukofsky D, Verebey K, et al: Detection of methaqualone in human urine by radioimmunoassay and gas–liquid chromatography after a therapeutic dose. *Clin Chem* 24:1425, 1978.

The Use of Psychiatric Rating Scales in Clinical Evaluation and Treatment

R. Michael Allen, M.D., and Mark S. Gold, M.D.

1. Introduction

From the time behaviorists first proposed that one could describe and quantify even complex human behavior by breaking it down into simple component units, attempts have been made to develop objective rating devices for the purpose of quantifying psychopathology. The most obvious use of such rating devices is the measurement of change in clinical drug trials and reduction of clinical events to numbers that are suitable for "crunching" for statistical analysis. With recent changes in the Joint Commission for Accreditation of Hospitals (JCAH) standards for psychiatric care requiring more objectivity in terms of treatment planning and outcome measurement, psychiatric rating scales have the potential of becoming useful tools in such documentation efforts.

It is important to define the scope of the discussion, as behavioral and psychiatric observation instruments range in sophistication from complex psychometrically designed and validated instruments such as the Minnesota Multiphasic Personality Inventory (MMPI)[1] to relatively unsophisticated but practical scales such as the Global Assessment Scale.[2] In addition, there are structured interview schedules such as the Schedule for Affective Disorders and Schizophrenia (SADS),[3] the Diagnostic Interview Schedule (DIS),[4] and the Present State Exam[5] that lie somewhere in between. I mainly want to address the use of traditional psychiatric rating scales in clinical settings from the point of view of how they can help the treating physician and the rest of the treatment team in assessing the patient's probable diagnosis and response to treatment.

2. Basic Concepts

For a complete discussion of the nature of behavioral rating, theoretical constructs, statistics, and psychometric history, the reader is referred to standard reviews

---

R. Michael Allen, M.D. • Neuropsychiatric Evaluation Unit, Psychiatric Institute of Fort Worth, Fort Worth, Texas 76104, and Department of Psychiatry, University of Texas Southwestern Medical School, Dallas, Texas 75235.   *Mark S. Gold, M.D.* • Research Facilities, Fair Oaks Hospital, Summit, New Jersey 07901, and Fair Oaks Hospital at Boca/Delray, Delray Beach, Florida 33445.

of the subjects.[6,7] Certain basic concepts must be understood before a meaningful evaluation of psychiatric rating scales and their usefulness in psychiatry can be made. The first factor to note is the way the scale is constructed; i.e., was it designed with a particular psychopathological theory in mind or simply designed from a general phenomenological point of view and derived by complex item analysis or more complicated mathematical techniques such as cluster analysis? For example, a rating scale to assess ego strength, superego development, or awareness of unconscious determinants of behavior has an obvious theoretical underpinning that has to be taken into account, and likewise for a scale that measures frequency of observed behaviors without reference to underlying anxiety, conflict, etc. Other issues that must be considered in deciding whether to use a rating scale are the following: Does it measure what you want it to measure accurately (concurrent and content validity)? Does it measure the things you want to measure reliably; i.e., are ratings performed by independent observers of similar skill consistent with each other, or is there demonstrated internal consistency in self-administered tests (split-half reliability)? Is there demonstrated test–retest reliability? Does it measure change to a sufficiently sensitive degree (incremental validity)? For some instruments, does it predict a criterion measure external to the scale at the time (predictive validity); e.g., does a new instrument measure a particular symptom complex or change in intensity of a symptom that is generally accepted and defined by previous (usually more complex and detailed) instruments or diagnostic criteria?

Other significant considerations about rating scales include mode of administration, i.e., self or interviewer; subject or informant for the rating, i.e., patient, family member, past records, or videotape; time period covered, e.g., past 2 weeks, year, life, or only at the present time; environmental setting, i.e., outpatient or inpatient; who is doing the rating, e.g., nurse, physician, nonprofessional staff; and, finally, how the scale is constructed, e.g., yes–no, multiple choice with defined gradations of severity, or a continuum for items involving subjective judgment on the part of the rater.

The use of a yes–no format and grading severity by asking specific questions about each degree of severity appears to increase the reliability of either an interviewer- or self-administered instrument. Requiring the interviewer or the patient to make global assessments of severity of symptomatology requires more sophisticated interviewers and patients.

The importance of some of the above considerations is as follows. Self-report rating scales tend to be more sensitive to the subjective distress of the patient as documented by Carroll *et al.* in their validation of the 52-item Carroll Rating Scale for depression (CRS)[8] but can also be inaccurate in certain types of patients who overreport or underreport their degree of distess as a variable of personality or of coping or personality styles as noted by Brown and Zung. In addition, the use of self-rating scales is limited by the patient population one is dealing with, e.g., socioeconomic. educational, cultural, and linguistic variables, as well as by the type of disorder one is attempting to rate (for example, psychotic versus nonpsychotic disorders).

Other issues such as impersonality, cost effectiveness in terms of professional time, and quality of data gathered are important determinants, as noted by Spitzer and Endicott.[7] Practically speaking, interviewer-administered scales vary from extremely structured interviews such as the SADS or DIS to extremely unstructured ones such as the Brief Psychiatric Rating Scale[10] with intermediate scales such as the Hamilton Depression (HAM-D) and Anxiety (HAM-A) scales.[11,12] In general, the structured diagnostic interviews require well-trained personnel but require less clinical judgment; the unstructured scales such as the BPRS require clinically skilled and experienced professionals, and the intermediate scales such as the HAM-D can be administered by moderately trained nonprofessional personnel.[13] Other scales such as the Nurses' Observation Scale for Inpatient Evaluation (NOSIE-30)[14] are designed to be administered by specific members of the evaluation team, e.g., the clinical nursing staff.

Other instruments that are not properly termed psychiatric rating scales include physical symptom checklists that are valuable in insuring a complete review of medical symptomatology, automated family and social histories, and computer-scored and standardized projective tests. These types of questionnaires are potentially great time-saving devices for the psychiatrist and clinical evaluation team. They, like any of the rating instruments, are not a substitute for a comprehensive psychiatric clinical interview but can improve the quality of the time spent with the patient by reducing the need to interrogate the patient about routine historical matters.

Specific psychiatric rating scales are discussed below according to mode of administration and type of psychopathology measured. When properly used, psychiatric rating scales and data inventories are among the most powerful and time-saving tools we have as both researchers and clinicians in objectively evaluating treatment outcome and severity of illness. It is a generally held opinion that one should use more than one type of rating instrument, e.g., a self-administered scale such as the CRS and an interviewer-administered scale such as the HAM-D for depression as well as a naturalistic one such as the NOSIE-30 to rate behavior and pathology, to balance and cancel out inherent sources of error in each type of instrument.

3. Rating Scales for Psychosis

There have been many attempts to develop objective, reproducible, and easy-to-administer rating scales for psychotic thought content, process, and behaviors. The gold standard in psychiatric research is the Brief Psychiatric Rating Scale developed by Overall and Gorham.[10] The BPRS consists of 18 items ranging from "excitement" to "depression," which are rated from 1 to 7 according to degree of severity (1 = not present to 7 = extremely severe). Thus, the minimum BPRS score is 18. On this form, the usual cutoff score for inclusion in antipsychotic studies is >40. Some investigators including the author prefer to rate from 0 to 6 and use 22 as a cutoff score, feeling that one should not assign a positive numeric value to an absent symptom. A shortcoming of the BPRS is the lack of agreed-on criteria for the various degrees of severity for each item. Thus, the BPRS is really a structured way of recording a clinical global impression for each of the 18 items with limits being set only in the range of possible ratings. Interestingly, when experienced clinicians or research assistants work together or cross rate even across the country with videotaped interviews, the interrater reliability is high. Overall has pointed to this fact as an objection to "criteria-basing" severity ratings, feeling that the way the scale is currently used is more valuable (J. E. Overall, personal communication). His group has developed complex cluster analysis computer programs that apparently are quite reliable in classifying clinical syndromes and have moderate predictive value in predicting outcome.

For clinical use, the concept of criterion-based severity ratings using a semistructured interview technique enables nonprofessional staff to produce reliable ratings and facilitates the development of interrater reliability. An example of this approach is the rating of hallucinations. If 0 = not present, then the severity may be graded in the following manner: 1 = very mild, the patient hears noises such as doors closing or footsteps occasionally; 2 = mild, the patient admits to hearing his name or words called out on occasion; 3 = moderate, the patient admits to hearing incomplete phrases that clearly sound as though they are coming from outside of his head or hears his thoughts aloud as if they were voices; 4 = moderately severe, the patient admits to hearing a voice or voices talking in complete sentences to him when no one else is in the vicinity; 5 = severe, the patient complains of command hallucinations or two or more voices carrying on a running commentary about his thoughts or behavior; 6 = extremely severe, the patient is obviously hallucinating to the point of responding to the hallucinations either actively by answering them or passively by attending almost exclusively to them, making the interview difficult to perform. One could likewise modify these criteria to include visual hallucinations or other types (somesthetic, olfactory). I have obviously borrowed heavily from Kurt Schneider's first-rank symptom definitions for this example and use DSM-III criteria for the depression, suspiciousness, and anxiety ratings. This approach renders the BPRS much more useful to the clinical staff as a tool to measure severity and change as treatment progresses. For clinical drug trials, however, one should use the scale as designed to insure compatability with other investigators and the previous literature.

Newer scales that have been developed to quantify and document the more fundamental signs of schizophrenia such as thought disorder and affect include Andreason's scales (Affect Rating Scale and Scale for the Assessment of Thought, Language, and Communication).[15-17] Recent work using a Raschian mathematical modeling approach by Lewine, Fogg, and Meltzer[18] has demonstrated that one can develop a rating scale for any symptom (in this case, positive and negative symptoms of schizophrenia) without having to field develop it using hundreds of patients.

The most widely used self-rating symptom checklist that queries the patient about psychotic symptoms is the Symptom Checklist-90 (SCL-90).[19] This scale has been used extensively in both inpatient and outpatient studies of drug response and psychotherapy outcome. Although the early studies demonstrate an impressive relilability and validity for the SCL-90, recent work has called its usefulness into question in outpatients.[20] Computer-administered interviews have been developed that almost qualify as self-rating scales,[21] and Fowler *et al.* have developed a problem-oriented computer interview that appears to be useful in quantifying change in such subtle signs as thought disorder.[22]

The last major approach to the diagnosis and rating of change of psychotic symptoms is the structured interview. The SADS-L[23] is widely used in psychopharmacological research to generate Research Diagnostic Criteria (RDC) diagnoses, and the SADS-C is used to measure response to treatment.[24] Spitzer and Endicott have even developed subscales of the SADS that yield Hamilton Depression scores.[24] The

Diagnostic Interview Schedule of the NIMH is now being piloted for research and is similar to the SADS except that it generates DSM-III diagnoses and can be modified to produce diagnoses based on the Feighner or RD Criteria.[4] These instruments have been developed according to the decision tree criteria-generating method and must be carefully administered if they are to produce reliable and valid results. The Present State Exam developed by Wing *et al.* is a British instrument that is most useful in assessing schizophrenia.[5] The disadvantages of the scheduled interview for the clinical evaluation unit or the clinician in practice are that they are tedious and time consuming, require highly trained personnel, may inappropriately lull one into a false sense of complacency concerning the accuracy of a diagnosis, and are awkward to administer to a patient whom one has seen before in a purely clinical setting. The DIS has been computerized and, although not yet suitable for total computer administration, greatly facilitates data entry for the meticulous clinician–interviewer.[25] Older psychopathology scales such as the Wittenborn are rarely used today.

4. Rating Scales for Affective Disorders

The variety and usefulness of rating scales for depression are much greater than those for schizophrenia and other psychotic disturbances. Also, with the exception of the extremes of the depressive spectrum (i.e., psychotic or stuporous and the atypical or very mild neurotic or hysteroid forms), self-rating scales have been developed that have been shown to have a high degree of reliability. The advantages and limitations of self-rating scales have been detailed above. Likewise, depression is the most treatable of the major psychiatric disorders, and objective measures of response to treatment are very useful in making treatment decisions.

The standard instrument for antidepressant drug studies is the HAM-D. This 17-point scale is heavily weighted with items that discern the somatic and neurovegetative components of the depressive syndrome. The Hamilton is a reasonably easy instrument to use and, as noted previously, is quickly learned by nonprofessional personnel. Normative and pathological data have been collected since its introduction in 1960, and it has even gained acceptance among some clinical psychometricians. It has defined criteria for each of the items and is quickly and easily administered. Although criteria have been developed for the definition of major depression (the usual lower range for inclusion in inpatient drug studies is 20–25 and for outpatients 15–20), it is not a diagnostic instrument like the SADS or DIS. It is sensitive to change and is easily quantified. Other interviewer-administered rating scales include the Raskin and other global scales, which add little to overall clinical global assessment.

The self-administered depression-rating scales that have gained the widest acceptance are the Beck Depression Inventory (BDI) and the Carroll Rating Scale for depression (CRS).[8,26] The Carroll was developed to correlate very closely with the HAM-D and consists of 52 yes–no questions that produce scores that can be correlated item for item with the Hamilton.[8] The CRS is likewise easily adapted for computer administration. Like the HAM-D, the CRS is not a diagnostic instrument and focuses on the somatic and neurovegetative components of the depressive syndrome. The BDI is designed to assess the cognitive component of depression and is more useful in nonendogenous patients and to measure outcome of cognitive behavioral therapy for depression. It is sensitive to change and has been correlated with the HAM-D. The Zung Depression Scale (ZDS) is not very useful in the research or inpatient setting, but its disadvantages in these settings (lack of specificity for major depressive symptoms, brevity, and less sensitivity to change) make it an excellent screening test in the outpatient setting, especially for use by nonpsychiatric physicians. It is easily administered and scored and is quite sensitive to the global manifestations of depression.

The most widely used rating scale for the assessment of mania is the Mania Rating Scale developed by Young et al.[27] Although mania is a difficult syndrome to objectively rate, this scale is useful in documenting response to lithium. The SADS-L is particularly useful in the differential diagnosis of mania from other psychotic illnesses. Manics are often better rated with a naturalistic scale such as the NOSIE-30, which is behaviorally and functionally oriented and covers a longer rating period than typical clinician-administered scales.

Another rating scale for the evaluation of mood states is the Profile of Mood States (POMS).[28] The POMS is a self-administered 65-item questionnaire that requires the patient to grade his mood state from 0 to 4 for each of the items. When scored, the POMS yields a scale for six symptom complexes: tension–anxiety, depression–dejection, anger–hostility, vigor, fatigue–inertia, and confusion–bewilderment. Since the patient serves as his own control, the POMS is often very useful in following the day-to-day or week-to-week response to treatment and is sensitive in detecting drug side effects such as akathisia, akinesia, and cognitive problems secondary to the anticholinergic side effects of most thymoleptic and neuroleptic agents. It is likewise useful in monitoring the response to nonpharmacological treatments such as biofeedback, relaxation training, cranial electrostimulation (CES), and psychotherapy.

5. Miscellaneous Scales

There are rating scales to rate almost every symptom, thought, somatic complaint, and clinical situation. Some of the major rating instruments and uses are as follows. The NOSIE-30 is a behavioral and functional scale that is completed by a research nurse in the research setting, and this instrument is almost universally used in drug trials. It is designed to be completed on a weekly basis, but more frequent ratings can be useful on an evaluation or acute care unit. It is easily learned, and interrater reliability is quickly developed. An advantage of the NOSIE on an evaluation unit is the valuable structured information it furnishes from the clinical nursing staff. The NOSIE is useful in almost all clinical populations including the geriatric patient.

The myriad of rating scales that are used in geriatric psychiatry are reviewed by Saltzman et al.[29] For the most part, the only rating scales other than those used for major psychiatric disorders and clinical situations already discussed are designed to assess cognitive and social function. The most widely used standardized instrument is the Mini-Mental-State. This is a quickly administered organic mental status examination that assesses most major areas of cognitive functioning except for abstract thinking.[30] It has been demonstrated to be sensitive in the assessment of rather rapid changes in cognitive status. Of course, there are several structured mental status examinations that are considerably more detailed, time consuming, and thus less practical for routine clinical use.[31,32]

Rating scales for symptomatic anxiety include the Hamilton Anxiety Scale (HAM-A), the Covi (usually paired with the Raskin depression scale in outpatient studies), and the phobia–anxiety inventory.[13,33,34] These instruments are mainly utilized in the outpatient setting.

Finally, psychiatrists should become more accustomed to objectively rating movement disorders, especially medication-induced extrapyramidal symptoms (EPS) and tardive dyskinesia. The recognition and treatment of the subtle EPS such as akathisia and akinesia are critical in terms of medication compliance and appropriate diagnosis and treatment. For example, akathisia is commonly diagnosed as anxiety, psychotic agitation, or even psychotic decompensation, and additional neuroleptics are prescribed. Akinesia is often misdiagnosed as depression, and antidepressant medication is prescribed needlessly. The simple application of a scale such as the one developed by Simpson and Angus[35] on a routine basis would raise the consciousness of the clinician.

Tardive dyskinesia is a serious problem that occurs most commonly in patients with affective disorder who are treated with a neuroleptic. It is incumbent on the clinician to recognize and quantify dyskinetic movements to avoid missing emerging dyskinesia early enough to prevent its progression and, perhaps more importantly, to avoid the overdiagnosis of this expensive and sometimes tragic consequence of neuroleptic therapy. Most cases of emergent dyskinesias are either withdrawal dyskinesia or even acute dyskinesias like the rabbit syndrome that are no cause for alarm if recognized and treated. The diagnosis of tardive dyskinesia written in a chart or spoken to a patient or his family without virtual certainty of the diagnosis is often more tragic for the clinician or a previous physician medicolegally than for the patient, who may be needlessly alarmed. Unfortunately, there are no easy-to-adminmister rating instruments to diagnose tardive dyskinesia. The best scale for the clinical assessment of dyskinetic movements by the inexperienced clinician is the modified Abnormal Involuntary Movement Scale (AIMS) provided by Sandoz pharmaceutical company. It is well constructed, and each item, as well as how the examination is to be conducted, is explained. The research AIMS from the NIMH[36] is used for research studies and is more detailed and specific than the Sandoz version. However, it is designed for use by research personnel who have been adequately trained in its administration. Unless the clinician is experienced in the assessment of movement disorders, he should consult one that is. Other, more comprehensive rating scales to assess tardive dyskinesia include the Simpson scale,[37] which is extremely detailed and tedious to perform but is a definitive assessment. Other movement disorders that can be detected using dyskinetic rating scales include Huntington's disease and Wilson's disease.

The last scales to be discussed are the so-called "magic" scales, which are derived from the old standby, the MMPI. For example, workers at the NIMH have developed pharmacological response research scales on the MMPI that are uncannily accurate at predicting imipramine and lithium responders.[38,39] The scale was discovered on cluster analysis of the MMPI results of hundreds of treatment-resistant patients who responded to imiprimine or lithium and not to amitriptyline; MMPIs can be scored for these and other research and clinical subscales by computer programs that are available for the Apple II series of personal computers.[40]

In conclusion, the use of psychiatric rating scales in the evaluation and treatment of psychiatric disorders has great potential usefulness to the clinician as well as to the clinical investigator. They are probably underutilized by clinicians because of the research mystique that surrounds their use in the academic training center. The potential benefit of the increasing use of objective rating scales has yet to be fully appreciated in the private world, but, as noted previously, the increasing demands of JCAH and government and third-party payment plans for objective documentation of need for treatment and of treatment outcome will increase the use of these instruments.

References

1. Hathaway SR, McKinley JC: *MMPI Manual,* Rev ed. New York, The Psychological Corporation, 1951.
2. Spitzer RL, Gibbon M, Endicott J: *Global Assessment Scale.* New York, New York State Department of Mental Hygiene. 1973.
3. Spitzer RL, Endicott J: *Schedule for Affective Disorders and Schizophrenia.* New York, New York State Department of Mental Hygiene, 1973.
4. Robins LN, Heltzer JE, Croughan J, et al: *The Diagnostic Interview Schedule,* version III. Washington, National Institute of Mental Health, Division of Biometry and Epidemiology, 1981.
5. Wing JK, Cooper JE, Sartorious N: *The Description and Classification of Psychiatric Symptoms: An Instructional Manual for the PSE and CATEGO System.* London, Cambridge University Press, 1974.
6. Hersen M, Bellack AS (eds): *Behavioral Assessment: A Practical Handbook.* New York, Pergamon Press, 1981.
7. Endicott J, Spitzer RL: Evaluation of psychiatric treatment, in Kaplan HI, Freedman AM, Sadock BJ (eds): *Comprehensive Textbook of Psychiatry/III.* Baltimore, Williams & Wilkins, 1980, pp 2391–2409.
8. Carroll BJ, Feinberg M, Smouse PE, et al: The Carroll Rating Scale for Depression I. Development, reliability and validation. *Br J Psychiatry* 138:194–200, 1981.
9. Brown GL, Zung WK: Depression scales: Self- or Physician rating? A validation of certain clinically observable phenomena. *Comp Psychiatry* 13:361–367, 1972.
10. Overall JE, Gorham DR: The Brief Psychiatric Rating Scale. *Psychol Rep* 10:799–812, 1962.
11. Hamilton M: A rating scale for depression. *J Neurol Neurosurg Psychiatry* 23:56–62, 1960.
12. Hamilton M: The assessment of anxiety states by rating. *Br J Med Psychol* 32:50–56, 1959.
13. O'Hara MW, Rehm LP: Hamilton Rating Scale for Depression: Reliability and validity of judgements of novice raters. *J Consult Clin Psychol* 51:318–319, 1983.
14. Honingfeld G, Klett CJ: The Nurses Observation Scale for Inpatient Evaluation. *J Clin Psychol* 21:65–71, 1965.
15. Andreasen N: Affective flattening and the criteria for schizophrenia. *Am J Psychiatry* 136:944–947, 1979.
16. Andreasen N: Thought, language, and communication disorders I. Clinical assessment, definition of terms, and evaluation of their reliability. *Arch Gen Psychiatry* 36:1315–1321, 1979.
17. Andreasen N: Thought, language, and communication disorders. II. Diagnostic significance. *Arch Gen Psychiatry* 36:1325–1330, 1979.
18. Lewine RRJ, Fogg L, Meltzer HY: Assessment of negative and positive symptoms in schizophrenia. *Schizophrenia Bull* 9:368–376, 1983.
19. Derogatis LR: *SCL-90: Administration, Scoring, and Procedures Manual.* Baltimore, Clinical Psychometric Research, 1977.
20. Kass F, Charles E, Klein DF, et al: Discordance between the SCL-90 and therapists' psychopathology ratings. *Arch Gen Psychiatry* 40:389–393, 1983.
21. Greist JH, Klein MH, Van Cura LJ: A computer interview for psychiatric patient target symptoms. *Arch Gen Psychiatry* 29:247–253, 1973.
22. Fowler DR, Finklestein A, et al: *The PIQE, a computer-administered problem-oriented interview.* Dallas V. A. Medical Center, Dallas, Texas.

23. Endicott J, Spitzer RL: A diagnostic interview: The schedule for affective disorders and schizophrenia. *Arch Gen Psychiatry* 35:837–844, 1978.
24. Spitzer RL, Endicott J: *Schedule for Affective Disorders and Schizophrenia: Change Version*. New York, Biometrics Research. 1978.
25. Commings D: A computerized version of the Diagnostic Interview Schedule. Duarte, CA, City of Hope Medical Center, 1984.
26. Beck AT, Beamesderfer A: Assessment of depression: The depression inventory: Psychological measurements in psychopharmacology, in Pichot P (ed): *Modern Problems in Psychopharmacology*. Basel, S Karger, 1974, p 151.
27. Young RC, Biggs JT, Ziegler VE, et al. A rating scale for mania. Reliability, validity, and sensitivity. *BR J Psychiatry* 133:429–435, 1978.
28. McNair DM, Lorr M, Droppleman LF: *Profile of Mood States*. San Diego, Education and Industrial Testing Services, 1971.
29. Saltzman C, Kochansky GE, Shader RI: Rating scales for geriatric psychopharmacology—a review. *Psychopharmacol Bull* 8:3–50, 1972.
30. Felstein MF, Felstein SE, McHugh PR: "Mini-Mental State": A practical method for grading the cognitive state of patients for the clinician. *J Psychiatr Res* 12:189–198, 1975.
31. Taylor MA: *The Neuropsychiatric Mental Status Exam*. New York, SP Medical and Scientific Books, 1981.
32. Strub RL, Black WF: *The Mental Status Exam in Neurology*. Philadelphia, FA Davis, 1977.
33. Lippman R, Covi L: Outpatient treatment of neurotic depression: Medication and group psychotherapy, in Spitzer R, Klein DL (eds): *Evaluation of the Psychological Therapies*. Baltimore, Johns Hopkins University Press, 1976, pp 178–218.
34. Alstrom AG, Nordlund CC: A rating scale of phobic disorders. *Acta Psychiatr Scand* 68:111–116, 1983.
35. Simpson GM, Angus J: A rating scale for extrapyramidal side effects. *Acta Psychiatr Scand [Suppl]* 212:11–19, 1970.
36. Guy W (ed): *National Institute of Mental Health Abnormal Involuntary Movements Scale. ECEDU Assessment Manual*. Washington, US Department of Health, Education and Welfare, 1976.
37. Simpson G. Hiliary L, Zoubok B, et al: A rating scale for tardive dyskinesia. *Psychopharmacology* 64:171–179, 1979.
38. Donnelly EF, Murphy DL, Waldman IN, et al: Prediction of antidepressant responses to imipramine. *Neuropsychobiology* 5:94–101, 1979.
39. Donnelly EF, Goodwin FK, Waldman IN et al: Prediction of antidepressant responses to lithium. *Am J Psychiatry* 135:552–556, 1978.
40. Aaronson AL: *MMPI Scoring Program*. Richland, WA, Psychological Software Specialists, 1983.

Evaluation of Affective Syndromes

Irl Extein, M.D., Mark S. Gold, M.D.,
and Frederick C. Goggans, M.D.

1. Diagnosis of Affective Disorders

The major affective syndromes—major depression and mania—are common psychiatric disturbances that, when present, cause significant morbidity but usually respond well to psychopharmacological treatments.[1-3] In medicine in general, physicians are more aggressive in trying to identify treatable conditions. Thus, there has been an appropriately increased emphasis since the advent of effective antidepressant medication and lithium over the last 25 years on the diagnosis of major depression and mania. In this chapter we discuss current clinical nosology of affective disorders, practical aspects of evaluation, and laboratory tests that may augment diagnosis and treatment planning. We focus on how evaluative procedures help to identify subgroups of patients likely to respond to specific pharmacological treatments and help to monitor and optimize treatment.

The DSM III[4] embodies much of what is best in contemporary nosology and appropriately emphasizes affective disorders in its diagnostic hierarchy. The DSM III defines major depression, mania, and other syndromes in terms of clear and operational descriptive criteria that are reliable, meaning that properly trained raters tend to agree on diagnoses.

2. Diagnostic Validity

Although the DSM III criteria are purely descriptive or phenomenological, there are other criteria that contribute to establishing the validity of the diagnostic categories.[5] These include course and outcome, family history, pharmacological response,

Irl Extein, M.D. • Fair Oaks Hospital at Boca/Delray, Delray Beach, Florida 33445.   *Mark S. Gold, M.D.* • Research Facilities, Fair Oaks Hospital, Summit, New Jersey 07901, and Fair Oaks Hospital at Boca/Delray, Delray Beach, Florida 33445.   *Frederick C. Goggans, M.D.* • Neuropsychiatric Evaluation Unit, Psychiatric Institute of Fort Worth, Fort Worth, Texas 76104, and Department of Psychiatry, University of Texas Health Science Center, Dallas, Texas 75235.

and biological markers. One would expect the DSM IV will include these other aspects of psychiatric diagnosis, which are particularly relevant to affective disorders.

The course and outcome of affective disorders are critical in characterizing these disorders. One of the hallmarks of affective disorders is their episodic nature. The natural course of major depressions and manias is to remit and then recur. Kraepelin[6] emphasized the episodic nature of manic–depressive illness in contrasting this disorder to the chronic downhill course of dementia praecox or schizophrenia.[7] Family history can be useful in diagnosing affective disorders. Affective disorders and schizophrenia "breed true," and genetic studies have helped establish bipolar affective disorder as a separate illness from unipolar depression.[8] Psychopharmacological response data help define affective disorders also. One could argue that response to antidepressants and lithium is the best—certainly the most practical—way to define an affective disorder. Thus, one might establish "lithium-responsive syndromes" rather than worrying about the intricacies of phenomenology. This has been of some practical importance. For example, periodic catatonia, schizophreniform disorder, and cyclothymic disorder have been shown to contain high proportions of lithium responders[1-3] and hence to be possible bipolar equivalents. As is discussed later, laboratory tests not only can serve to confirm the diagnosis of depression or mania but may go beyond being diagnostic markers and define biological subgroups that have characteristic treatment response.

3. Organic Affective Disorders

The DSM III has established a diagnostic "hierarchy" of organic disorders, then affective disorders, then schizophrenia. This is very important for evaluation purposes. Perhaps the most important aspect is that a psychiatrist cannot make the diagnosis of a primary psychiatric disorder until any possible organic cause of the syndrome has been ruled out. As psychiatrists became more medically sophisticated, more medical causes of "secondary" affective syndromes are being identified. The DSM III dignified such syndromes with the title of "organic affective disorders" but left the criteria quite vague. There are many examples. Many medical problems can lead to, exacerbate, or complicate affective disorders.[10] Certainly, major depressions that complicate the course of serious medical illness, such as postmyocardial infarction or chronic neurological disease, must be considered carefully from a medical viewpoint. Affective syndromes may be a *forme fruste* of a variety of medical illnesses, including endocrine diseases. Recent work has suggested that early or "subclinical" hypothyroidism (diagnosed by the TRH stimulation test, not by base-line thyroid function) may present to the psychiatrist as depression before classic signs and symptoms of hypothyroidism develop. Similarly, the early stages of Cushing's disease may be difficult to distinguish from depressive disorder clinically and biochemically. Vitamin and other nutritional deficiencies may lead to or exacerbate depression. The incidence of folate deficiency in depressives (without necessarily showing full-blown megaloblastic anemia) has been shown to be high. Medications, antihypertensives in particular, can lead to or exacerbate depression.

The interplay of affective syndromes and drug and alcohol abuse is complex and a research frontier. Several basic principles are emerging. First, evaluation for major depression (clinical and laboratory) must be done after detoxification to have real significance for treatment planning.[9] Many drug intoxication and withdrawal states can cause affective changes. Second, some substance abusers have two illnesses, e.g., alcoholism and bipolar disorder, and need to be treated aggressively for both, e.g., lithium and Alcoholics Anonymous. Third, the physiological sequelae of chronic drug abuse can cause affective syndromes, such as the protracted abstinence syndrome of recently detoxified methadone addicts or the depressive syndromes seen in some heavy cocaine users after withdrawal. These may reflect persistent deficits in brain endorphin and norepinephrine systems, respectively. Affective disturbances are common in patients with dementia and related organic brain syndromes. Lability and affective disinhibition are common, as is depression. It is often difficult to tell whether depression in the elderly is part of an organic brain syndrome or is an independent depressive disorder. A thorough medical assessment and empirical antidepressant medication trials are often indicated.

4. The Spectrum of Affective Syndromes

The DSM III hierarchy clearly encourages a broad view of affective disorders in the face of what used to be thought of as characterological disturbances or schizophrenia. Affective disorders must be ruled out before schizophrenia can be diagnosed. Thus, major depression or mania with psychosis (mood congruent or mood incongruent) can be diagnosed so long as the full-blown affective syndromes are present. Longstanding "subaffective" syndromes such as dysthymic disorder and cyclothymic disorder are considered affective disorders rather than personality disorders. This broad view of affective disorder is based on validity criteria mentioned above.

Multiple factors impinge on affective syndromes, including personality characteristics, medical illness, and life stress.[11] The DSM III appropriately sets these factors as separate diagnostic axes independent of the presence or absence of the affective syndrome on axis 1. This acknowledges the reality that, for example, a patient with a major depressive episode may or may not have a longstanding personality disorder and may or may not have been under unusual life stress or loss prior to the beginning of the

Table 14-1. Summary of DSM III Criteria for a Major Depressive Episode

A. Dysphoric mood or loss of interest or pleasure in all or almost all usual activities
B. At least four of the following present nearly every day for at least 2 weeks:
    1. Poor or increased appetite or significant weight loss or gain
    2. Insomnia or hypersomnia
    3. Psychomotor agitation or retardation
    4. Loss of interest or pleasure or decreased sexual desire
    5. Loss of energy
    6. Feelings of worthlessness, self-reproach, or inappropriate guilt
    7. Diminished ability to think or concentrate, indecisiveness
    8. Thoughts of death or suicide or suicide attempt
C. Not caused by certain specified psychotic or organic disorders

depression. The diagnosis of major depression (Table 14-1) is based on the presence or absence of the full-blown medical syndrome of depression with autonomous depressed mood and associated neurovegetative symptoms such as sleep and appetite disturbance, not on the other diagnostic axes. Studies have suggested that stress and loss can serve as precipitants to major depression and mania, but only in patients genetically predisposed. Patients with bipolar affective disorder reportedly have no more personality disorder than a control group of people not psychiatrically ill when the bipolar patients are tested between episodes of illness.

5. Practical Aspects of Evaluation

The diagnostic criteria discussed above are only as good as the data base from which diagnoses are made. As a practical matter, an optimal neuropsychiatric evaluation should be done during a drug- and medication-free evaluation period of 1–2 weeks. The evaluation should follow the biopsychosocial model and evaluate psychological, social, and biological functions. Often a multidisciplinary team approach is the most thorough. A crucial matter is to gather information from sources other than the patient. These sources may be able to give a more objective and detailed history. Depressed and manic patients are notoriously poor historians because their ill state impairs thinking and their mood colors their recollections of the past. The drug-free period is important in weeding out iatrogenic problems and placebo or milieu responders and allowing for uncontaminated psychiatric, medical, and laboratory assessment (see Table 14-2). Such simple variables as history of previous medication response, which is a powerful predictor of future response, sometimes takes painstaking detective work, contacting multiple sources, and requires the structure and time of an evaluation period to be documented properly. Given the high incidence of inadequate antidepressant medication trials,[12] it is very important to take pains to document medication history exactly.

6. Descriptive Predictors of Response to Antidepressant Treatment

The DSM III definition of major depressive disorder is an effort to define reliably the depressive syndrome most likely to require and respond to pharmacotherapy. This depression represents a clearly altered mental state compared to the patient's usual self,

Table 14-2. Clinical Advantages of Medication-Free Neuropsychiatric Evaluation of Patients with Affective Disorders

1. Observation of patient without influence of drugs or medications
2. Identification of iatrogenic problems
3. "Rule out" medical and neurological illnesses
4. Obtaining thorough history and family assessment
5. Identification of "placebo" or milieu responders

has a definite onset, causes a clear impairment of functioning, and has a definite duration. The important point is that patients manifest not only a relatively fixed, autonomous depressed mood but also a cluster of symptoms that involve multiple body systems, such as those regulating sleep, appetite, sexual drives, and gastrointestinal and other visceral functions (see Table 14-3). For depressed patients with no syndrome or endogenous elements and for whom depressive feelings seem entirely explicable in terms of neurotic character and/or life situation, psychotherapy alone may seem to be the treatment of choice. For patients at the other end of the spectrum who have the medical syndrome of major depression seemingly unrelated to psychological conflicts or life events, pharmacotherapy alone would be indicated. For the many patients who fall between these extremes, there is a place for psychotherapy as well as pharmacological treatment.[11] Generally, antidepressant medications are indicated to the extent that syndromal elements are present independent of the degree to which reactive features or neurotic traits may also be evident. Psychotherapy is usually indicated in depressed patients when reactive or neurotic features are present without severe symptoms of the medical syndrome or when these features persist after improvement in the medical syndrome.

Thus, the question of psychotherapy versus drugs is often a false one. Rather, the questions that should be asked are: For what symptoms or incapacities is this patient being treated? At what stage of the illness are different treatments most effectively used? The answers may result in a treatment plan that includes an initial attempt to deal with environmental stress, then antidepressant medication to relieve the neurovegetative symptoms and depressed mood, followed by psychotherapy when the patient has improved enough to be able to explore the issues that may have precipitated the depression. The continued use of medications as prophylaxis against recurrent episodes of depression or mania must be considered in a separate category.

Various investigators have studied depressed patients in the hope of finding whether specific symptoms are predictors of response to antidepressant treatment.[1-3,13-15] Table 14-3 contains a summary of the symptoms found to be associated with good and poor response to antidepressant treatment. Good premorbid functioning, autonomy of depression, and changes in sleep, appetite, and psychomotor status are

Table 14-3. Descriptive Predictors of Response
to Antidepressant Medications

Good Outcome	Poor Outcome
Good premorbid functioning	Chronicity
Clear onset of depressive episode	Delusions or hallucinations[a]
Anorexia	Prominent anxiety
Middle and late insomnia	Hypochondriacal or histrionic traits
Psychomotor changes	Reactivity of mood
Emotional withdrawal	
Inability to experience pleasure	
Autonomy of depression	

[a]Respond better to combined antidepressant/neuroleptic or ECT.

probably the most helpful clinical predictors of good outcome. Bipolar depression is defined as a major depression in a patient with a history of mania. Such a patient is said to have manic–depressive illness or bipolar affective disorder. Such a patient is likely to benefit from treatment with lithium carbonate both for the acute depression and as prophylaxis against recurrent depressive and manic episodes. Bipolar depressions tend to be more likely to be associated with low energy, hypersomnia, and psychomotor retardation, though these features are not diagnostic.

Bipolar depressed patients can be missed if they have histories of mild mania—called hypomania—only or if they are in their first few episodes of affective illness. This latter group of patients, who have had one or several depressions but have yet to develop a hypomania or mania, are called in retrospect "false unipolars" who will go on to show a hypomania or mania later. Psychotic depression often responds poorly to antidepressant medication alone.[16] Combination antipsychotic–antidepressant treatment or ECT may be required. Hypochondriacal, hysteroid, or anxious symptoms were shown to be associated with a poor outcome in one study.[15] The presence of these symptoms, however, should not preclude a trial of antidepressant medication if there are clinical and laboratory data to support the diagnosis of major depressive disorder. So-called "atypical depressions" marked by anxiety, hypersomnia, hyperphagia, mood reactivity, and characterological features are reported by some to respond well to MAO inhibitors, particularly if panic attacks are associated.[17] As was noted above, depressed patients with these symptoms may be treated optimally with a combination of pharmacotherapy and psychotherapy.

Although patients with major depressive episodes are the most likely to need and respond to antidepressant medications, the use of antidepressants in other categories of depression warrants attention. Many patients suffer from chronic low-grade depression, dysthymic disorder in DSM III terminology. In patients who develop major depressive episodes superimposed on such chronic low-grade depression—so-called "double depression"—the likelihood of successful response to treatment of the major depressive episode is reduced. Akiskal et al.[18] have distinguished early-onset characterological depressions from late-onset chronic depressions that complicate the course of major (unipolar) depressions and nonaffective illnesses. The characterological depressives include both "character spectrum disorders," often complicated by substance abuse, who have a generally unfavorable outcome, and "subaffective dysthymias," which tend to respond to tricyclics or lithium. Clearly, some patients with less severe depressions benefit from antidepressants. However, a recent study of tricyclic treatment of depressed outpatients found that the category of major depression largely accounted for the drug–placebo difference found for the entire sample.[19] Some clinicians find MAOIs the best pharmacological treatment for the chronic characterological depression.[17]

Patients diagnosed as cyclothymic by DSM III, with manic and depressive features but not sufficient for the diagnosis of bipolar disorder, have many features similar to bipolar patients. Perhaps most important was the finding that the cyclothymic patient has a pattern of response to tricyclics, including precipitation of mania, similar to the bipolar patient.[20] The heterogeneous group of patients diagnosed as schizoaffective includes many who respond well to antidepressants and/or lithium.

Many women with puerperal (postpartum) psychosis are suffering from an affective illness by most criteria.[21] In fact, postpartum psychosis should not be viewed as a disease in its own right. Women with affective disorders do, however, seem at greater risk for developing a depressive or manic episode in the postpartum period. Such episodes should be treated like any other episode, though with caution in regard to transmission of psychotropic medications to the newborn via breast milk.

7. Biological Predictors of Response to Antidepressant Treatment

As outlined in other chapters of this volume, there are a number of neuroendocrine and other biological markers[22] that are associated with major depressive disorders (see Table 14-4). These diagnostic tests, such as the dexamethasone suppression test (DST)[23] and thyrotropin-releasing hormone (TRH) test,[24] have confirmatory utility in identifying primary psychiatric major depression and help to identify candidates for psychopharmacological treatment or ECT. A shortened REM sleep latency has been shown to be a sensitive and relatively specific marker for major depression.[25] Investigators have hypothesized that a biological rhythm disturbance may be a fundamental component of the pathophysiology of depression.[26]

Neuroendocrine tests such as the DST and TRH test seem to have significance in treatment planning beyond mere correlations with DSM III diagnosis and are an important aspect of the evaluation of depressed patients. Identification of early or subclinical hypothyroidism[27] may identify a subgroup of depressives who respond to thyroid replacement alone or who require and respond to thyroid hormone potentiation (T_3 potentiation) of tricyclic antidepressants.[28] The association between early or subclinical hypothyroidism (identified by TRH tests or elevated base-line TSH) and rapid mood cycling (spontaneous or tricyclic induced)[29] suggests that thyroid testing can help identify patients at risk for the difficult problem of rapid mood cycling and may suggest avenues for treatment such as thyroid hormone treatment. Failure to normalize on the DST[30] or TRH[31] test after a successful course of antidepressant medication or ECT is associated with a much higher likelihood of relapse, which may be partially counteracted by aggressive follow-up treatment with antidepressants. These last two uses of neuroendocrine tests to define likely response to treatments and prognosis are

Table 14-4. Neuroendocrine Abnormalities in Patients with Major Depressions

Hormone	Basal	Challenged
GH	—	L-Dopa, insulin, amphetamine, and clonidine stimulation ↓; TRH stimulation ↑
PRL	↑	TRH stimulation ↓ Opioid stimulation ↓
LH	↓	LHRH stimulation ↑
TSH	—	TRH stimulation ↓ (unipolars)
ACTH/cortisol	↑	Dexamethasone, nonsuppresion; amphetamine stimulation ↓
MHPG	↓ (bipolars)	

examples of laboratory parameters giving information useful in treatment planning that simply could not be obtained by descriptive methods.

Some biological predictors have been identified for antidepressants that preferentially inhibit the uptake of norepinephrine (NE). These include the observation of an individual's mood response to a single dose of amphetamine and the level of daily excretion of biogenic amine metabolites such as 3-methoxy-4-hydroxyphenylglycol (MHPG). Studies by his group and others led Maas to hypothesize that there were at least two broad types of biological depressions—termed type A and Type B.[32] Type A depressions were felt to be associated with relatively low 24-hr excretion of MHPG, an acute euphoria or behavioral activation in response to 30 mg oral *d*-amphetamine, and a positive clinical response to a trial of imipramine, desipramine, or other norepinephrine-augmenting antidepressant. Type B depressions, on the other hand, were felt to be associated with a lack of response to imipramine, a relatively moderate or high MHPG excretion, and a positive response to amitriptyline or agents that were more likely to affect serotonin-containing neurons.

Patients with bipolar depression were noted to have the lowest MHPG excretion of any clinical subgroup.[33] Such patients have been shown to be particularly likely to respond to imipramine and other noradrenergic antidepressants.[1-3]

Recently, the National Collaborative Study on the Psychobiology of Depression examined the relationship between pretreatment neurotransmitter metabolites and the response to imipramine or amitriptyline treatment.[34] Eighty-seven patients who met research diagnostic criteria for major depression of either the unipolar or bipolar type were included in the study. There were no significant differences in the therapeutic effectiveness of the two antidepressant drugs in the group of patients as a whole. Low compared to normal or high pretreatment MHPG was associated with better response to imipramine. No significant relationships were found, however, between urinary MHPG levels and the subsequent response or lack of response to amitriptyline.[30] Low levels of CSF 5-HIAA, a metabolite of serotonin, were not related to outcome of amitriptyline therapy, but low pretreatment CSF 5-HIAA was correlated with response to imipramine.

Although the National Collaborative Study suggests revision of some of the earlier theories of Maas, the validity of the notion that low MHPG predicts imipramine responsiveness was confirmed by this study.

Given the clinical and biological heterogeneity of DSM-III-diagnosed patients along the depressive spectrum, it is not surprising that there is much variation in response rates of different subgroups of depressives to antidepressants. There is a high rate of spontaneous remission as well as placebo response in depressive illness.[1-3] Up to 50% of a mixed group of depressives will improve over several months without specific treatment. Thus, there is much "noise" in any systematic evaluation of antidepressant efficacy. In populations well defined by DSM III diagnoses and neuroendocrine tests, there is no doubt less. One clinically useful approach to the problem of variability in response is to apply, when practical, a drug-free "washout" or evaluation period when initially assessing the depressed patient. Not only does this allow for a careful psychiatric and medical assessment and relief from the ill effects of medication, but it also insures that patients with spontaneous remissions or response to psychosocial support will be spared unnecessary labeling and medication. This process also maximizes the probability that patients treated with antidepressants will be true pharmacological responders.

8. Target Symptoms for Antidepressant Treatment

In order to prescribe antidepressants properly, it is important to define target symptoms for the treatment.[1-3] In many clear-cut cases of major depressive episodes with good premorbid functioning, one can aim for virtually an absolute and complete remission of the depressive syndrome. In cases that are less clean cut, especially where there have been characterological and other longstanding problems that may be difficult to sort out from the depression in question, one may aim for improvement and symptom reduction without expecting remission from all the depressive symptomatology. The physician, as a general rule, can expect antidepressants at best to return the patient to his or her base-line level of functioning before the depression but seldom to affect base-line character structure or functioning. Well-designed studies of female outpatients with major depression have shown that antidepressant medications and psychotherapy have additive benefits, but on different target symptoms.[35] The antidepressants were necessary to alleviate depression symptoms, whereas psychotherapy was necessary to improve social functioning.

The neurovegetative symptoms of depression are useful target symptoms to use in adjusting dosage and monitoring response. Full benefits for antidepressants are not seen until patients have achieved therapeutic levels for 3–4 weeks. However, improvement in sleep can often be seen much earlier. If sleeplessness or severe anxiety or agitation are problems, the temporary addition of sedative–hypnotics or a low dose of a neuroleptic, particularly at bedtime, can be helpful during the first few weeks of treatment. There is almost no place for use of a barbiturate or barbituratelike hypnotic in the treatment of depression in light of the availability of alternative medications and risk of addiction and lethal overdosage. Improvement in appetite, weight gain, and improvement in energy, concentration, and libido are important targets in monitoring response to antidepressants as well as changes in the mood itself. Note that depressive cognition, marked by hopelessness, helplessness, worthlessness, and suicidality, can accompany the depressed mood and needs to be assessed. It is also important to interview the patient's family to monitor progress. Depressed patients are notoriously negative in reporting and are often the last to notice their improvement.

It is the severity of symptoms such as poor nutritional status, psychosis, suicidality, and presence of family supports and cooperativeness of the patient that go into the decision of whether to treat the patient as an outpatient or inpatient. In view of the generally favorable response to treatment of depression, it is best in uncertain cases to err on the side of hospitalization.

9. The Differential Diagnosis of Mania

The differential diagnosis of a manic episode is just as complex and important as the differential diagnosis of a major depression. Manic–depressive patients in the manic state can display florid psychosis, including paranoia, auditory hallucinations, and Schneiderian "first-rank" symptoms indistinguishable from psychotic symptoms of schizophrenic psychosis.[36,37] Likewise, patients with schizophrenic disorder in the acutely psychotic state can manifest hyperactivity, irritability, and grandiosity suggestive of a manic state. The ability to differerentiate these two disorders is crucial for several reasons, including the more optimistic prognosis of affective illness and of antipsychotic medication in schizophrenia and the risk of tardive dyskinesia in misdiagnosed bipolar patients treated for many years with antipsychotic medication. Knowledge of the longitudinal course of a patient's, illness can improve the clinician's ability to distinguish mania from schizophrenia but in many cases does not eliminate the need to make treatment decisions, such as whether to use lithium carbonate, based on ambiguous cross-sectional clinical presentations.

In general, studies of acutely psychotic patients have shown that the presence of affective symptomatology predicts good outcome.[1–3,37] The presence or absence of first-rank psychotic symptoms alone has little prognostic significance. There are a number of good-prognosis psychotic illnesses that tend to have affective features: "good-prognosis" schizophrenia, schizoaffective disorder, schizophreniform disorder, atypical psychosis, brief reactive psychosis, cyclic psychosis, and periodic catatonia. There are studies that suggest that all of these related conditions contain significant subgroups of patients who respond to lithium. Genetic studies have demonstrated that schizoaffective and related disorders are closer to affective disorder than to schizophrenia.[38] The important questions still remain as to whether there is a true "third psychosis" independent of affective disorders and schizophrenia and how a psychiatrist can accurately identify from all excited psychotic patients the true manic patients who have a good prognosis and high proportion of lithium responders.

Several biological markers have been suggested for mania. Though urinary MHPG tends to be low in bipolar depression and to increase in the manic phase, MHPG in mania is not usually above normal. Blunted TSH response to TRH has been demonstrated in about 60% of acute manics and has been suggested as a marker that can distinguish mania from schizophrenia.[39] A high rate of DST nonsuppression has been reported in mania also. A blunted growth hormone response to apomorphine has been reported in mania compared to schizophrenia and schizophrenifrom disorder.[40] Higher erythrocyte lithium ratios (intracellular to extracellular) have been reported in bipolar depression and mania compared to other psychiatric disorders and controls.[41] Higher growth hormone responses to apomorphine and higher lithium ratios reportedly predict lithium response in schizophrenia and schizophreniform disorder.[42] Though initial reports of cerebral ventricular enlargement in chronic schizophrenia raised the possibility that this might be a specific finding, recent studies showed ventricular enlargement in some patients with affective disorder and no differences on this measure among schizophrenic, schizoaffective, and bipolar patients.[43] It has been suggested that there is a subgroup of schizophrenics, defined by enlarged ventricles on CAT scan and organic deficits on neuropsychological testing, who show poor response to neuroleptics and poor prognosis in general.[44]

References

1. Klein DF, Gittelman R, Quitkin F, et al: *Diagnosis and Drug Treatment of Psychiatric Disorders.* Baltimore, Williams & Wilkins, 1980.

2. Goodwin FK: Drug treatment of affective disorders: General principles, in Jarvik ME (ed): *Psychopharmacology in the Practice of Medicine*. New York, Appleton-Century-Crofts, 1977, pp 241–253.
3. Baldessarini RJ: *Chemotherapy in Psychiatry*. Cambridge, Harvard University Press, 1979.
4. American Psychiatric Association, Committee on Nomenclature and Statistics: *Diagnostic and Statistical Manual of Mental Disorders*, ed 3. Washington, American Psychiatric Association, 1980.
5. Robins E, Guze S: Establishment of diagnostic validity in psychiatric illness: Its application to schizophrenia. *Am J Psychiatry* 126:983–987, 1970.
6. Kraepelin E: *Manic Depressive Insanity and Paranoia*. Edinburgh, E & S Livingstone, 1921.
7. Kraepelin E: *Dementia Praecox and Paraphrenia* (Barclay RM, trans). Edinburgh, E & S Livingstone, 1919.
8. Winokur G, Morrison J, Clancy J, et al: The Iowa 500: A blind family history comparison of mania, depression, and schizophrenia. *Arch Gen Psychiatry* 27:462–464, 1972.
9. Dackis CA, Pottash ALC, Gold MS, et al: The dexamethasone suppression test for major depression among opiate addicts. *Am J Psychiatry* 141:810–811, 1984.
10. Hall RCW, Popkin MK, Devaul RA, et al: Physical illness presenting as psychiatric disease. *Arch Gen Psychiatry* 35:1315–1320, 1978.
11. Goodwin FK, Extein L: The biological basis of affective disorders, in Cancro R, Shapiro L, Kesselman M (eds): *Progress in the Functional Psychoses*. New York, Spectrum Publications, 1979, pp 129–152.
12. Keller MB, Kleman GL, Lavori PW, et al: Treatment received by depressed patients. *JAMA* 248:1848–1855, 1982.
13. Bielski RJ, Friedel RO: Prediction of tricyclic antidepressant response: A critical review. *Arch Gen Psychiatry* 33:1479–1489, 1976.
14. Charney DS, Nelson JL: Delusional and nondelusional unipolar depression: further evidence for distinct subtypes. *Am J Psychiatry* 138:328–333, 1981.
15. Kupfer DJ, Spiker DG: Refractory depression, prediction of nonresponse by clinical indicators. *J Clin Psychiatry* 42:307–312, 1981.
16. Glassman AH, Roose SP: Delusional depression—a distinct clinical entity? *Arch Gen Psychiatry* 38:424–427, 1981.
17. Liebowitz MR, Quitkin FM, Steward JW, et al: Phenelzine *v.* imipramine in atypical depression. *Arch Gen Psychiatry* 41:669–677, 1984.
18. Akiskal HS, Rosenthal TL, Haykal RF, et al: Characterological depressions. *Arch Gen Psychiatry* 37:777–783, 1980.
19. Stewart JW, Quitkin FM, Liebowitz MR, et al: Efficacy of desipramine in depressed outpatients. *Arch Gen Psychiatry* 40:202–207, 1983.
20. Akiskal HS, Djenderedjian AH, Rosenthal RH, et al: Cyclothymic disorder: Validating criteria for inclusion in the bipolar affective group. *Am J Psychiatry* 134:1227–1233, 1977.
21. Brockington IF, Cernick KF, Schofield EM, et al: Puerperal psychosis. *Arch Gen Psychiatry* 38:829–833, 1981.
22. Gold MS, Pottash ALC, Extein L: Diagnosis of depression in the 1980's. *JAMA* 245:1562–1564, 1981.
23. Carroll BJ, Feinberg M, Greden JF, et al: A specific laboratory test for the diagnosis of melancholia. *Arch Gen Psychiatry* 38:15–22, 1981.
24. Extein I, Pottash ALC, Gold MS: The thyrotropin-releasing hormone test in the diagnosis of unipolar depression. *Psychiatry Res* 5:311–316, 1981.
25. Kupfer DJ: REM latency: A psychobiological marker for primary depressive disease. *Biol Psychiatry* 11:159–174, 1976.
26. Rosenthal NE, Sack DA, Gillin JC, et al: Seasonal affective disorder. *Arch Gen Psychiatry* 41:72–80, 1984.
27. Gold MS, Pottash ALC, Extein I: Hypothyroidism and depression. *JAMA* 245:1919–1925, 1981.
28. Targum SD, Greenberg R, Harmon R, et al: Adjunctive thyroid hormone in refractory depression, in: *New Research Abstracts, 136th Annual Meeting of the American Psychiatric Association*. Washington, American Psychiatric Association, 1982, p NR38.
29. Cowdry RW, Wehr TA, Zis AP, et al: Thyroid abnormalities associated with rapid cycling bipolar illness. *Arch Gen Psychiatry* 40:414–420, 1983.
30. Greden JF, Gardner R, King D, et al: Dexamethasone suppression test in antidepressant treatment of melancholia. *Arch Gen Psychiatry* 40:493–500, 1983.
31. Kirkegaard C, Bjorum N, Cohn D, et al. Studies on the influence of biogenic amines and psychoactive

drugs on the prognostic value of the TRH stimulation test in endogenous depression. *Psychoneuroendocrinology* 2:131–136, 1977.

32. Maas JW: Clinical and biochemical heterogeneity of depressive disorders. *Ann Intern Med* 88:556–563, 1978.

33. Schildraut JJ, Orsulak PJ, Schatzberg AF, et al: Toward a biochemical classification of depressive disorders I: Differences in urinary MHPG and other catecholamine metabolites in clinically defined subtypes of depressions. *Arch Gen Psychiatry* 35:1427–1433, 1978.

34. Maas JW, Kocsis JH, Bowden CL, et al: Pre-treatment neurotransmitter metabolites and response to imipramine or antriptyline treatment. *Psychol Med* 12:37–43, 1982.

35. Klerman GL, DiMascio A, Weissman J, et al: Treatment of depression by drugs and psychotherapy. *Am J Psychiatry* 131:186–191, 1974.

36. Carlson G, Goodwin F: The stages of mania—a longitudinal analysis of the manic episode. *Arch Gen Psychiatry* 28:221–228, 1973.

37. Pope HG, Lipinski JF: Diagnosis in schizophrenia and manic–depressive illness. *Arch Gen Psychiatry* 35:811–828, 1978.

38. Pope H, Lipinski J, Cohen B, et al: Schizoaffective disorder—an invalid diagnosis? A comparison of schizoaffective disorder, schizophrenia, and affective disorder. *Am J Psychiatry* 137:921–927, 1980.

39. Extein I, Pottash ALC, Gold MS, et al: Using the protirelin test to distinguish mania from schizophrenia. *Arch Gen Psychiatry* 39:77–81, 1982.

40. Hitzemann R, Hirschowitz J, Hitzemann B, et al: The prolactin response in schizophrenic, schizophreniform, and manic disorders. *Biol Psychiatry* 19:913–918, 1984.

41. Ramsey TA, Frazer A, Mendels J, et al: The erythrocyte lithium–plasma lithium ratio in patients with primary affective disorders. *Arch Gen Psychiatry* 36:457–461, 1979.

42. Hirschowitz J, Zemlan FP, Garven DL: Growth hormone levels and lithium ratios as predictors of success of lithium therapy in schizophrenia. *Am J Psychiatry* 139:646–649, 1982.

43. Rieder RO, Mann LS, Weinberger DR, et al: Computed tomographic scans in patients with schizophrenia, schizoaffective, and bipolar affective disorder. *Arch Gen Psychiatry* 40:735–739, 1983.

44. Crow TJ: Molecular pathology of schizophrenia—more than one disease process. *Br J Med* 280:1, 1980.

Evaluation of Psychotic Syndromes

David E. Sternberg, M.D., and A. L. C. Pottash, M.D.

1. Introduction

Psychosis is used here to refer to a clinical state characterized by impairment of reality contact (i.e., presence of delusional ideation and/or hallucinatory perceptions) and, by implication, a major disruption of functioning. A psychotic state is not specific to any diagnosis. Multiple pathways lead to a psychotic state. Table 15-1 lists those disorders, both "organic" and "functional," in the DSM III diagnostic classification that are either always or occasionally associated with a psychotic state.

A significant percentage of people presenting in a psychotic state will, on proper evaluation, be found to have an underlying medical illness that is responsible for their symptoms. In some instances, the organic factor that produces the psychotic state may constitute a life-threatening medical illness. It follows that the first concern of the clinician in assessing the acutely psychotic patient is to rule out a life-threatening medical condition. Having ruled out potentially fatal conditions, the evaluator next considers other serious medical illnesses that, though not imminently life threatening, need prompt medical attention.

The DSM III classification requires that prior to assuming a "functional" psychotic disorder, the clinician must rule out a "known organic factor by history or medical laboratory examination." Obviously, the more thorough the search for an organic factor in psychotic states, the more frequently will one be found. In a large study, Hall and co-workers reported that an organic illness was the absolute or presumed cause of the psychotic state in over 9% of the patients.

Because of the importance of early and accurate diagnosis of medical disease producing a psychotic state, the evaluation and differential diagnosis of "organic" psychosis is discussed first, followed by the "functional" psychoses.

2. Medical Causes of Psychosis

The causes of organic brain syndromes that can produce psychotic states are numerous. Table 15-2 provides an extensive list of medical conditions that can produce

David E. Sternberg, M.D. • Falkirk Hospital, Central Valley, New York 10917, and Department of Psychiatry, Yale University School of Medicine, New Haven, Connecticut 06508.   ***A. L. C. Pottash, M.D.*** • Fair Oaks Hospital at Boca/Delray, Delray Beach, Florida 33445, and Fair Oaks Hospital, Summit, New Jersey 07901.

Table 15-1. Disorders in DSM III Classification Associated with Psychosis

Organic mental disorder
  Dementias
    Primary degenerative dementia
    Multi-infarct dementia
  Substance induced
    Alcohol intoxication, idiosyncratic intoxication, withdrawal, withdrawal delirium, hallucinosis, dementias
    Barbiturate withdrawal, withdrawal delirium
    Cocaine intoxication or other sympathomimetic
    Amphetamine intoxication, delirium, delusional disorder
    Phencyclidine (PCP) intoxication, delirium, mixed organic disorder
    Hallucinogen hallucinosis, delusional disorder
    Cannabis delusional disorder
    Other or unspecified substance intoxication, withdrawal, delirium, delusional disorder, hallucinosis, mixed organic mental disorder
  Organic brain syndromes
    Delirium
    Dementia
    Organic delusional syndromes
    Organic hallucinosis
    Atypical or mixed organic brain syndrome
Schizophrenic disorders
Paranoid disorders
  Paranoia
  Shared paranoid disorder
  Acute paranoid disorder
  Atypical paranoid disorder
Other psychotic disorders
  Schizophreniform disorder
  Brief reactive psychosis
  Schizoaffective disorder
  Atypical psychosis, e.g., postpartum psychosis
Affective disorder
  Major affective disorders
    Bipolar disorder
    Major depression
  Atypical affective disorders
    Atypical bipolar disorder
    Atypical depression
Personality disorders
  Paranoid personality disorder
  Schizotypal personality disorder
  Borderline personality disorder

psychosis. Dysfunction of brain tissue may either occur because of a primary pathology within the brain itself or be secondary to pathological conditions arising outside the central nervous system.

A number of diseases such as Alzheimer's, Pick's, Huntington's, and Parkinson's disease cause loss or degeneration of neurons in the substance of the brain. Trauma, infections, and tumors may also damage brain tissue. In epilepsy, there are abnormal

Table 15-2. Medical Disorders Associated with Psychosis[a]

Primary brain dysfunction
  Parenchymatous disease of the CNS
    Alzheimer's disease
    Huntington's chorea*
    Marchiafava disease (degeneration of corpus callosum)
    Parkinsonism
    Pick's disease
  Epilepsy
    Postictal state
    Psychomotor epilepsy*
  Brain tumors, primary and metastatic*
  Trauma
    Extradural hematoma
    Subdural hematoma
  CNS infections and postinfectious states
    Cerebral abscess
    Cerebral malaria*
    Encephalitis (e.g., herpes*)
    Jakob–Creutzfeldt disease*
    Meningitis
    Neurosyphilis*
    Rabies*
    Syndenham's chorea*
  Vascular
    Aneurism
    Atherosclerosis
    Collagen vascular disease*
    Embolus*
    Hypertensive encephalopathy
    Subarachnoid hemorrhage
  Normal-pressure hydrocephalus
  Other noninfective cerebral disease
    Multiple sclerosis
    Neurofibromatosis (Von Recklinghausen's)
    Pellagra*
    Tuberous sclerosis*
    Wernicke's encephalopathy*
Secondary brain dysfunction
  Systemic infections with fever and/or sepsis
  Hypoxic, hypoperfusion, and acid–base imbalance states
    Acidosis (respiratory)
    Alkalosis (respiratory or metabolic)
    Anemia (severe primary or secondary)
    Blood loss
    Cardiac arrhythmia
    Cardiac failure
    CO_2 narcosis
    Hypotension
  Endocrinopathies
    Corticosteroid disorders (Cushing's syndrome,* Addison's disease–adrenal cortical hypofunction)
    Pancreatic disorder (diabetic ketosis)

(continued)

Table 15-2. (*Continued*)

Parathyroid disorder (hyperparathyroidism–hypercalcemia, hypoparathyroidism–hypocalcemia)
Pituitary hypofunction
Postpartum psychosis*
Thyroid dysfunction (thyrotoxicosis, hypothyroidism, myxedema*)
Endogenous intoxication
  Hepatic encephalopathy
  Hypomagnesemia
  Porphyria*
  Uremia
  Wilson's disease* (hepatolenticular degeneration)
Exogenous drugs and toxins
  Alcohol (intoxication and withdrawal*)
  Amantadine*
  Amphetamines* and other sympathomimetics
  Anticholinergics* (atropine)
  Anticonvulsants (phenytoin and cogeners)
  Antihistamines
  Antihypertensives* (glutethimide, methyldopa, propranolol)
  Antiparkinsonian drugs* (L-dopa, anticholinergics)
  Baclofen*
  Barbiturates and other sedative/hypnotics (intoxication and withdrawal)
  Bromides*
  Cannabis
  Cimetidine (Tagamet)
  Cocaine*
  Colchicine
  Digitalis and cardiac glycosides
  Disulfiram* (Antabuse)
  Hallucinogens* (LSD, mescaline, PCP)
  Heavy metals* (lead, manganese, mercury, thallium)
  Insecticides (organophosphates)
  Isoniazid*
  Mushroom poisoning*
  Nutmeg
  Opiates
  Phencyclidine* (PCP and other arycyclohexylamine)
Heatstroke

*a*Conditions in which psychosis is especially common are marked by an asterisk (*).

electrical discharges of neurons within the brain. Vascular disorders such as subarachnoid hemorrhage adversely affect brain tissue function. There are also disorders of the cerebrospinal fluid system, as in normal-pressure hydrocephalus, that cause organic deficits.

The brain depends on the rest of the body for its nourishment and internal environment. If an inadequate supply of blood reaches the brain, or if that blood is deficient in oxygen or glucose, the brain cannot function properly. Endocrine and metabolic disturbances, infections with fever and sepsis, and electrolyte and acid–base imbalances may provide an improper internal environment for brain tissue functioning. Similarly, drugs, alcohol, poisons, heavy metals, and other toxins may impair brain tissue directly or impair other organs that the brain depends on for adequate functioning. Certain nutrients, such as vitamin B_{12}, folate, and thiamine, are also essential for the operation of the central nervous system.

2.1. Life-Threatening Conditions

Anderson has identified seven not uncommon medical causes of acute psychosis that are potentially fatal.[1] These include (1) cerebrovascular accident, (2) hypertensive encephalopathy, (3) hypoglycemia, (4) hypoxic and hypoperfusion states, (5) meningitis and encephalitis, (6) poisoning, and (7) Wernicke–Korsakoff syndrome. Other life-endangering conditions that might be added to the list are diabetic ketoacidosis, nonketotic hyperosmolar states, hyperthermia, acute adrenal inefficiency, thyroid storm, subdural hematoma, and drug-withdrawal state.

2.2. Examination for Organic Factors

Clearly, evaluating clinicians ought to rule out organic etiology of a psychotic state as part of the initial evaluation. There is much information that can be gathered in the initial interview that will alert the clinician to the possibility of underlying medical illness (Table 15-3).

2.2.1. Initial Interview

Primary is the need for the clinician to maintain a high index of suspicion that medical illness is a potential underlying cause of the psychotic state. Age of onset of psychosis can be an aid in differential diagnosis. Since, by definition, schizophrenia does not begin after age 40, a first episode of psychosis in a person over 40 without an affective syndrome is most likely organic in origin. A rapid onset of psychotic symptoms suggests an organic etiology. Whereas "functional" psychoses are generally preceded by a prolonged prodromal period, such organic psychoses as drug (e.g., hallucinogens or toxins) intoxications, drug withdrawals, or the psychosis of temporal lobe epilepsy are characterized by rapid onset. Since some medical and psychiatric disorders have a hereditary basis, a careful family history of illness should be obtained.

Table 15-3. Clues to an Organic Cause of Psychosis

---

1. Onset of symptoms after age 40
2. Rapid onset of symptoms (without prodromal period)
3. Family history of degenerative brain disease (e.g., Wilson's, Huntington's) or inherited metabolic disease (e.g., diabetes, porphyria)
4. Visual, tactile, or gustatory hallucinations
5. Psychotic symptoms develop during a major medical illness, while taking medically prescribed drugs, or in a patient with a diagnosed medical disorder
6. History of alcohol or drug abuse, multiple over-the-counter drug use, or exposure to occupational toxins
7. Signs of "organicity" on mental status testing: cognitive impairment, altered level of consciousness

---

Such inherited disorders as Wilson's disease and Huntington's chorea often first present with psychotic symptoms. Visual hallucinations or distortions should be considered of organic etiology until ruled out. Hall and co-workers[2] reported that 20% of patients with an organic psychosis experienced visual hallucinations or distortions, whereas only 0.5% of nonmedically impaired psychiatric patients presented these symptoms. Development of a psychotic state in a patient with a diagnosed medical illness is most often related to either complications of the disease itself or to the medications being used to treat the illness. It is essential that the clinician inquire about every substance that the patient ingests. This must include over-the-counter medications, laxatives, illicit drugs, exposure to fumes, toxins, or insecticides, and alcohol.

2.2.2. Mental Status

A careful mental status examination should be performed, as it can often suggest an organic illness. Inability to sustain attention, memory deficits, fluctuating levels of consciousness, and disorientation to time, person, or place are sensitive indicators of organic states. A valuable, rapid, and easily learned test that Folstein[3] showed to be a reliable method for distinguishing organic from functional disorders is the Mini Mental State Examination shown in Table 15-4.

2.3. Physical Examination

An attentive physical examination is essential in evaluating the psychotic patient. McIntyre and Romano[4] studied the practices of psychiatric residents in emergency rooms. They found that 59% of residents failed to perform physicals, but when phys-

Table 15-4. The Mini Mental State Examination[a]

Part I

a. What is the year, season, date, day of the week, month? (5 points)

b. Where are we: country, state, city or town, hospital, floor of building? (5 points)

c. The examiner names three objects, taking 1 sec to say each. The patient is asked to repeat all three objects after the examiner has said them. (3 points)

d. Serial sevens. One point for each correct answer. Stop after five answers. Or, spell the word "world" backwards. (5 points)

e. Recall the three objects named in c. (3 points)

Part II

a. The patient is shown a pencil and a watch and asked to name them. (2 points)

b. The patient is asked to repeat: "No ifs, ands, or buts." (1 point)

c. The patient is handed a sheet of paper and asked to carry out a three-state command: "Take this paper in your right hand, fold it in half, and put it on the floor." (3 points)

d. The patient is shown a sign that reads "Close your eyes" and is asked to read and obey the sign. (1 point)

e. The patient is asked to write a sentence. (1 point)

f. The patient is asked to copy a Bender–Gestalt figure. (1 point)

[a]Interpretation of results of Mini Mental State Examination: Demented patients averaged 9.7 points out of 30. Cognitively impaired depressed patients scored an average of 19 out of 30 points. The average score for normal subjects was 27.6 out of 30. Scores of 12 or less out of 30 indicate a high probability of organic illness. Adapted from Folstein *et al.*[3]

ical examinations were done, the results proved useful in 92% of the cases. Sometimes physical examinations are not performed on the psychotic patient because of actual or assumed lack of cooperation. Usually, a sympathetic but firm and straightforward approach will gain cooperation. Occasionally, use of a high-potency antipsychotic (e.g., i.m. haloperidol) or restraints are necessary because of agitation. Reliable vital signs should always be obtained. There is absolutely no excuse for failing to obtain complete vital sign measurements. In addition, a careful neurological examination is invaluable, with special attention to cranial nerves, cerebellum, and motor systems.

A variety of easily observed physical signs and symptoms are important indicators of organic illness. A fever may be a clue to a systemic infection or meningitis. A rapid pulse may be seen with infections, hypoglycemia, hypoperfusion, anemia, and hyperthyroidism among many other conditions. Hypertensive encephalopathy is suggested by markedly elevated blood pressure, whereas in hypoperfusion states blood pressure tends to be low. Headache and a stiff neck may be signs of meningitis or intracranial hemorrhage. Pupillary size may be a clue to a drug-induced delirium. Markedly dry skin suggests dehydration, especially in the elderly, or the possibility of an anticholinergic delirium. Needle marks on the skin suggests drug abuse. A confused alcoholic with nystagmus, ophthalmoplegia, and ataxia is likely to be suffering from Wernicke–Korsakoff syndrome and needs parenteral thiamine to prevent permanent neurological damage.

2.4. Laboratory Testing

The absolute minimum laboratory testing that should be used in all cases to evaluate a potential organic basis of a psychotic state includes SMA-22 (i.e., electrolytes, glucose, liver function, renal function), CBC with differential, urinalysis, complete toxicologic screen (preferably by a methodology other than thin-layer chromatography), and endocrine profile (thyroid, cortisol). Depending on other findings, chest and skull X rays, LP, and EEG should also be considered. Although the percentage of positive findings will be small, nevertheless, because some frontal lobe tumors can produce mental changes including psychosis prior to the development of any other neurological symptoms, this author recommends a CT scan of the head in all first-onset psychotic states. Additional laboratory testing (e.g., vitamin levels) is usually indicated in order to provide a complete evaluation to rule out organic etiologies. Because of the frequency with which these factors are associated with psychotic states, a special focus is made on endocrinologic, drug-induced, and alcohol-induced psychoses.

3. Endocrinopathy and Psychosis

Neuroendocrinologic research has increasingly emphasized the interaction between CNS function and hormonal regulation, pointing out both the influence of hormones on human behavior and the important impact of psychological state on endocrinology. Psychosis characterized by endocrine disturbance can be classified into three subgroups: (1) primary endocrine disease with psychotic manifestations, (2) life cycle physiological hormonal changes associated with increased risk of psychosis, and (3) hormonal treatment resulting in iatrogenic psychosis.

3.1. Thyroid Dysfunction

The thyroid hormones and their regulating hormones interact with a multitude of metabolic processes and probably have some neurotransmitter qualities themselves. The brain is thus exceedingly vulnerable to the adverse effect of thyroid hormone dysregulation.

3.1.1. Thyrotoxicosis

Excess thyroid hormone almost invariably leads to alterations of brain function, usually seen as anxiety, emotional lability, and hyperactivity.[5] However, psychosis with manic and schizophrenic features often undistinguishable from a functional psychosis is also seen. Indeed, acute psychotic delirium usually accompanied by fever is noted in "thyroid storm" and is a medical emergency requiring immediate treatment. Furthermore, it appears that a psychosis can be precipitated by rapid iatrogenic alteration, going from excess to normal thyroid levels as well as from severe deficiency to euthyroid states.[6]

3.1.2. Hypothyroidism and Myxedema

Deficiency of thyroid hormone beginning in adulthood is characterized by intellectual slowing with memory deficit, lethargy, and depression. Often such mental symptoms are the first indicator of thyroid deficiency. In the past, 50% (now 10%) of patients with myxedema presented with psychotic symptoms. The psychosis of "myxedema madness" is usually of a paranoid quality and can have florid delusions and hallucinations.[7] Treatment of myxedema with thyroid replacement usually results in complete resolution of the psychotic symptoms. Patients with bipolar illness characterized by rapid mood cycles who are often unresponsive to lithium treatment have a high incidence of hypothyroidism (often of subtle degrees) and benefit from thyroid replacement.[8]

3.2. Parathyroid Disease

Parathyroid hormone regulates levels of circulating calcium and the metabolism of phosphate. Excess hormone results in hypercalcemia and low phosphate, whereas hormone deficiency results in hypocalcemia and high phosphate. Since the balance of these minerals is essential for normal nervous function, disorders of parathyroid hormone often produce mental disorders.

3.2.1. Hyperparathyroidism

Although physical changes are usually predominant, mental symptoms are common. Occasionally, such mental changes as anergia with irritability and rage are the first manifestations of disease.[9] Psychosis is rare but is associated with the acute delirium of "parathyroid crisis."[10] Resolution of the mental symptoms coincides with the decrease in serum calcium levels.

3.2.2. Hypoparathyroidism

Many psychiatric manifestations accompany hypoparathyroidism, including impaired concentration, labile affect, depression, irritability, crying, anxiety, and panic attacks.[11] However, psychotic states are extremely rare in this disorder.

3.3. Corticosteroid Disorders

Cortisol both has profound impact on mental states and is profoundly affected by various mental states. Acute psychosis is associated with elevated levels of plasma cortisol. Patients with major depression have more frequent secretory cortisol spikes, higher absolute plasma levels of cortisol, and increased 24-hr secretion of cortisol.[12] Thus, elevated plasma cortisol levels alone do not necessarily imply the presence of Cushing's syndrome.

3.3.1. Cushing's Syndrome

Cushing's syndrome is defined as a state of sustained elevated levels of cortisol and (often) adrenal androgens, usually arising via an adrenal cortical disorder but possibly by a CNS defect resulting in excess corticotrophin-releasing factor (CRF) or excess ACTH secretion from the pituitary or an ectopic tumor. Major mental symptoms are noted in about 40% of patients with spontaneous Cushing's syndrome, often antedating physical stigmata.[13] Depression is most frequent. A depressive psychosis with delusions, hallucinations, and overt paranoid ideation is more common than a schizophrenialike psychosis.[14] Interestingly, the occurrence and severity of mental changes have not been shown to have any relationship to the clinical severity of the Cushing's syndrome.

3.3.2. Addison's Disease

Addison's disease is a state of low output of adrenal steroids arising from either a disorder of the adrenal cortex or impaired ACTH secretion from the pituitary. Mental abnormalities are invariably present, usually depression and apathy, memory deficit, and often irritability and anxiety. Such mental symptoms often occur prior to the impaired consciousness of an Addisonian crisis. Psychotic states associated with Addison's disease usually have a paranoid quality but can vary in type and can appear with affective (depressive or manic) features or can mimic a disorganized schizophrenialike state.[15,16]

3.3.3. Iatrogenic Psychoses: Corticosteroid and ACTH Induced

Minor affective changes are induced in most patients given corticosteroids or ACTH in therapeutic doses. However, major mental disturbances are produced in nearly 3% of patients when the prednisone dose is below 40 mg/day, 6% of patients when the dose is between 40 and 80 mg/day, and 18% of patients when the dose is over 80 mg/day.[12] About a fourth of these are psychotic states resembling either manic or paranoid schizophrenialike syndromes. The psychotic disorders associated with corticosteroid or ACTH administration may develop at any time during treatment and, although more common at high doses, show no consistent relationship to dosage. Recovery usually follows a decrease in dose or discontinuation, but it may be gradual. For patients who require continued high-dose treatment, lithium may provide prophylaxis of steroid-induced psychosis.[17]

3.4. Physiological Hormonal Changes and Psychosis

3.4.1. Puberty

The transitional period between childhood and adulthood is characterized by rapid changes in hormone levels resulting in a growth spurt, the appearance of secondary sexual characteristics, and possibly the profound psychological and behavioral changes of puberty (e.g., increased aggression, labile mood, sexual drive). Although not identified by DSM III, a rare clinical entity, "periodic psychosis of puberty," has been described.[18,19] Much more common in girls, the syndrome is characterized by severe psychotic symptoms becoming apparent during the luteal phase and resolving at the onset of menstrual bleeding. Curiously, in boys the cycles are also 4 weeks apart.

3.4.2. Postpartum Psychosis

The postpartum period is a time of "high risk" for various degrees of mental disturbance, with recent studies reporting some disturbance in about one-third of women.[20,21] Authorities conflict over whether labor and delivery act simply as stress factors precipitating disorders belonging to the major psychiatric categories or whether the major postpartum syndromes are specific and unique. Whereas mild depression appearing post-partum is so common as to be considered normal, at the other end of the spectrum lie severe psychotic depressions or manic psychoses and schizophrenialike psychoses with prominent Schneiderian symptoms.[22,23] Patients with such syndromes often have no family history of the major psychoses and no episodes of illness outside the postpartum period. Some authorities relate such syndromes to the acute drop in fetoplacental hormones, thyroxin, and cortisol after delivery,[24] but studies have failed to correlate these changes to the clinical findings.[25] The severe disorders tend to respond to the same pharmacological and other treatments as used in the disorders they mimic (e.g., antipsychotics, antidepressants, ECT, lithium). Some authors report an excellent antidepressant response to high-daily-dose progesterone. When the illness is acute and specific to the postpartum period, the prognosis is good.

4. Psychosis Associated with Drugs

After ruling out a medical illness etiology of the psychotic state, the physician should consider whether the psychosis might be caused by a drug of abuse, a drug withdrawal, or an idiosyncratic drug reaction. Such drug-associated psychotic states are common given the current prevalence of drug use in this society. Four general types of drug-associated psychotic states (i.e., adrenergic, anticholinergic, hallucinogen, phencyclidine) can be distinguished by their clinical presentations.[26]

4.1. Adrenergic Psychosis

This type of psychosis and its clinical picture result from excess sympathetic nervous activity. It may present with a paranoid schizophreniform reaction consisting of a florid psychotic state and a clear sensorium, mania or hypomania, and/or sterotypic behavior such as lip biting, skin picking, or bruxism. Marked insomnia is invariably present. Hallucinations can be both auditory and visual. Indeed, when caused by amphetamine toxicity, the psychosis can have multiple Schneiderian first-rank symptoms and be virtually indistinguishable from a schizophrenic episode.[28]

Adrenergic psychosis can be caused by ingestion of sympathomimetic stimulants (e.g., amphetamine, methylphenidate, cocaine) or by withdrawal from CNS depressants such as alcohol or sedative–hypnotic drugs (e.g., barbiturates, benzodiazepines, glutethimide, methaqualone). Hyperthyroidism also can present with an adrenergic psychosis. Withdrawal from CNS depressants is a medical emergency because of the appearance of status epilepticus and a potentially fatal course. The timing for development of an adrenergic psychosis following CNS depressant drug withdrawal depends on the degree of drug tolerance and especially on the half-life of the specific abused drug. The longer the drug's half-life, the later is the onset of the syndrome. Thus, addiction to diazepam with the long half-life of its active metabolites may not develop into an adrenergic psychosis for over a week after drug discontinuation or dosage decrease, whereas the delirium tremens of alcohol withdrawal occurs within 1 to 3 days.

Individuals with preexisting psychotic syndromes appear to be especially sensitive to psychostimulant drugs, and remitted patients can have a recurrence of psychotic symptoms following low-dose ingestion of these drugs.[29] High doses of virtually all psychostimulants will produce a psychotic state in all individuals, including those assessed to be normal.[30] The most common psychotic reaction to high-dose psychostimulant is a paranoid psychotic state with auditory hallucinations that resembles paranoid schizophrenia.[31,32] Additionally, cocaine-induced psychosis often is marked by formism, hallucinations of bugs on or under the skin.

Signs of sympathetic excess on physical examination include tachycardia, hypertension, elevated temperature, tremor, and hyperreflexia. Pupils tend toward mydriasis with increased reactivity to light.

4.2. Anticholinergic Psychosis

This type of psychosis and its clinical picture arise from blockade of the parasympathetic nervous system. It tends to present with bizarre mental and neurological symptoms, psychomotor agitation, hallucinations (usually visual), confusion with disorientation, and impaired short-term memory.[33]

Among the over 600 drugs with anticholinergic properties are such psychiatric medications as tricyclic antidepressants, antiparkinsonian drugs (abused for euphoriant effects), and neuroleptics. Others include antihistamines, belladonna alkaloids (atropine, scopolamine), antispasmodics, and over-the-counter preparations (cold remedies, motion sickness pills, cough medicines, and sleeping pills).

Decreased cholinergic tone promotes an increase in pupil size, decreased salivary and sweat gland secretion, decreased intestinal and urinary motility, and increased heart rate. Thus, physical examination will reveal dilated, sluggishly reactive pupils, blurred near vision, dry mouth, dry flushed skin with fever, decreased bowel sounds (constipation), urinary retention, and a rapid weak pulse. Whereas both psychostimulants and anticholinergics cause mydriasis and tachycardia, in contrast to the desiccation of the anticholinergics, the psychostimulants cause salivation and sweating.[33] The EKG may reveal an increased Q–T interval with heart block and potentially fatal arrythmias.

Because of the potentially fatal course of anticholinergic drug toxicity, although the clinician should attempt to identify the anticholinergic agent by history or laboratory examination, if parasympathetic shutdown is suspected, one cannot wait for laboratory results to initiate treatment. Physostigmine, 1–2 mg i.v., can be used to confirm the diagnosis and to treat the syndrome. The physician should observe for clinical improvement versus a breakthrough of peripheral parasympathetic signs. Clearing of the syndrome usually occurs rapidly (i.e., less than 1 hr). Because physostigmine is very short acting, if clinical improvement occurs, physostigmine may be repeated every 30 min.

4.3. Hallucinogen-Induced Psychosis

Acute psychosis following psychedelic drug intoxication generally presents with illusions, hallucinations, and other perceptual distortions (especially visual ones) including increased vividness, synesthesia, and body image changes. Mood changes, either euphoria or depression, anxiety and panic states, and depersonalization or derealization are also seen. The drugs vary markedly in their rate of onset, peripheral side effects, duration of action, and potency. Some psychedelic drugs (e.g., mescaline, STP, nutmeg) have significant sympathomimetic properties and thus present with the signs of an adrenergic psychosis, whereas other drugs do not (e.g., the indole type: LSD, psilocybin, DMT).[34] Ingestion of tetrahydrocannabinol via marijuana can activate psychotic symptoms in patients with a history of psychosis and, if ingested in sufficient dosage, produce a full hallucinogen-induced psychosis in normal subjects. The acute reaction to hallucinogens is relatively short-lived, depending on the dose ingested and the half-life of the specific drug, and can usually be managed supportively (e.g., "talking down"). When a psychotic reaction lasts longer than a day, one should suspect the ingestion of other drugs and/or the exacerbation of a preexisting psychotic disorder.

4.4. Phencyclidine Psychosis

Phencyclidine (PCP, angel dust) is a drug with unusual properties that is increasingly being abused and deserves special consideration. Depending on the dose ingested, it can act as a depressant, stimulant, anesthetic, or hallucinogen.[35] A growing proportion of patients presenting with acute psychosis show evidence of PCP intoxication.[36] Phencyclidine affects multiple neurotransmitter systems, particularly potentiating central dopamine neurotransmission and profoundly blocking the muscarinic cholinergic receptor.[37]

Phencyclidine intoxication may present as mania, schizophrenia, depression, or organic delirium, and its symptomatology may be indistinguishable from such syndromes. The psychosis of PCP intoxication may last for days to months and may closely mimic the negative psychotic symptoms of chronic schizophrenia. Phencyclidine's effects are dose related but extremely variable and unpredictable. The low-dose syndrome follows within 2 hr of ingesting approximately 5–10 mg of PCP (serum level 20–30 ng/ml) and is associated with a variable presentation including a blank stare, agitation, disorientation, misperceptions and hallucinations, bizarre behavior and catatonia, paranoid ideation, and an unusually marked tendency to hostility and frank violence. Physical signs at this dose include rapid pulse, ataxia, horizontal and vertical nystagmus, paresthesias and analgesia, excess salivation, and vomiting. Moderate doses (10–20 mg) produce a more stuporous state with stereotyped movements, fever, hyperreflexia, and hypertension. Higher doses lead to labored breathing, seizures, and prolonged coma. Doses over 100 mg are usually lethal.

Because of PCP's high affinity for adipose and brain tissue, it remains in those tissues long after it is undetectable in the blood, where its half-life is only 1 hr. However, the recent development of a capillary gas chromatograph–nitrogen detector method has allowed PCP to be found in the urine days after ingestion.[38] Given the recent prevalence of PCP abuse, its danger, and its ability to mimic psychiatric disorders, PCP intoxication should be suspected in all patients with unusual psychotic presentations, and their urine should be assayed for PCP.

4.5. Psychosis Caused by Medically Prescribed Drugs

A large number of medications prescribed in the practice of medicine can cause psychotic states. These include antihypertensives, anticonvulsants, oral contraceptives, antiarrhythmics, some antibiotics, and a variety of hormones (listed in Table 15-2). Medically prescribed drugs with an especially high incidence for producing psychotic states include L-DOPA, corticosteroids, and ACTH, the antituberculosis antibiotics iproniazid and cycloserine, the antihypertensives α-methyldopa and all β blockers, and the cardiotropics digitalis, aprindine, and lidocaine. Psychosis developing secondary to medically prescribed drugs may arise via a dose-related phenomenon (e.g., L-DOPA, corticosteroids), an idiosyncratic vulnerability (e.g., β blockers), or both (e.g., disulfiram).

4.6. Laboratory Evaluation of Drugs of Abuse

Drug intoxication and most drug withdrawal diagnoses require identification of the drug in exhaled breath, blood, or urine. Routine "drug screens" may not have the sensitivity necessary to measure psychiatrically relevant quantities of these drugs, and more specific, antibody-based tests may need to be ordered. The psychiatrist can test specifically for additional abusable substances on the basis of the patient's signs, symptoms, history, and age and the family's description of the phenomenology and assessment of drug use/abuse. A negative history of drug use or abuse, however, is not sufficient to replace negative specific tests for drugs of abuse.

Newer urine drug abuse screens that use enzymatic assays are sensitive to concentrations of drugs in the abuse range, as opposed to the older thin-layer chromatographic assays, which are less sensitive. Even more sensitive and accurate gas chromatograph–mass spectroscopy (GC–MS) assays for all major drugs of abuse in blood are now available and can aid diagnosis when urine testing is inconclusive or is not capable of detecting psychoactive quantities of the drug(s) in question or when the drug in question has a known blood level–behavior relationship.

As soon as the patient has been interviewed and the physical examination has been performed, samples of blood and urine should be sent to the laboratory for identification and quantification of the drugs of abuse. One may use antibody-based urine assays for most drugs of abuse, including alcohol. Quantitative capillary-column GC, or GC–MS analysis of blood for specific drugs not easily detectable in urine (e.g., gluthethimide, PCP, cocaine, Δ^9-THC) are ordered when clinically indicated. When urine is used to detect drug abuse, a supervised first-void morning urine is essential. Concurrent urine specific gravity is used to insure that the sample is the unadulterated concentrated first-void morning urine.

5. Psychosis Related to Alcohol Abuse

Psychotic symptoms, both transient and long lasting, develop in alcoholic patients. The symptoms are aspects of specific clinical entities and not merely part of the clinical continuum toward delirium tremens. Unless these discrete conditions are correctly diagnosed, they will remain poorly treated. Alcoholic patients are also prone to a host of medical diseases related to malnutrition, hepatic infections, and trauma. Psychosis in an alcoholic patient requires careful evaluation of associated medical disorders. The different syndromes associated with psychosis and related to alcoholism are defined and listed below by their occurrence during states of (1) intoxication, (2) withdrawal, or (3) chronic alcoholism organicity.

5.1. Intoxication States

5.1.1. Alcohol Idiosyndratic Intoxication (Pathological Intoxication)

This is a rare transient (lasting a few hours) state of acute excitation during intoxication marked by major impulsivity and dyscontrol and leading to violent outbursts of aggressive, destructive, and irrational behavior. It occurs after drinking an amount of alcohol so small as to be insufficient to induce intoxication in most people. Furthermore, the behavior is atypical of the person when not drinking (e.g., the person may, when not drinking, be gentle and mild mannered). Usually, during the episode, the person appears out of contact, and after the episode the patient has no memory of the behavior.

The syndrome appears to be secondary to an idiosyndratic reaction to alcohol and recurs consistently with intake. Some of these patients appear to have a subclinical form of temporal lobe epilepsy, as they develop temporal lobe spikes on EEG after ingesting small amounts of alcohol. Furthermore, patients with preexisting brain injuries suffered via trauma or encephalitis are especially prone to this syndrome. Thus, when a patient develops this disorder, full neurological evaulation is indicated.

5.1.2. Psychosis Developing in Functional States during Alcohol Intoxication

Many patients with various functional psychiatric disorders abuse alcohol. Alcohol can clearly precipitate an acute psychotic relapse in a schizophrenic patient.[39] Patients with schizophrenic-spectrum-disorder-type personalities (e.g., schizoid, schizotypal) may, on ingestion of alcohol, reveal psychotic worsening. Patients with a borderline personality disorder frequently abuse drugs and alcohol. These patients are predisposed to very short-lived ("micro") psychotic states, which are often precipitated by both alcohol intoxication and withdrawal.

5.2. Withdrawal States

5.2.1. Alcohol Withdrawal Delirium (Delirium Tremens)

This disorder is discussed as a sympathetic syndrome in Section 4 of this chapter. Briefly, the syndrome is characterized by the symptoms of the full sympathetic syndrome developing usually 2–4 days after cessation or reduction of alcohol consumption in an individual who drank excessively and steadily for many years.[40] Delusions (usually paranoid) and hallucinations (usually visual) develop, often accompanied by agitated behavior. Patients always become markedly confused and fully disoriented. The presence of an underlying medical illness predisposes to a fatal outcome. Thus, such disorders as subdural hematoma, meningitis, electrolyte abnormality, dehydration, and severe hepatic disease should be investigated.

5.2.2. Alcohol Hallucinosis

This condition is a distinct clinical entity usually occurring within 48 hr after cessation or reduction of alcohol intake in an alcohol-dependent person.[41] It is characterized by vivid auditory hallucinations. In the context of a falling blood alcohol level, the syndrome usually begins with an illusionary stage characterized by misinterpretation of sounds and sights and progresses to voices, often of a threatening nature, and then paranoid ideation. Although tremulousness is usually present, in contrast to alcohol withdrawal delirium, there is no clouding of consciousness, and the patient remains oriented. In fact, it only rarely progresses to delirium but rather tends to resolve spontaneously. There is no evidence that schizophrenia predisposes to this disorder.

5.3. Chronic Alcoholism Organicity: Alcohol Amnesic Disorder (Korsakoff's Psychosis)

This syndrome occurs in chronic alcoholics as a result of repeated episodes of a thiamine deficiency.[42] It is characterized by an acute phase (Wernicke's disease) characterized by a profound confusional state with disorientation, apathy, and drow-siness. There are associated neurological symptoms such as the ocular disturbances of lateral gaze paralysis and nystagmus, cerebellar ataxia, and peripheral polyneuropathy. Administration of thiamine leads to resolution of these symptoms in the vast majority of patients. A few patients continue to have severe residual deficits of short-term memory, leading to an inability to make sense out of events and a tendency to fabricate stories (i.e., confabulation). These patients, with alcohol amnesic disorder, appear to suffer from an irreversible structural defect of the CNS. Because of the routine admin-istration of thiamine during alcohol detoxification, the syndrome is now rare.

6. Functional Psychotic Disorders

Having ruled out medical disorders (including drug intoxications, reactions, and withdrawals) causing the patient's psychotic state, the clinician can then turn to the "functional" psychotic disorders. The psychiatric syndromes of the DSM III that can be associated with psychosis are listed in the latter half of Table 15-1. Whereas in past years American psychiatrists tended to overdiagnose schizophrenia in psychotic pa-tients, the advent of the DSM III, with its criteria for each diagnostic category, has led to a more careful consideration of psychotic diagnoses other than schizophrenia. This has made schizophrenia essentially a diagnosis of exclusion. However, the DSM III's overreliance on phenomenological characteristics, as is discussed below, may continue to bias diagnostic specificity.

A number of factors critically influence the differential diagnostic categorization of psychotic features according to DSM III.

6.1. Duration of Illness and Age of Onset

Duration of illness is an important determinant in the assignment of diagnosis in DSM III. For example, when psychotic symptoms are of less than 2 weeks' duration, the psychosis is considered either a brief reactive psychosis or an atypical psychosis (determined by the presence or absence of a major environmental stress, respectively). The diagnosis of schizophrenia requires a duration of at least 6 months (including prodomal and active phases). A syndrome with symptoms of schizophrenia with a duration of under 6 months is designated schizophreniform. Transient psychotic symp-toms can occur in schizotypal, borderline, schizoid, and paranoid personality disor-ders, but the psychotic symptoms resolve rapidly (hours or days), and the patients returns to the usual level of functioning. With regard to age of onset, for psychotic symptoms to be considered schizophrenic in origin, the patient must have developed such symptoms prior to age 45. These criteria are based on epidemiologic data.

6.2. Specific Psychotic Symptoms

The DSM III renders the psychotic phenomenology an important factor in the diagnostic criteria. For example, on the basis of the work of the German psychiatrist

Kurt Schneider,[43] who believed that certain psychotic symptoms (e.g., delusions of control, thought broadcasting, insertion, or withdrawal, hallucinations of voices commenting on the patient's behavior) may be pathognomonic for schizophrenia, the DSM III assigned such symptoms a prominent place in the diagnosis of schizophrenia (plus that of schizophreniform and schizoaffective disorders). Recent investigations find, however, that many psychotic patients with either affective disorder (e.g., mania) or postdrug (e.g., amphetamine) intoxication present with such Schneiderian symptoms.[44,45]

6.3. Presence of an Affective Syndrome

The presence or absence of a major affective syndrome (i.e., depressive or manic) is an important decision point in the differential diagnosis of psychotic states according to DSM III. However, the criteria for an affective syndrome, partially because of the reliance on clinical phenomenology, may be relatively nonspecific. For example, criteria for mania, including expansive or irritable mood, restlessness, decreased need for sleep, and distractibility, or for depression, including depressed mood, insomnia, feelings of worthlessness, inappropriate guilt, and impaired concentration, may be present in any psychotic state, even those clearly medically or drug induced.

Like the process of ruling out an organic factor in psychotic states, the more thoroughly the clinician searches for alternative functional diagnoses, the more frequently will an alternative diagnosis be found correct. This is especially relevant to the question of the presence/absence of an affective syndrome. The importance of accurate diagnosis of these syndromes is emphasized by their beneficial and occasionally curative pharmacological treatments. The development of biological tests for affective illness adds a further degree of specificity to the diagnostic evaluation of the psychotic patient.

6.3.1. Biological Tests for the Presence of Affective Illness

Research into the neurobiology of major depression, mania, and schizophrenia has produced a growing body of evidence suggesting that some of the biological alterations associated with these syndromes may serve as biological markers of the disease. A good biological marker has many clinical applications. For the purpose of evaluation, if a test successfully marks the presence, absence, or degree of a pathology, it may be used to confirm or exclude a diagnosis and to identify latent clinical cases (e.g., to identify biological depression in a borderline personality disorder). The tests discussed here have proven clinically useful for the evaluation process, especially for confirming the presence of affective illness in the psychotic patient.

6.3.2. Dexamethasone Suppression Test

The dexamethasone suppression test (DST), introduced in 1960 for the diagnosis of Cushing's disease, has become the most widely used biological test in psychiatric disorders. Carroll and co-workers, expanding on earlier observations by Sachar and others that cortisol levels were elevated in many depressed patients, systematically studied DST results in a variety of psychiatric patient groups and standardized the DST procedure. Application of the DST to patients with major depression reveals a more subtle disturbance in depressed patients than that noted in patients with Cushing's disease, who have complete nonsuppression of cortisol. That is, following the administration of dexamethasone, many depressed patients have either only partial suppression or early recovery ("escape") from suppression of cortisol output.

The standardized methodology for the DST suggested by Carroll and co-workers is to administer 1 mg of dexamethasone orally at 11 p.m. or midnight and to determine plasma cortisol concentrations at 4 p.m. and 11 p.m. the following day by radioimmunoassay or competitive protein binding assay. If either postdexamethasone plasma cortisol concentration is 5 μg/dl or more, the test is considered positive, that is, a failure to suppress. Factors that can affect the validity of the DST are listed in Table 15-5.

In the many studies reported, escape from dexamethasone suppression occurs in 26 to 81% of patients with a clinical diagnosis of major depression. On the average, these studies suggest that 45% of major depressed patients have an abnormal DST. In contrast, very few healthy control subjects (approximately 6%) show an abnormal DST. On the basis of these data, the sensitivity of the DST is 45%, and the specificity of the test is 96%, figures that compare favorably with those recorded for laboratory tests used in standard medical practice. No difference in the proportion of unipolar versus bipolar depressives with abnormal DST results is noted. Patients with delusional depression tend to have unusually high (greater than 15 μg/dl) postdexamethasone cortisol levels.

The specificity of the test in psychiatric control groups depends on the diagnosis of the patients studied. Very few schizophrenic or manic patients have DST nonsuppression. On the other hand, certain clinical syndromes, which may actually be phenotypic variants of depressive illness, show a significant proportion of patients with DST abnormality. These include schizoaffective disorders, catatonia, borderline character disorders, chronic pain syndromes, and bulimia. Treatment trials suggest that such patients with abnormal test results respond preferentially to antidepressant medication. Similarly, a recent follow-up study of patients initially diagnosed as having a

Table 15-5. Factors Affecting Validity of Dexamethasone Suppression Test

False-positive tests
Cushing's disease
Pregnancy, high-dose estrogens
Severe weight loss
Phenytoin, barbiturates, carbamazepine, meprobamate, α-methyldopa, reserpine
Uncontrolled diabetes mellitus
High fever, dehydration
Acute alcohol withdrawal
False-negative tests
Addison's disease
Hypopituitarism
Steroid treatment
High-dose benzodiazepines

schizophreniform disorder found that the patients with DST nonsuppression on admission tended subsequently to have a probable affective disorder on the basis of their full remission and antidepressant medication response.[47] In this study, the DST results proved more useful diagnostically than did the assessment of the clinical phenomenology alone.

In summary, then, a DST abnormality appears useful in diagnosing major depression or a variant of affective illness in settings with a high prevalence of major depression. A negative test result is not very valuable diagnostically, as more than 50% of patients with major depression show normal suppression.

6.3.3. Thyrotropin-Releasing Hormone Test

The thyroid-stimulating hormone (TSH) response to thyrotropin- releasing hormone (TRH), the TRH test, is a neuroendocrine challenge originally developed for the diagnosis of endocrinologic diseases of the hypothalamic–pituitary–thyroid axis. A serendipitous finding in experimental trials of TRH treatment for depression was a lesser release of TSH after TRH infusion in depressed patients than in controls.[48]

The method for administering the TRH test used by most investigators is as follows. After an overnight fast, in the morning at bedrest, give 500 μg of TRH by intravenous push over 30 sec. Take blood samples for measurement of TSH by radioimmunoassay from the indwelling catheter at base line (pre-TRH push) and at 15-min intervals up to 90 min after administration of TRH. Calculate the maximal TSH increment from base line, ΔTSH, by subtracting the base-line TSH from the peak TSH level. A ΔTSH of less than 5 or 7 μg/nl is considered abnormal by most sources. A ΔTSH greater than 25 may also be abnormal. The TRH test can be administered to inpatients or outpatients, is safe, and has only mild and short-lived side effects (nausea, headache, urge to urinate). Factors that can influence the TSH response include thyroid hormone abnormalities, other endocrine diseases, hepatic or renal failure, advanced age, weight loss, alcohol intoxication or withdrawal, and treatment with steroids, estrogens, phenytoin, carbamazepine, or lithium.[48]

Depending on the ΔTSH criterion used (less than 5 or 7 μg/nl), a blunted TSH response to TRH infusion is found in 25 to 56% of patients with major depression across all studies. In contrast, few nonendogenously depressed patients, schizophrenic patients, or healthy controls show this neuroendocrine abnormality.[48,49] Thus, for the diagnosis of major depression, the TRH test has reasonable sensitivity and high specificity. Alcoholic subjects, even when abstinent for years, have a high incidence of TSH blunting. Thus, the test may be useful in diagnosing alcoholism but not in evaluating depressive illness in alcoholic subjects.[50] Evidence that TRH test abnormalities are relatively independent of DST nonsuppression implies that using both tests can enhance the identification of major depression (the sensitivity of combined tests is 86%).

As discussed previously, the clinical presentation of agitated schizophrenic patients and manic patients can be virtually identical. Yet differentiating these syndromes is extremely important given the clear-cut efficacy of lithium in treating mania. The TRH test may prove useful in making the difficult differential diagnosis of mania versus schizophrenia. One study reports a blunted TSH response significantly more frequently in manic patients (60%) than in schizophrenic patients (27%).

6.3.4. Platelet Serotonin Transport and Platelet Imipramine Binding

The brain neurotransmitter serotonin (5-HT) may be involved in the etiology of depressive illness. Transport (uptake) of 5-HT in the blood platelets of depressed patients is decreased. The maximal velocity of 5-HT transport is significantly decreased in both unipolar and bipolar depressed patients. However, it is normal in manic and schizophrenic patients.[52] Moreover, recent reports describe a receptor site on blood platelets that binds radioactively labeled imipramine that is closely associated with 5-HT transport. There is a highly significant decrease in the number of these imipramine binding sites on the platelets of depressed patients.[53] The number of imipramine binding sites on platelets from schizophrenic patients is not different from those from normal controls.

6.4. Positron-Emission Tomography

Although this is still a research procedure, results of recent studies suggest that tests for the diagnosis of schizophrenia may be forthcoming in the near future. The recent development of positron-emission tomography (the PET scan) has permitted the study of cerebral glucose utilization similar to the use of the CAT scan to study brain tissue. As cerebral glucose utilization is believed to reflect the activity of various parts of the brain, this advance permits the observation of the actual functional activity of various brain regions. Ingvar and Franzen,[54] using xenon radiography, had observed reduced blood flow to the frontal lobes of older chronic schizophrenic patients during mental activation. In a later review of this research, Ingvar postulated that this hypofrontal activity in deteriorated schizophrenic patients might be related to malfunction of dopaminergic projections to this region.[55] This finding was dramatically verified with the development of the PET scan. Buchsbaum and colleagues[56] measured glucose metabolism in the brains of schizophrenics and normal controls. They also found that the frontal cortex of schizophrenics was less active than that in normal persons. This area of the brain is believed to be the center for goal-directed behavior. Thus, low activity in the frontal cortex may explain the lack of goal-directed behavior and deteriorated motor ability that are characteristic negative symptoms of schizophrenia. The researchers also found reduced activity in the left central gray matter in schizophrenic brains, an area thought to be involved in various schizophrenic symptoms such as perceptual–cognitive disorders and motor–behavioral deterioration.

7. Conclusion

Effective and specific treatments are established for many of the diseases that present with psychotic symptoms. The importance of accurate diagnosis is emphasized by such beneficial and often curative treatments, for correct diagnosis is essential to correct treatment. In effect, diagnosis is prognosis.

In evaluating the psychotic patient, the psychiatrist must be a medical specialist who carefully considers the differential diagnosis and weighs alternative diagnoses rather than assuming one by habit. Historically, too many psychotic patients have been quickly labeled schizophrenic when, more appropriately, that diagnosis should remain a diagnosis of exclusion. Although the criteria of DSM III are a step in the right direction, more rigorous criteria, with less emphasis on pure phenomenology, are needed.

The psychiatrist must be alert to the fact that diverse causative factors can lead to nearly identical psychotic symptoms. As this chapter points out, encephalitis, hypothyroidism, head trauma, or an environmental catastrophy can lead to psychotic disturbances that appear identical, yet each of these conditions also lead to many other symptoms, signs, and laboratory findings. Clearly, a valid diagnosis cannot be based on the patient's psychotic symptoms alone but requires the psychiatrist's medical knowledge for an aggressive investigation.

References

1. Anderson WH, Kuehnle JC: Strategies for the treatment of acute psychosis. *JAMA* 229:1884–1889, 1974.
2. Hall RCW, Popkin MK, Devaul RA, et al: Physical illness presenting as psychiatric disease. *Arch Gen Psychiatry* 35:1315–1320, 1978.
3. Folstein MF, Folstein SE, McHugh PR: Mini-mental state—a practical method for grading the cognitive state of patients for the clinician. *J Psychiatr Res* 12:189–198, 1975.
4. McIntyre JS, Romand J: Is there a stethescope in the house? *Arch Gen Psychiatry* 34:1147–1151, 1977.
5. Whybrow PC, Prange AJ, Treadway CR: Mental changes accompanying thyroid gland dysfunction. *Arch Gen Psychiatry* 20:48–63, 1969.
6. Josephson AM, Mackenzie TB: Appearance of manic psychosis following rapid normalization of thyroid status. *Am J Psychiatry* 136(6):846–847, 1979.
7. Easson WM: Myxedema with psychosis. *Arch Gen Psychiatry* 14:227–283, 1966.
8. Extein I, Pottash ALC, Gold MS: Does subclinical hypothyroidism predispose to tricyclic induced rapid mood cycles? *J Clin Psychiatry* 43(7):290–291, 1982.
9. Peterson P: Psychiatric disorders in primary hyperparathyroidism. *J Clin Endocrinol Metab* 28:1491–1495, 1968.
10. Mikkelsen E, Reider A: Post parathyroidectomy psychosis: Clinical and research implications. *J Clin Psychiatry* 40:352–357, 1979.
11. Denko JD, Kaelbling R: The psychiatric aspects of hypoparathyroidism. *Acta Psychiatrica Scand* 164(Suppl):1–70, 1962.
12. Sachar EJ (ed): *Hormones, Behavior, and Psychopathology.* New York, Raven Press, 1976.
13. Cohen SI: Cushing's syndrome: A psychiatric study of 29 patients. *Br J Psychiatry* 136:120–126, 1980.
14. Hickman JW, Atkinson RP, Flint LD, et al: Transient schizophrenic reaction as a major symptom of Cushing's syndrome. *N Engl J Med* 264:797–800, 1961.
15. Cleghorn RA: Adrenal cortical in sufficiency: Psychological and neurological observations. Can Med Assoc J 65:449–454, 1951.
16. McFahrland T: Addison's disease and related psychoses. *Compr Psychiatry* 4:90–95, 1963.
17. Falk WE, Mahnke MW, Poskanzer DC: Lithium prophylaxis of corticotropin-induced psychosis. *JAMA* 241:1011–1013, 1979.
18. Atschule MD, Bren J: Periodic psychosis of puberty. *Am J Psychiatry* 119:1176–1178, 1963.
19. Berlin FS, Bergey GK, Money J: Periodic psychosis of puberty: A case report. *Am J Psychiatry* 139:119–120, 1982.
20. Kendell RE, Wainwright S, Hailey A, et al: Influence of childbirth on psychiatric morbidity. *Psychol Med* 6:297–302, 1976.
21. Cox JL, Connor Y, Kendell RE: Prospective study of the psychiatric disorders of childbirth. *Br J Psychiatry* 140:111–117, 1982.
22. Kadrmas A, Winokur G, Crowe R: Post-partum mania. *Br J Psychiatry* 135:551–554, 1979.

23. Katonah CLE: Puerperal mental illness: Comparisons with non-puerperal controls. *Br J Psychiatry* 141:447–452, 1982.
24. Hamilton JA: Model utility in post-partum psychosis. *Psychopharmacol Bull* 18(3):184–187, 1982.
25. Nott PN, Franklin M, Armilage C, et al: Hormonal changes and mood in the puerperium. *Br J Psychiatry* 128:379–383, 1976.
26. DiSclafani A, Hall RCW, Gardner ER: Drug induced psychosis: Emergency diagnosis and management. *Psychosomatics* 22(10):845–855, 1981.
28. Janowsky DS, Risch C: Amphetamine psychosis and psychotic symptoms. *Psychopharmacology* 65:73–78, 1979.
29. Janowsky DS, El-Yousef MK, Davis JM, et al: Provocation of schizophrenic symptoms by intravenous administration of methylphenidate. *Arch Gen Psychiatry* 28:185–191, 1973.
30. Bell DS: The experimental reproduction of amphetamine psychosis. *Arch Gen Psychiatry* 29:35–40, 1973.
31. Ellinwood EH: Amphetamine psychosis: Descriptions of the individuals and process. *J Nerv Ment Dis* 144:273–283, 1967.
32. Griffith JD, Cavanaugh J, Held J: Dextroamphetamine: Evaluation of psychotomimetic properties in man. *Arch Gen Psychiatry* 26:97–100, 1972.
33. Perry P, Wilding, DC, Juhl RP: Anticholinergic psychosis. *Am J Hosp Pharm* 35:725–728, 1978.
34. Martin W, Sloan J: Pharmacology and classification of LSD-like hallucinogens, in Martin W (ed): *Drug Addiction II: Amphetamine, Psychotogen and Marijuana Dependence. Handbuch der Experimentellen, Pharmakologie,* vol 45. Berlin, Springer-Verlag, 1977, pp 129–144.
35. Ayd FS: Phencyclidine. *Int Drug Ther Newslett* 14(5):17–20, 1979.
36. Luisada PV: The phencycliding psychosis—phenomenology and treatment, in Petersen RC, Stillman RC (eds): *Phencyclidine (PCP) Abuse: An Appraisal. NIDA Research Monograph, 21.* Washington, NIDA, 1978, pp 241–253.
37. Johnson KM: Neurochemical pharmacology of phenocyclidine, in Petersen RD, Stillman RC (eds): *Phencyclidine (PCP) Abuse: An Appraisal. NIDA Research Monograph 21.* Washington, NIDA, 1978, pp 44–52.
38. Pitts FN, Yago LS, Aniline O, et al: Capillary GC–nitrogen detector measurement of phencyclidine (PCP) ketamine and other arylcycloalkylamines in the picogram range. *J Chromotogr* 193:157–159, 1980.
39. Schuckit MA: The history of psychotic symptoms in alcoholics. *J Clin Psychiatry* 63:53–57, 1982.
40. Brown CG: ⁀he alcohol withdrawal syndrome. *Ann Emerg Med* 11:276–280, 1982.
41. Surawicz FG: Alcoholic hallucinosis: A missed diagnosis: Differential diagnosis and management. *Can J Psychiatry* 25:57–63, 1980.
42. Victor M. Adams RD, Collins GH: *Wernicke–Korsakoff Syndrome.* Philadelphia, FA Davis, 1971.
43. Schneider K: *Clinical Psychopathology.* New York, Grune & Stratton, 1959, pp 88–144.
44. Janowsky DS, Risch C: Amphetamine psychosis and psychotic symptoms. *Psychopharmacology* 65:73–78, 1979.
45. Carpenter WT, Strauss JS, Mulch S: Are there pathognomic symptoms in schizophrenia: An empirical investigation of Schneider's first rank symptoms. *Arch Gen Psychiatry* 28:847–852, 1973.
46. Carroll BJ, Feinberg M, Greden F, et al: A specific laboratory test for the diagnosis of melancholia. *Arch Gen Psychiatry* 38:15–22, 1981.
47. Targum SD: Neuroendocrine dysfunction in schizophreniform disorder: Correlation with 6-month clinical outcome. *Am J Psychiatry* 140:309–313, 1983.
48. Prange AJ, Wilson IC, Lara PP, et al: Effects of thyrotropin-releasing hormone in depression. *Lancet* 2:999–1002, 1972.
49. Extein I, Pottash ALC, Gold MS: Relationship of thyrotropin-releasing hormone test and dexamethasone suppression test abnormalities in unipolar depression. *Psychiatry Res* 4:49–53, 1981.
50. Loosen, PT, Prange AJ: TRH in psychiatry patients. *N Engl J Med* 303:224–225, 1980.
51. Extein I, Pottash ALC, Gold MS, et al: Using the protirelin test to distinguish mania from schizophrenia. *Arch Gen Psychiatry* 39:77–81, 1982.
52. Meltzer HY, Arora RC, Baber R, et al: Serotonin uptake in blood platelets of psychiatric patients. *Arch Gen Psychiatry* 38:1322–1326, 1981.

53. Paul SM, Rehavi M, Skolnick P, et al: Depressed patients have decreased binding of tritiated imipramine to platelet serotonin transporter. *Arch Gen Psychiatry* 38:1315–1317, 1981.
54. Ingvar DH, Franzen G: Abnormalities of cerebral blood flow in patients with chronic schizophrenia. *Acta Psychiatr Scand* 50:425–462, 1974.
55. Ingvar DH: Abnormal distribution of cerebral activity in chronic schizophrenia: A neurophysiological interpretation, in Baxter C, Melnechuck KT (eds): *Perspectives in Schizophrenia Research.* New York, Raven Press, 1980, pp 107–125.
56. Buchsbaum MS, Ingvar DH, Kessler R, et al: Cerebral glucography with positron tomography. *Arch Gen Psychiatry* 39:251–259, 1982.

16

Evaluation of Anxiety Disorders

Cary L. Hamlin, M.D., and A. L. C. Pottash, M.D.

1. What Is Anxiety?

Anxiety, the term, comes to English from the German word *Angst,* meaning fear. Anxiety, the concept, is an emotional state very much like fear, actually a subset of fearful events. To understand anxiety as a particular kind of fear, it is necessary to understand that fear may be normal or abnormal. Normal fear is the mood component of a nervous system reflex that attempts to cope with possible noxious exposure.[1] The experience of noxious exposure causes fear, which in turn causes avoidance of the object and/or situation that caused the noxious exposure. If the avoidance is successful, then the fearful mood is inhibited by a burst of euphoria and a sigh of relief. If the avoidance attempt is unsuccessful, then the fearful mood is further stimulated, and avoidance behaviors become more frenetic. Very high-intensity states of fear can be normal if one is unable to escape significant noxiousness.

It should be noted that for complex tasks any significant level of anxiety impairs performance, perhaps by disruption of temporal lobe cortical activation; thus, more anxiety often means less chance to avoid.[2,3] Any stimulus that is reliably a predictor of the noxious exposure can take on the response of that exposure in the manner of classical conditioned avoidance.[4]

Anxiety is abnormal fear. There are three types of anxiety experiences: exogenous, chronic, and endogenous.[5] Exogenous anxiety is, like normal fear, a reaction to a real external threat, but the amount of fear experienced is inappropriately high given the real present danger. Chronic anxiety is present constantly and often develops in response to unpredictable noxious exposures.[5] Endogenous anxiety attacks occur spontaneously and may be caused by a neurochemical imbalance in the fear–avoidance reflexes.[6,7] Anxieties are pathological experiences of fearful mood.

2. Differential Diagnosis of Anxiety

A complete syndromal classification of anxiety disorders probably does not exist yet, but recent advances in taxonomy are beginning to approximate that goal. The

Cary L. Hamlin, M.D. • Outpatient Research Unit, Fair Oaks Hospital, Summit, New Jersey 07901. ***A. L. C. Pottash, M.D.*** • Fair Oaks Hospital at Boca/Delray, Delray Beach, Florida 33445, and Fair Oaks Hospital, Summit, New Jersey 07901.

important first step was provided by the *Diagnostic and Statistical Manual of Mental Disorders,* third edition (DSM III).[8] In this document, for the first time, specific diagnostic criteria in terms of duration, type, and intensity of symptoms present for diagnosis are set down (see Table 16-1). The sections on anxiety and phobic disorders were authored by experienced, careful clinical investigators of these disorders. Robert Spitzer, who was the nosologist who collaborated with them, and Janet Williams have compiled DSM III Revised (DSM IIIR), which eliminates the inappropriately rigid separation between panic disorder and agoraphobia with panic attacks and makes three stages of the same disease: panic disorder, uncomplicated; panic disorder with limited phobic avoidance; and panic disorder with agoraphobia.[9] Also, as commonly happens if the panic attacks are in remission for a time, the diagnosis becomes panic disorder with agoraphobia (panic attacks in remission). The DSM III is thus evolving to better and better approximate the real clinical material.

David Sheehan has taken issue with the DSM III syndromes. He complains that they are degenerate because individual patients can meet inclusion criteria for multiple anxiety disorders simultaneously.[10] He has proposed a syndromal classification that focuses on the presence of endogenous-type anxiety experiences and avoidance behavior.[11] We have lauded Sheehan's efforts to focus on endogenous anxiety and the responses to it but questioned if his system does not ignore important clinical complexity and leave some patients undiagnosed.[7] Using data from the National Institute of Mental Health's Epidemiologic Catchment Area Program, Boyd *et al.* noted that the presence of almost any DSM III syndrome increased the chances of other DSM III syndromes.[12] This seems to confirm the idea that overlapping syndromes between taxonomic classes result in diagnostic confusion.

Clearly, the outline of an accurate taxonomic classification of anxiety and phobic disorders exists in DSM III, and time, experience, and debate will result in progressively more complete and accurate diagnostic criteria. The importance of this work for the development of biological methods of psychopharmacology cannot be overestimated.

The correct diagnosis of a patient's anxiety symptoms is important because we think that label determines how a patient can optimally be treated psychopharmacologically.[7] There was a time in psychiatric practice when the blanket application of psychotherapy was the treatment for anxiety disorders. At that time, it made little difference in practice what the patient was called since the response was stereotyped. Likewise, a generation ago in psychopharmacology, when nonspecific sedatives were also stereotypically applied to anxiety symptoms, there was no reason for a complicated differential diagnosis of anxiety. Those days are gone. Advances in psychopharmacology since then, specifically the development of drugs that are selective in their actions on specific neurotransmitter mechanisms, have increased the need for accurate differential diagnosis of anxiety disorders.

In reality, there are opposite responses to the same medication in different anxiety disorders [e.g., desipramine in panic disorder versus complex partial (temporal lobe) epilepsy, an organic anxiety disorder], and recent research has suggested some specific anxiolytics as more effective than other specific anxiolytics in certain DSM III disorders (e.g., chlomipramine versus nortriptyline in obsessive–compulsive disorder).[13,14] Perhaps different anxiety disorders have different but characteristic abnormalities of reticulolimbic neurotransmitter dynamics that could determine opposite responses to the same medications in different disorders. These facts emphasize that in psychiatry no less than the rest of medicine, successful treatment requires correct diagnosis.

The clinical anxiety disorders must be differentiated from normal fear and from other psychiatric and medical conditions. The mood of fear, including anxiety, is so ubiquitous among the sick that it sometimes appears to be a constant, patients differing in it only by intensity. On closer study, there appear to be quantized states of anxiety that have characteristic pictures, the anxiety disorder syndromes.

The DSM III notes that the anxiety disorders include the phobic disorders (simple phobia, social phobia, agoraphobia, panic disorder with agoraphobia), the anxiety states (panic disorder, obsessive–compulsive disorder, generalized anxiety disorder), posttraumatic stress disorder, and atypical anxiety disorder.[8] The DSM III (axis 1) adjustment reaction (anxiety), affective disorders (major depression, bipolar depression, dysthymic disorder), dissociative disorder (depersonalization disorder) and somatoform disorder (hypochondriasis), organic affective disorders, and drug abuse disorders (intoxications and withdrawals) have prominent anxiety symptoms. The clinical scope of anxiety is broad because any normal person can, and usually at some time in life's tribulations does, experience adjustment anxiety. There is likely to be even more anxiety experienced by psychiatric patients, exclusive of anxiety disorders and the disorders just mentioned, because their perceptions of events are frequently distorted, producing more stressful events.

In a recently published book, we noted a total of over 50 conditions based on a review of the literature that can present with prominent anxiety symptoms.[7] Using data from a patient's history, mental status examination, physical examination, and laboratory tests and knowing the diagnostic criteria of DSM III and ICD-IX, one is supposed to be able to make an accurate diagnosis of the patient's disorder. As Sheehan has pointed out, this is not a straightforward process because by inclusion criteria alone, the taxonomic categories are degenerate.[10] The recent revision of DSM III by Spitzer and Williams, which permits multiple DSM III diagnoses in a given patient, may help to better define the anxiety disorders than the old criteria, but even that system may be degenerate; e.g., the patient with panic disorder followed years later by major depression with generalized anxiety is not really the same as the one who first develops major depression with generalized anxiety and then develops panic attacks.[15]

At the 1984 American Psychiatric Association meeting, Spitzer noted their development of a structured clinical interview for DSM III (SCID), which may help to assign diagnoses to anxiety disorder patients. However, the relationship of neuroendocrine, metabolic, and cardiac syndromes to DSM III diagnostic groups (organic anxiety disorders) is not well understood. More detailed information, particularly about pertinent negatives, is necessary to differentiate the etiologies that generate anxiety syndromes.

This chapter is about how to go from data to diagnosis of anxiety disorders. The taxonomic system that we will employ is DSM III as recently modified by Spitzer and Williams. The phenomenon of endogenous anxiety that forms the basis of Sheehan's taxonomy figures prominently in our differential diagnostic paradigm. The longitudinal development of anxiety, avoidance behaviors, associated moods, and other symptoms in their relationships to stressful external events provides data that may provide

Table 16-1. Diagnostic Parameters in Anxiety States and Phobias

Diagnosis	Symptoms	Stimuli	Response	Other
Panic disorder uncomplicated	Dizziness Palpitations Dyspnea Chest pain Faintness Choking Flushing Trembling Derealization Paresthesias Apprehension	None Vistas (?) Hot / humid (?) Novelty (?) Lactate IV	Hypochondriac	3 Attacks / 3 weeks 4 Symptoms / attacks Switchlike on Subpanics also Females > males Asthenic body Mitral prolapse
Limited phobia		β-Adrenergic α_2-Adrenergic Crowds Driving Elevators Public transportation Waiting lines	Social avoidant If necessary Takes stairs	Gradual onset Anticipatory Fears > avoids
Agoraphobia	Chronic fear	Separation Distance home	Avoids alone Housebound	High anxiety Panic stops (?)
Obsessive–compulsive behavior	Obsessions Compulsions Chronic fear Chronic guilt	Control loss "Germs" Unprepared Did wrong	Noxious ideas Washings Listmaking Checking Rituals	Ego alien Glove erythema Restore control Preoccupation
Generalized anxiety disorder	Trembling Restlessness Tics Palpitations Flushing / chills Nausea / diarrhea Total worry	Startle Anxiety increases	Jumpiness Strained face Fatigue Tachycardia Cold hands / feet Vomiting Hypervigil	Chronic 1 month Age > 18 yrs. Sxs of 3 of 4: 1. Hypertonous 2. Hypersympathetic 3. Apprehension

Disorder				
Social phobia	Nil threats Distractibility Blushing Shame Apprehension Tremor Palpitations Sweating Dry mouth Avoids eye contact	Scrutiny Authority Peers	Disorganization Hypervigilance Hides out Graded response Response Unconditioned, usually	4. Hypervigilance Critical Projection No spontaneity Panic
Agoraphobia (only)	Chronic fear Low threat tolerance	Separation Trapped Distance	Onset childhood Avoids alone Housebound Home	Minor panic Rare
Simple phobia	Apprehension Hypersympathetic	Conditioned Noxiousness Reptiles graded Response Thunder Enclosure Heights		Common Treat if disabling

Posttraumatic stress disorder
 	
Acute
  Onset < 6 mos.
  Duration < 6 mos.
Chronic
  Duration > 6 mos.
Delayed
  Onset > 6 mos.
	Psychic numbing
	Constricted affect
	Distractibility
	Chronic intense fear
	Survivor guilt
	Irritability
	Obsessive recollection
	Insomnia
	Recurrent nightmares
		Extreme noxious exposure
		  e.g. War, Murder)
		Reminders
			Potentiated
			Startle
			
			Increase fear
			Avoidance behaviors
			Explosiveness
			
			Paranoia	

criteria for DSM III diagnosis, axis I. Physical evaluation, including examination and laboratory tests, can provide evidence for diagnostic assessments on DSM III, axis III. In addition, we have recently noted that certain laboratory evaluations can be diagnostically useful, and we include them on axis III.[7,16,17] The resultant biaxial taxonomy seems to us to have a predictive value for responses to selected anxiolytics.

A general model of the noxious-avoidance reflex in man permits organization of the features that must be considered to classify a patient's anxiety symptoms with a diagnosis. Normal fear is a response to the threat of noxious exposure. What kind of threatened exposures cause anxiety symptoms in the patient? The anxiety response is partly dependent on a person's past exposures to similar threats. What is the patient's conditioning history with respect to threats associated with the patient's symptoms? The anxiety response is affected by one's emotional state at the time of the threat stress. What is the patient's mood state: anxiety, distress, shame, anger, attention, surprise, joy? What is the time course of the patient's anxiety symptoms? What other moods are associated with the patient's anxiety? What defense mechanisms and avoidance behaviors does the patient display, and how successful are they to elude the threatened stress? What associated historical features are also relevant to the diagnosis? Consideration of these historical data usually permits a DSM III axis I diagnosis to be reached.

3. What Is the Threat?

The kind of threatened exposure that cause anxiety symptoms in various anxiety disorder patients are as follows:

1. In uncomplicated panic disorder, there is no perceived threat at all often enough that we think no conscious or unconscious threat causes these patients' panic and subpanic anxiety attacks; i.e., they are endogenously caused. Nemiah has postulated that some patients with panic attacks have alexithymia, e.g., no consciousness of their mood state or words to describe it; thus, the patient's threat-generated but unconscious anxiety breaks through as somatic anxiety symptoms apparently out of the blue.[18] In spite of using compulsive isolation of affect as an anxiety-defensive maneuver, the typical patient who describes unprovoked somatic and other anxiety symptoms is not alexithymic. In conversion disorder, the patient is unaware of the threat and anxiety that result in somatic symptoms; however, the psychiatrist usually is aware of it. There is a large group of patients, including those with uncomplicated panic disorder, who perceive their anxiety symptoms to arise spontaneously, and the consulting psychiatrist can perceive no unconscious causation. These patients have a syndrome of endogenous anxiety, whereas if conscious or unconscious threats produce the symptoms, then those have exogenous anxiety.[11] It should be noted that the phenomenological definition "endogenous anxiety" introduced by Sheehan to describe the core feature of panic disorder is found in several disorders and is then not alone pathognomonic of panic disorder.

2. The nature of the exogenous threat in relationship to anxiety symptoms is

important to distinguish anxiety from normal fear. In normal fear, if the potential noxiousness is little, then the anxiety generated is also small. If the noxiousness is great, then so too is the anxiety generated. Also, anxiety varies as a function of one's temporal relationship to the noxious exposure, and in normal fear, events with a low probability of occurrence produce little fear.

3. In adjustment anxiety, an exogenous threat not previously associated with great noxiousness produces greater than expected levels of anxious mood, which often interfere with successful avoidance of the threat.[8]

4. In simple phobia, an exogenous threat, usually one that has been previously conditioned by significant real noxious exposure, that in itself is potentially not very noxious provokes anxiety and sustained avoidance.

5. In posttraumatic stress, the exogenous stress is "outside the range of usual human experience" and includes such events as murder, rape, accidents, natural disasters, war, etc., where the magnitude of the real noxiousness is extremely high.[8] Melick notes that about 15% of the population exposed to a natural disaster developed severe anxiety.[19]

6. In obsessive–compulsive disorder, the anxiety-generating perceived threat is loss of control, although patients complain of various things such as contamination, leaving the gas on, vomiting after eating, and so forth. Patients are afraid not to do certain ritualistic protective things such as avoiding the cracks in the sidewalk, performing the sign of the cross three times, or washing their hands.

7. In social phobia, patients fear and avoid the scrutiny of others, often authority figures, sometimes peers, seldom subordinates.[8]

8. In agoraphobia, patients fear incapacitation and thus being alone, in a crowd, in a wide-open space, in a tunnel, elevator, car, plane, bus, train, on a bridge, ladder, etc. The term agoraphobia (*agora,* Greek for marketplace) to describe these extensive phobic threats is a little misleading because much more than the "marketplace" produces fear.[20]

9. In hypochondriasis, patients are afraid that they suffer from some serious illness, and events perceived as symptoms are responded to with great foreboding.

10. In depersonalization disorder, there is anxiety about that symptom.

11. In dysthymic disorder, threats to self-esteem produce anxiety symptoms.

12. In chronic sympathomimetic abuse, patients fear that others are trying to harm them and respond to selected aspects of interactions with others in a paranoid way.

A careful assessment of what objects or situations are productive of each type of anxiety that the patient experiences is necessary to formulate a DSM III axis I diagnosis.

4. What Is the Patient's Temperament?

The examination of the patient's temporal patterns of emotional experience (e.g., emotional traits) is essential to the classification of the patient's anxiety disorder.

Anxiety was previously noted to be abnormal fear, and it occurs in three forms, which can be differentiated on phenomenological grounds.

1. Anxiety as it usually occurs in response to exogenous threats is a continuous function of the temporal proximity of noxious exposure and the intensity of such exposure, just as it is in normal fear. However, the intensity of the perceived threat may be greater than that of the real threat depending on the internal condition of the patient.
2. Endogenous anxiety does not have a graded relationship to threats but rather occurs discontinuously in a switchlike, on–off manner.[11] The intensity of an endogenous attack depends on the number of symptoms that occur together, but for any given symptom the intensity is maximal within seconds, like a flash.
3. The third form is chronic anxiety, and its symptoms can be appreciated by reading the criteria for generalized anxiety disorder. When the net production of anxiety exceeds its dissipation, chronic anxiety results. In generalized anxiety disorder, chronic anxiety is continually present to some degree for a month. Generalized chronic anxiety is an end state, a syndrome analogous to congestive heart failure that can be produced by a number of anxiety illnesses.

Some authors have advocated typing anxiety symptoms by the somatic systems that are involved: cardiorespiratory, gastrointestinal, muscular. Anxiety symptoms occur in all these symptoms in different proportions, and it is unclear to us that labeling according to which is most affected is meaningful taxonomically.

Appreciating the temporal order of development of endogenous, exogenous, and chronic–generalized anxiety forms does seem to us to be taxonomically useful, and we now discuss this approach for the anxiety disorders and some others. The "trait" qualities of the patient's other moods (e.g., anger, shame, guilt–distress, surprise, joy) and avoidance habits are also helpful to classification.

In uncomplicated panic disorder, patients experience endogenous anxiety attacks, initially in the absence of exogenous or chronic anxiety. The DSM III criteria require any four of a list of 12 anxiety symptoms—apprehension of impending death, insanity, or uncontrol, trembling, choking, palpitations, chest pain, dyspnea, paresthesias, hot or cold flashes, dizziness, derealization, faintness, sweating—to occur during the attack.[8] They last minutes. We consider only one, two, or three symptoms to be an attack if a person also has polysymptom attacks. The DSM III also requires a minimum of three attacks in 3 weeks for the diagnosis, but patients with less frequent attacks may also have the disorder.[8,11] This corresponds to Sheehan's stages 1 and 2 of the illness.[21]

Sooner or later the symptoms that are associated with these attacks condition exogenous anxiety: hypochondriacal anxiety is set off by the symptoms themselves, social anxiety is set off by the headlong flight the attacks can unexpectedly produce, agoraphobic anxiety is set off by the places one has been when the attacks occur and a tendency for the patients to "what if" themselves into the safest places to have an attack (i.e., with doctor, husband, at home, etc.). These exogenously conditioned anxieties include Sheehan's stages 3 to 6.[21] Always when the patient first develops agoraphobic anxiety and avoidance, the patient also displays chronic–generalized anxiety. Sometimes this develops as early as the hypochondriasis stage. Chronic–generalized anxiety is usually associated with fatigue, distress, anhedonia, and distractability that would meet criteria for atypical depression. Quite often patients at this stage develop sleep and appetite disturbances as well, and they fulfill criteria for major depression, Sheehan's stage 7 of panic disorder. Throughout the development of this disease, the endogenous attacks continue and may even be facilitated by exogenous and chronic anxiety. When patients have restricted their exogenous threats by extreme agoraphobic avoidance, the patients often note that the endogenous attacks remit completely.

The presence of hypochondriacal, social, or agoraphobic anxiety that is associated with little behavioral avoidance is to us panic disorder with limited phobic avoidance; however, the line between limited and extensive may be difficult to draw. In DSM IIIR, a diagnosis of major depression no longer preempts a diagnosis of panic disorder with agoraphobia or generalized anxiety disorders.[15] However, agoraphobia presupposes the presence of generalized anxiety; thus, the diagnosis is major depression and panic disorder with agoraphobia.[8,15] An additional diagnosis of generalized anxiety disorder is not made. The diagnosis in a case of panic disorder with limited phobic avoidance and criteria for generalized anxiety disorder has not been clearly spelled out to our knowledge. Given that some patients with limited phobic avoidance have, and some have not, chronic generalized anxiety, both diagnoses are meaningful. As noted before, the patient with panic disorder with agoraphobia may have the endogenous attacks in remission. However, the generalized chronic anxiety may also be in remission, and if this is true, then the presumption in DSM III that agoraphobia means generalized anxiety is false. We suggest an axis I diagnosis that is an *Anlage* of all the syndromes present: panic disorder with agoraphobia, generalized anxiety disorder, and major depression.

A major associated disorder that should be looked for in all cases of panic disorder is sedative abuse, and Sheehan noted at the 1984 annual meeting of the American Psychiatric Association that there frequently are benzodiazepines in the urines of patients who said they were not taking any.[22]

Any endogenous anxiety attack patient who describes ever having had hallucinations in any sensory modality or illusions or fugue states that did not occur associated with drug intoxication or withdrawal or classical migraine should be assumed not to have panic disorder. Also, the patient should have a family medical history of anxiety or phobia without a history of thyroid disorders.

The situation in agoraphobia without panic attacks is different from that in panic disorder with agoraphobia. This has been called "nonspecific insecurity syndrome," and there is a high trait anxiety, which is to say that standard stress produces more anxiety in these patients than in normals.[7] This is a chronic illness that begins in childhood, unlike panic disorder, which begins in young adult life. These polyphobic patients fear independent action and have the agoraphobic avoidances from exogenous stimuli and a great deal of anxiety. They do not seem to have spontaneous attacks ever, although Klein has suggested that they have minor endogenous attacks.[23] In none of the cases we have seen did the patients note spontaneous anxiety symptoms, nor did they report depersonalization or derealization that is so common in panic disorder. This is a rare disease, a fact that has led DiNardo to deny its existence.[24] We believe, however, that about 1% of those with agoraphobia have this separate disorder.

In generalized anxiety disorder, there is the chronic presence for a month of symptoms of three of four categories: increased muscle tonus, sympathetic autonomic hyperactivity, apprenhensive anticipation, and viligant hyperattention that fatigues concentration and produces difficulty falling asleep.[8] This syndrome is usually associated with chronic fatigue and atypical depressive symptoms. Endogenous anxiety attacks are not supposed to occur, but in the generalized anxiety that is associated with major depression, they are common.[25,26] There may be a subtype of panic disorder in which generalized anxiety precedes the development of endogenous attacks rather than follows them, and whether this is a variant of the presentation of panic disorder, generalized anxiety disorder, or a separate taxonomic class awaits further study.

The class of social phobics does not experience endogenous anxiety attacks, and the personalities of these individuals are remarkable for high trait shame.[7] This is in contrast to patients with endogenous-anxiety-conditioned social phobia.[11] These people are highly self-critical and shy. They often avoid accidental contacts with acquaintances; e.g., seeing a friend who did not see them, they might duck into a store to avoid being seen. Anxiety is generated by the perception that they have done something inadequate relative to the friend; thus, they can not face up to contact. Actual contact is often associated with blushing, stammering, and avoidance of eye contact. Usually the real reasons for shame are minimal, but the aversivness of the shame produced by the scrutiny of others conditions anticipatory exogenous anxiety and avoidance of certain individuals and particularly groups. In certain situations, e.g., public speaking, the level of anxiety can render the person mute. There is often the development of generalized–chronic anxiety in these patients. The onset of high trait shame can usually be traced into childhood.

Usually obsessive–compulsive patients do not experience endogenous anxiety attacks, and the presence of such, we think, should alert one to the presence of a major depression. Typically, these patients experience intense guilt if events render them out of control, and this guilt is associated with intense anxiety. The anxiety often becomes chronic and generalized, and it is associated with derealization and depersonalization. Obsessions (recurrent, ego–alien, intrusive, senseless thoughts) and compulsions (stereotypic avoidance rituals, e.g., handwashing to rid imaginary germs) accomplish some reduction in state anxiety but preoccupy the patient to the point of functional impairment. Symptoms usually wax, wane, and interchange repeatedly over years.[26–28] The presence of hallucinations, fugue states, or a family history of thyroid disease should alert one to organic conditions or schizophrenia.[29]

The anxiety experienced in posttraumatic stress disorder is chronic and generalized, and its onset may be immediately after the trauma or delayed until years later.[30,31] There are no endogenous attacks. Thoughts or situations that remind the patient of the trauma are associated with marked increases in anxiety level. These reminders occur repeatedly and have an intrusive quality. Guilt about having been somehow responsible for the event and about having survived is prominent, and distress is also prominent. Patients often have recurrent nightmares about the trauma. Paranoid anxiety is common. Shortly following the trauma, there is a ''punch drunk'' quality to the patients' behavior that has been called psychic numbing. Perhaps this occurs because concentration is exhausted and attention is poor. Yet patients are hypervigilant in that they have potentiated startle. There is distractability, which disorganizes an orderly orientation to novelty. Trait anger is also high, and explosive violent acts are often present. Pleasurable states of mind are seldom seen. Avoidance of reminders of the trauma is often seen. The occurrence of paranoid psychotic states after posttraumatic-stress-level trauma is common, and these cases have been diagnosed as complex partial epilepsy, hallucinogen abuse, and schizophrenia.[32–35] These observations may mean that, as with chronic sympathomimetics, stress can cause psychosis in normals. However, the possibility that posttraumatic stress psychosis only occurs in patients with preexisting vulnerability has not been ruled out.

The DSM III classification "organic affective disorder" requires the presence of criteria for major depression or mania and causality by an organic condition.[8] According to these criteria then, organic panic disorder does not exist as an organic affective disorder except in association with the criteria for major depression. We think this is incorrect in our clinical experience. We have noted the presence of autoimmune thyroiditis, complex partial (temporal lobe) epilepsy, Parkinson's disease, and pheochromocytoma in patients who presented complaining of endogenous anxiety, as others have also described.[16,35–39] In our cases, criteria for major depression or mania to permit a diagnosis of organic affective disorder were not present when the patients presented. Often these patients went through the same stages of hypochondriasis, social phobia, agoraphobia, generalized anxiety, to major depression that occur in panic disorder. Sometimes during other episodes of emotional illness such patients had episodes of major depression or mania (none of the Parkinson's patients).[40] Thus, the criteria for classification as organic affective disorder should be enlarged to include criteria for panic disorder without major depression as sufficient. Such a situation may occur in hypoglycemia, hypoparathyroidism, carcinoid, and acidosis.[36] We would prefer enlarging the classification of organic affective disorder rather than creating a classification of organic anxiety, which MacKenzie and Popkin suggested, because of the association of anxiety and other affective disorder at some point in the course of most patients.[41]

We have often seen organic affective disorder presenting with inclusion criteria for panic disorder in patients with complex partial (temporal lobe) epilepsy. This disorder accounted for about 25% of our outpatient sample of patients, which made it second only to panic disorder as a cause of endogenous attacks. There have been reports of complex partial epilepsy as a cause of panic attacks, and recent reports note the presence of epilepsy associated with refractory anxiety.[36,38,39,42] Usually, but not invariably, we found associated historical features that permitted differentiation. Sensory hallucination was the most consistent difference between this disorder and other causes of endogenous anxiety syndrome. Visually, these patients had hallucinations of white, black, or colored spots that may flash or oscillate while the patient has one or both eyes open or closed. There were sometimes silent cartoonlike moving picture hallucinations. There were visual illusions of the movement of objects in the visual field, usually in the left periphery. Episodic loss of depth perception, vision, or hearing were reported. Auditory hallucinations occasionally included ego–alien voices but usually were of music, tonal or staticlike noises, and marked variation in the intensity of constant-intensity sound sources. These could be differentiated from tinnitus by the patient's perception that they were coming from outside the head. Olfactory or gustatory hallucinations were less frequently reported. Spontaneous vertigo that was not associated with auditory deficit or nystagmus but associated with nausea was seen.

Fugue states occured briefly in some patients. Usually there were other kinds of affective syndromes present at other times, including intermittent explosive disorder, mania, atypical mania, major depression, and organic personality. Paranoid anxiety was common in these patients. Often the hallucinations and endogenous attacks occured cotemporally, but sometimes these symptoms occured independently in time. Sexual promiscuity, bisexuality, and homosexuality were usual in this patient group, and these same behaviors were rare in patients with panic disorder. School histories of learning disabilities in either visual–spatial or verbal tasks were common. We think complex partial epilepsy is a common cause of endogenous panic anxiety.

The histories of patients later diagnosed as having autoimmune thyroiditis (e.g., Hashimoto's or Grave's diseases) are often remarkable for being indistinguishable from histories obtained from patients having panic disorder.[16] When we reported this observation at the 1984 Annual meeting of the American Psychiatric Association, Donald Klein noted that he had found (and later published) an unexpectedly high incidence of elevated plasma TSH or T_3 concentrations in phobic patients.[37] Features that this organic affective disorder and panic disorder share include (1) the onset of endogenous anxiety attacks that are followed after variable periods of time by hypochondriasis, social phobia, agoraphobia, generalized anxiety, and major depression, (2) an onset in young adult life, and (3) when an adequate sample of first and second degree relatives can be assessed, a family history of similar nervous disorder. Eventually, the development of physical signs of thyroid excess or deficiency would serve to differentiate thyroiditis from panic disorder, but by then the thyroiditis patient would have gone through years of suffering that could result in severe impairment or even suicide. Any patient with these historical features needs a laboratory evaluation for autoimmune thyroiditis. Subclinical autoimmune thyroiditis patients comprised approximately 10% of all patients who complained of endogenous anxiety.

The histories of patients later diagnosed as having Parkinson's disease in the early stages can appear quite similar to those of panic disorder, but there are some differential points.[40] The onset of endogenous attacks in old age, and their frequent onset when the patient is trying to initiate ambulation, seemed useful to separate them. The presence of an observable tremor that is seldom as pronounced in panic disorder, stooped posture, shortened stride, and an affect that is more flat than anxious or frowning are the main mental status examination differences.

5. Physical Testing in the Diagnosis of Anxiety Disorders

Physical testing plays an essential role in the differentiation of organic affective disorders from anxiety disorders. We have had success using certain biochemical parameters as markers that can differentiate certain anxiety disorders from each other (see Table 16-2 and Figure 16-1). We expect the role of biological markers in the diagnosis of anxiety and other affective disorders to grow, and we note the recent demonstration by Gershon and his collaborators of supranormal numbers of muscarinic receptors on the skin cells of patients with bipolar affective disorder as an example of that growth.[43] Studies of the molecular biology of psychiatric patients have given birth

Table 16-2. Norepinephrine Catabolism in Anxiety States and Major Depression[a]

Diagnostic group	Number	Mean age (range)	Sex	Norepinephrine (μmoles/day $\pm$ S.E.)	MHPG (mg/day $\pm$ S.E.)	VMA (mg/day $\pm$ S.E.)
Panic disorder (PD)	97	37 (18–68)	37m, 60f	36.82098 $\pm$ 1.0	1.455 $\pm$ 0.6	5.679 $\pm$ 0.2
General anxiety disorder (GAD)	13	36 (23–49)	7m, 6f	59.15637 $\pm$ 5.6**	2.173 $\pm$ 0.4*	8.733 $\pm$ 0.9**
Obsessive compulsive disorder (O–C)	7	32 (22–49)	3m, 4f	54.52674 $\pm$ 4.6**	2.233 $\pm$ 0.4*	8.066 $\pm$ 0.7**
Major depression (MD)	15	43 (26–63)	4m, 11f	38.78086 $\pm$ 3.5	1.665 $\pm$ 0.2	6.044 $\pm$ 0.5

[a]Difference from PD: *$p < 0.05$; **$p < 0.01$.

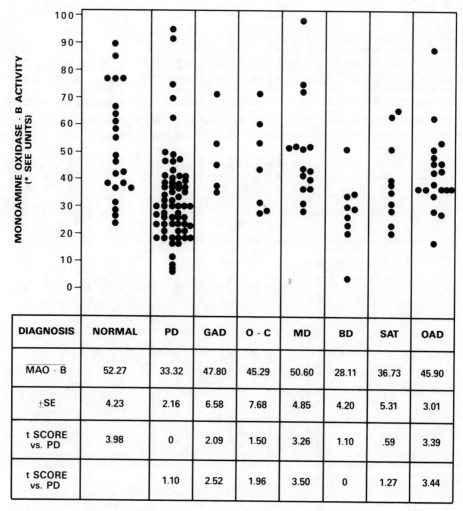

DIAGNOSIS	NORMAL	PD	GAD	O - C	MD	BD	SAT	OAD
MAO - B	52.27	33.32	47.80	45.29	50.60	28.11	36.73	45.90
±SE	4.23	2.16	6.58	7.68	4.85	4.20	5.31	3.01
t SCORE vs. PD	3.98	0	2.09	1.50	3.26	1.10	.59	3.39
t SCORE vs. PD		1.10	2.52	1.96	3.50	0	1.27	3.44

Figure 16-1. Monoamine oxidase B activity in anxiety and depressive states. Units are nanomoles iodobenzylamine per hour per milligram protein.

to a scientific psychiatry that promises to become as fully sophisticated as any other area of medicine.

Given the need to rule out organic affective disorder in patients who complain of endogenous anxiety, and being aware of no systematic study of how much workup is sufficient to do this, we attempted to use physical and laboratory examinations that to some might appear to be "looking for zebras with a fine-tooth comb."

Significant numbers of organic affective-depressed patients with objective evidence of autoimmune thyroiditis had (1) normal free tetraiodothyronine and (2) normal base-line TSH and also (3) met symptom criteria for major depression.[44] We have observed something similar in patients without major depression but having panic disorder criteria and a TRH test ΔTSH of 20 or greater. The majority of these patients had antimicrosomal thyroid antibodies in titer greater than 1 : 200, and often the titers were greater than 1 : 1,000,000 and/or thyroid radionuceotide scan had shown abnormally increased or decreased uptake. The majority of these patients had normal baseline TSH levels but experienced some relief of panic attacks when treated with enough exogenous thyroid hormone to normalize the TRH test's ΔTSH. Generalized chronic anxiety responds less completely to thyroid hormones, and present evidence does not permit a conclusion to be reached on the question "Does thyroid replacement eliminate the emotional pathology in autoimmune thyroiditis?" We conclude that autoimmune thyroiditis produces affective disorders, including panic attacks, long before the thyroid index falls or the basal TSH rises. Physical examination of the thyroid was the least accurate parameter to find these cases. Any patient who complains of endogenous anxiety attacks should get a TRH test, and if the ΔTSH is greater than 20, then antithyroid antibodies and a radionuceotide scan should be obtained.

Neurologists and psychiatrists used to assume that if the patient's history suggested complex partial (temporal lobe) epilepsy and the patient's EEG was negative, then the patient was having dissociative symptoms rather than epilepsy. This overreliance on a 20-min sample of brain electrical activity may have resulted in the misdiagnosis of the majority of cases of complex partial temporal lobe epilepsy.

In a pilot study, we (C. Hamlin, C. Heliksson, and G. Tucker, unpublished data, 1976) examined the hallucinatory experiences of patients with EEG-documented temporal lobe epilepsy. The sensory hallucinations we found then served as the basis for information we looked for in patients' answers to questions about their vision, hearing, smell, etc. All patients who reported such symptoms without directed questioning in the endogenous anxiety attack group, regardless of the presence of fugue states, received a nasopharyngeal-lead EEG (eight lead) after sleep deprivation. Some patients received 24-hr EEG telemetry on no medications, and some received a 24-hr EEG after a therapeutic trial of desipramine was complicated by persistent hyperautonomic side effects, fugue states, rage attacks, or failure of the panic attacks to respond to a plasma level of 200 ng/ml. In only one case was an EEG abnormality found with the nasopharyngeal-lead EEGs, and that one was seen retrospectively after the desipramine-challenge 24-hr EEG was markedly abnormal. Several of the patients had abnormal unmedicated 24-hr EEGs (temporal lobe spike abnormalities) even though the nasopharyngeal-lead EEGs were normal. The majority of patients who reported sensory hallucinations or illusions or explosive episodes with endogenous attacks could not tolerate a therapeutic level of desipramine, and some had temporal lobe spiking on 24-hr EEG telemetry. We conclude that patients having a history that suggests the organic affective disorder/complex partial epilepsy syndrome that we previously described should receive a therapeutic trial of desipramine and a 24-hr EEG telemetry while at a therapeutic level of that medication to attempt to document an epileptic disorder.

Jacob *et al.* at Pitt noted abnormal vestibular and audiologic testing in panic disorder with agoraphobia patients who reported dizziness during their panic attacks.[53] We found a patient, who noted vertigo as part of his panic attacks, who had abnormal caloric testing, positional vertigo, and normal audiometry. This patient exhibited markedly worse panic attacks on therapeutic window desipramine and he improved when the medication was withdrawn. Evaluation of vestibular and audiologic reflexes may be therapeutically useful.

Gorman *et al.* have noted no hypoglycemia in a sample of patients with endogenous attacks.[45] We found abnormal glucose tolerance tests infrequently in our endogenous anxiety patients, the criterion being an anxiety attack occuring in association with a lower than 50 mg/dl glucose concentration during the test. A small minority of endogenous attack patients may have them caused by hypoglycemia, but doing glucose tolerance tests was not diagnostically useful most of the time.

It is well known that valvular heart disease is a potential cause of tachyarrhythmias, which can cause an endogenous anxiety attack.[46] As well, minor degrees of mitral valve prolapse are often seen noncausually associated with endogenous anxiety attacks in patients.[47] We think that auscultation of the chest is sufficient to rule out symptomatically significant mitral valve prolapse, but it may not detect the minor prolapse that is often associated with true panic disorder.

We examined 24-hr urines for methoxyhydroxyphenylglycol (MHPG) and for methoxyhydroxymandelic acid (VMA) in the majority of our endogenous anxiety patients. One case of pheochromocytoma was found associated with endogenous anxiety, headaches, and hypertension. That diagnosis was suggested by MHPG and VMA results. This patient had an MHPG of about 4500 µg per 24 hr and a VMA of 15,000 µg, and he received abdominal CAT scan and chest tomograms and a phentolamine challenge test, which documented the tumor.

Platelet monoamine oxidase (B) was normal at 41 (see Fig. 16-1); MHPG and VMA urinary excretion seems valuable to subtype anxiety patients. Patients with panic disorder had significantly less norepinephrine catabolites than those with obsessive–compulsive disorder or generalized anxiety disorder (see Table 16-2).[17] We reported at the 1984 American Psychiatric Association meeting that nonmajor depressed panic disorder patients had significant blunting of ΔTSH compared to normals and that blunting of the TRH test did not differentiate major depressed patients from panic disorder patients (see Fig. 16-2).[16] A ΔTSH greater than 20 was seen in our agoraphobia-only patients and in organic affective disorder/temporal lobe epilepsy in the absence of antithyroid antibodies.

We also reported at the 1984 American Psychiatric Association meeting that platelet monoamine oxidase isoenzyme B (using benzylamine as substrate) activity was abnormally low in panic disorder, and there was a significant difference between panic disorder and major depression that was followed by generalized anxiety and endogenous anxiety attacks (see Fig. 16-1).[16] Low monoamine oxidase B activity may be a marker of panic disorder, and we observed normal activities in major depression, organic affective disorder/TLE, and obsessive–compulsive disorder (see Fig. 16-1). The MAO-B was also low in autoimmune thyroiditis and in bipolar depression. We think that MAO-B activity is a useful diagnostic marker to differentiate anxiety and depressive disorders.

The presence of a DSM III criteria panic attack is seen following intravenous sodium lactate infusion in about 90% of panic disorder patients versus about 10% of normals.[48,49] Liebowitz *et al.* reported a normal lactate infusion response in social phobia, significantly less often positive than in panic disorder.[54] We have seen the normal rate of lactate response in generalized anxiety, obsessive–compulsives, social phobics, and patients with major depression followed by generalized anxiety and endogenous attacks. About 50% of autoimmune thyroiditis patients have a positive lactate response, and they often have anxiety symptoms for hours after the end of the

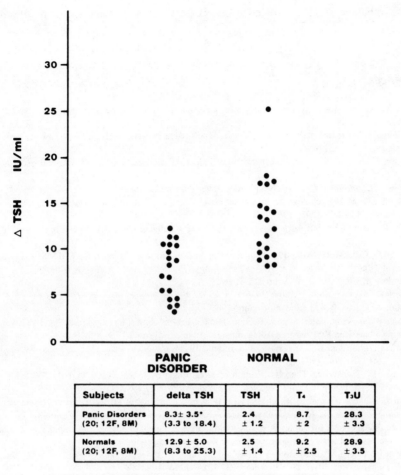

Subjects	delta TSH	TSH	T₄	T₃U
Panic Disorders (20; 12F, 8M)	8.3± 3.5* (3.3 to 18.4)	2.4 ± 1.2	8.7 ± 2	28.3 ± 3.3
Normals (20; 12F, 8M)	12.9 ± 5.0 (8.3 to 25.3)	2.5 ± 1.4	9.2 ± 2.5	28.9 ± 3.5

Figure 16-2. ΔTSH in panic disorders. *, t score = 3.3p < 0.01.

infusion. Base-line and positive lactate infusion response increases in epinephrine and tribulin plasma concentrations have been reported to be significantly greater than normal in panic disorder.[50,51] A 1-mg dexamethasone suppression test usually showed suppression of cortisol concentration below 5 μg for 24 hr afterward in cases of panic disorder unless biological signs of major depression supervened. The finding of abnormally decreased left parahippocampal gyrus metabolic rate (positron in 7 patients with positive responses to emission tomography) i.v. lactate infusion in panic disorder, if confirmed, promises the emergence of neuroradiological diagnosis of panic disorders.[52]

Are physical and laboratory examinations useful in the differential diagnosis of anxiety and phobic disorders? Our experience has shown to us that they are useful to differentiate panic disorder, generalized anxiety disorder, obsessive–compulsive disorder, organic affective disorders, major depression, and bipolar depression from each other. More importantly, these observations can begin the task of objectively defining which anxiety states are caused by neurochemical imbalances and the specific natures of those imbalances. This knowledge is necessary for the rational use of psychotropic drugs.

References

1. Mowrer A: Stimulus response analysis of anxiety and its role as a reinforcing agent. *Psychol Rev* 46:553–565, 1939.
2. Broadhurst P: The interaction of task difficulty and motivation: The Yerkes Dodson law revived. *Acta Psychol (Amst)* 16:321–342, 1959.
3. Hamlin C, Goldstein L: Ischemic pain stress: Effect on lateralization of EEG amplitudes. *Adv Biol Psychiatry* 9:39–43, 1982.
4. Pavlov I: *Conditioned Reflexes.* New York, Dover Publishing, 1960.
5. Kandell ER: Metapsychology to molecular biology: Explorations into the nature of anxiety. *Am J Psychiatry* 140:1277–1293, 1983.
6. Klein D, Rabkin J (eds): *Anxiety: New Research and Changing Concepts.* New York, Raven Press, 1981.
7. Hamlin C, Gold MS: Anxiolytics: Predicting response/maximizing efficacy, in Gold MS, Lydiard RB, Carman J (eds): *Advances in Psychopharmacology: Predicting and Improving Treatment Response.* Boca Raton, CRC Press, 1984, pp 225–276.
8. American Psychiatric Association: *Diagnostic and Statistical Manual of Mental Disorders,* ed 3. Washington, American Psychiatric Association, 1980.
9. Spitzer R: New approaches to classification: Panic disorders clinical update. Presented at 137th annual meeting, American Psychiatric Association, Los Angeles, Abstract 12B, May 1984.
10. Sheehan D, Sheehan K: The classification of anxiety and hysterical states, Part I. *J Clin Psychopharmacol* 2(4):235–244, 1982.
11. Sheehan D, Sheehan K: The classification of anxiety and hysterical states, Part II. Toward a more heuristic classification. *J Clin Psychopharmacol* 2(6):386–393, 1982.
12. Boyd J, Burke J, Gruenberg E, et al: The diagnostic hierarchies of DSM-III. Paper presented at the Annual Meeting of the American Psychiatric Association, New York, Abstract 40, 1983.
13. Thoren P, Asberg M, Cronholm B, et al: Clomipramine treatment of obsessive–compulsive disorder: A controlled clinical trial. *Arch Gen Psychiatry* 37:1281–1285, 1980.
14. Thoren P, Asberg M, Bertilsson L, et al: Clomipramine treatment of obsessive–compulsive disorder: Biochemical aspects. *Arch Gen Psychiatry* 37:1289–1294, 1980.
15. Spitzer R, Williams J: Proposed revisions in the DSM III classification of anxiety disorders based on research and clinical experience. Paper presented at Anxiety and the Anxiety Disorders, National Institute of Mental Health sponsored conference, Tuxedo Park, New York, Abstract 40, September 12–14, 1983.
16. Hamlin C, Dackis C, Martin D, et al: Blunted thyrotropin release hormone stimulation test in panic disorders. Diagnosis and treatment of panic and phobic disorders-session. Paper presented at the Annual Meeting of the American Psychiatric Association, Los Angeles, Abstract 13, May 8, 1984.
17. Hamlin C, Lydiard RB, Martin D, et al: Urinary excretion of noradrenaline metabolite decreased in panic disorder. *Lancet* 2:470–471, 1983.
18. Nemiah J: Alexithymia and psychosomatic illness. *J Cont Ed Psychiatry* 10:25–37, 1978.
19. O'Melick M, Logue J, Fredrick C: Stress and disaster, in Goldberger L, and Shlomo B (ed): *Handbook of Stress.* New York, Free Press, 1982, pp 613–630.
20. *Webster's Seventh New Collegiate Dictionary.* Springfield, G & C Merriam, 1970.
21. Sheehan D: Strategies for diagnosis and treatment of anxiety disorders, in Pasnau R (ed): *Diagnosis and Treatment of Anxiety Disorders.* Washington, American Psychiatric Press, 1984.
22. Quitkin F, Rifkin A, Kaplan J, et al: Phobic anxiety syndrome complicated by drug dependence and addiction. *Arch Gen Psychiatry* 27:159–162, 1972.
23. Klein D: Medication in the treatment of panic attacks and phobic states. *Psychopharmacol Bull* 18:85–90, 1982.
24. DiNardo P, O'Brien G, Barlow D, et al: Reliability of DSM III anxiety disorder categories using a new structured interview. *Arch Gen Psychiatry* 40:1070–1074, 1983.

25. VanValkenburg C, Winokur G, Behar D, et al: Depressed women with panic attacks. *J Clin Psychiatry* 45(9):367–369, 1984.

26. Leckman J. Weissman M, Merikangas K, et al: Panic disorder and major depression. *Arch Gen Psychiatry* 40:1055–1060, 1983.

27. Pollitt J: Natural history of obsessional states. *Br Med J* 1:194–198, 1957.

28. Kringler E: Obsessional neurotics: A long term follow up. Br J Psychiatry 111:709–722, 1965.

29. Mayer-Gross W, Slater E, Roth M: *Clinical Psychiatry,* Chapter 3. London, Bailliere Tindall Cassel, 1974.

30. Coleman J, Butcher J, Carson R: *Abnormal Psychology and Modern Life.* Glenview, Scott Foresman, 1980, pp 171–203.

31. Bartemeier L, Kube L, Menninger K: Combat exhaustion. *J Nerv Ment Dis* 104:385–525, 1946.

32. VanPutten T, Emory W: Traumatic neurosis in Vietnam returnees. *Arch Gen Psychiatry* 29:695–698, 1973.

33. Tausk V: Diagnostic considerations concerning the symptomatology of the so called war psychoses. *Psychoanal Q* 38:382–405, 1969.

34. Jaffe R: Dissociative phenomena in former concentration camp inmates. *Int J Psychoanal* 49:310–312, 1968.

35. Friedman M: Post-Vietnam syndrome: Recognition and management. *Psychosomatics* 22(11):931–943, 1981.

36. Rosenbaum J: Anxiety, in Lazare A (ed): *Outpatient Psychiatry: Diagnosis and Treatment.* Baltimore, Williams & Wilkins, 1979, p 252.

37. Lindemann C, Zitrin C, Klein D: Thyroid dysfunction in phobic patients. *Psychosomatics* 25(8):603–606, 1984.

38. Dietch J: Diagnosis of organic anxiety disorders. *Psychosomatics* 22:661–669, 1981.

39. Dietch J: Cerebral tumor presenting with panic attacks. *Psychosomatics* 25:861–863, 1984.

40. Schwab R, Fabing H, Pritchard A: Psychiatric symptoms in Parkinson's disease. *Am J Psychiatry* 107:901–907, 1951.

41. Mackenzie T, Popkin M: Organic anxiety syndrome. *Am J Psychiatry* 140:342–344, 1983.

42. Brodsky L, Zuniga J, Casenas E, et al: Refractory anxiety: A masked epileptiform disorder. *Psychiatr J Univ Ottawa* 8:42–45, 1983.

43. Nadi NS, Nurnberger JI, Gershon S: Muscarinic receptor super-sensitivity in bipolar skin. *N Engl J Med* 311:225–230, 1984.

44. Gold MS, Kronig M, Pottash ALC, et al: Subclinical hypothyroidism in depressed patients. Presented at the 137th annual meeting, American Psychiatric Association, Los Angeles, Abstract 22A, May 5–11, 1984.

45. Gorman J, Martinez J, Liebowitz M, et al: Hypoglycemia and panic attacks. *Am J Psychiatry* 141:101–102, 1984.

46. Crowe R, Pauls D, Kerber R, et al: Panic disorder and mitral valve prolapse, in Klein D, Rabkin J (eds): *Anxiety: New Research and Changing Concepts.* New York, Raven Press, 1981, p 103–116.

47. Gorman J, Fyer A, Gileklich J: Mitral valve prolapse and panic disorder: Effect of imipramine, in Klein D, Rabkin J (eds): *Anxiety: New Research and Changing Concepts.* New York, Raven Press, 1981, p 317–340.

48. Pitts F, McClure J: Lactate metabolism in anxiety neurosis. *N Engl J Med* 277:1329–1336, 1967.

49. Rifkin A, Klein D, Dillion D: Blockade by imipramine or desipramine of panic induced by sodium lactate. *Am J Psychiatry* 138(5):676–677, 1981.

50. Sandler M, Glover V, Elsworth J, et al: Tribulin output in anxiety and panic. Symposium on neurobiology of agoraphobia. Presented at the 137th annual meeting, American Psychiatric Association, Los Angeles, Abstract 30A, May 1984.

51. Shader R, Goodman M, Gever M. Panic disorders: Current perspectives. *J Clin Psychopharmacol* 2(6):25–265, 1982.

52. Reiman E, Raichle M, Butler K, et al: A focal brain abnormality in panic disorder, a severe form of anxiety. *Nature* 310:683–685, 1984.

53. Jacob R, Moller M, Turner S, et al: Otoneurological examination in panic disorders and agoraphobia with panic attacks. *Am J Psychiatry* 142:715–720, 1985.

54. Liebowitz M, Fyer A, Gorman J, et al: Specificity of lactate infusions in social phobia versus panic disorders. *Am J Psychiatry* 142: 947–950, 1985

Evaluation of the Substance Abuser

Lawrence DeMilio, M.D., Mark S. Gold, M.D., and David Martin

1. Introduction

The evaluation of patients abusing legal or illicit substances is a complicated clinical task. Although the process includes basic elements common to all comprehensive psychiatric evaluations, many specialized avenues of questioning and data collection are added. This unique evaluation also calls for specific shifts in interview format, approach to the patient, interpretation of behaviors and symptoms reported, diagnostic procedures utilized, and initial management decisions.

In terms of general approach, it is crucial to quickly foster active patient involvement in the evaluation and treatment processes. Early focus on this issue can direct patients away from ultimately counterproductive "passive participant" roles.

2. The Clinical Interview

Interview technique must shift to a more directive style. Initially, it is best to allow the patient to take the lead in describing his personal background, recent events, and reasons for seeking treatment. However, the clinician must collect certain crucial data in the first interview (e.g., specific recent drug intake, current withdrawal symptoms, medical history). Therefore, the interviewer must shift to specific, direct questions about certain areas fairly early.

In reporting their drug use, patients often feel threatened by concerns over confidentiality. Therefore, clinicians working with these patients must be familiar with regional disclosure laws and discuss these issues openly.

Obtaining a comprehensive and detailed drug history is crucial. This history should cover each of the following categories: alcohol, including form and amounts used; stimulants, including cocaine and amphetamines; narcotics, including heroin,

Lawrence DeMilio, M.D. • Stony Lodge Hospital, Ossining-on-Hudson, New York 10562. *Mark S. Gold, M.D.* • Research Facilities, Fair Oaks Hospital, Summit, New Jersey 07901, and Fair Oaks Hospital at Boca/Delray, Delray Beach, Florida 33445. *David Martin* • Psychiatric Diagnostic Laboratories of America, Inc., Summit, New Jersey 07901.

methadone, codeine, and meperidine; cannabis, and whether used as marijuana or hashish; CNS depressants (other than alcohol), especially barbiturates, benzodiazepines, methaqualone, and glutethimide; hallucinogens, including LSD and PCP; inhalants, most frequently glue or paints; psychotropic prescription medications, including neuroleptics and tricyclic and MAOI antidepressant medications.

In each category, there are several important facts to cover. Record amounts used and routes of use. Ask about which drug combinations the patient has used. Detail the date and circumstances of first use and outline the lifetime period of heaviest use. Closely detail the pattern of recent use, especially the 3 to 4 weeks preceding evaluation; this will best predict the likely course of detoxification. Ask about the development of tolerance and obtain specifics about previous withdrawal experiences (e.g., did convulsions, significant depression, or delirium occur?).

Certain aspects of personal medical history should be covered at initial interview. Prescription medications utilized for current medical conditions must be recorded. Ask about known neurological, endocrinologic, or cardiovascular conditions, each of which may complicate the detoxification period.

Interviewers should attempt to outline the general current role of substance use in the patient's life. Patients continue to "use" for a variety of reasons. For example, many continue purely for the pleasurable effects of their drug(s) of choice. Some, farther along a drug use cycle, continue primarily to avoid painful aspects of "rebound" or overt withdrawal. Some use drugs to form social contacts, often because of serious social skills deficits. Certain patients describe a life style totally devoid of pleasurable activities except for drug use. Occasionally, special life circumstances dictate patterns of use: for example, some female patients have periods of heavy use only when involved in relationships with male users or dealers.[1] Knowing a patient's individual pattern will help in forming an optimal treatment plan.

"Staging" is another aspect of drug evaluation advocated by many authorities.[2-4] Basically, it implies that patients will pass through recognizable stages of use prior to complete "chemical dependency." For example, among adolescents, occasional, unplanned weekend use of beer or marijuana with peers is labeled the earliest, "experimental" stage. The next stage includes occasional solitary use, use on school days, and development of early tolerance. The following stage includes frequent solitary use, "dealing" or stealing for drug funds, and school or minor legal complications from use. The final, "dependency" stage is characterized by daily use, difficulty skipping days, physical problems, occasionally, initial use of injected drugs, and (often denied) loss of control over use.

Evaluation of psychiatric symptomatology should be completed at initial interview, including a temporal sequence of symptoms reported and substance use. However, diagnostic impressions must be considered provisional, pending sequential reexamination as detoxification and stabilization proceed.

Once the pertinent medical, psychiatric, and historical data have been obtained, certain initial management decisions must be made. In general, continued evaluation of the serious substance-abusing patient is best accomplished in a controlled, inpatient setting. This decision immediately and effectively removes the patient from his drug supplies. It interrupts the previously reinforcing behavioral cycle of drug seeking, purchase, and use and removes the patient from secondarily reinforcing environmental "cues" (e.g., prior drug acquaintances, neighborhoods where drugs had previously been purchased). These cues can provide serious threats to continued recovery.[5] This management decision also introduces patients to a new peer group with developing values strongly antithetical to their prior drug use. This can become an important "bridge" to aftercare group programs. Further, it allows for close monitoring during detoxification and efficient coordination of the neurological, medical, and psychological components of continued comprehensive evaluation.

3. Physical Examination

Physical examination provides further important data. Examiners should look for the common medical complications of substance abuse, many of which stem from drug adulterants, use of unsterile needles, or deficiencies in nutritional or immunologic status. Examination of the skin may reveal damage from i.v. use or cigarette burns stemming from the analgesic and soporific effects of sedatives. Cardiac examination may reveal arrhythmias or valvular damage, especially among intravenous users. Abdominal examination frequently identifies RUQ tenderness accompanying active hepatitis. Ophthalmologic examination may show retinal vascular emboli in i.v. users. Neurological examination should screen for peripheral neuropathies, ataxia, and encephalopathy. Among intravenous users, common infections include skin abscesses, cellulitis, endocarditis, hepatitis, meningitis, tuberculosis, and pneumonia.[6-9] Hypertension, tachycardia, and arrhythmias are common in stimulant abusers.[10] In some i.v. users, cerebrovasular accidents can occur on the basis of sudden shifts in blood pressure or from arterial emboli.[11,12]

In patients with histories of heavy alcohol abuse, close physical assessment is crucial. Hydration needs to be assessed through daily weights and urine specific gravity, providing renal function is normal. Potassium and magnesium balance should be closely monitored and deficits corrected. Erythrocyte indices and iron stores should be assessed. Prothrombin time should be measured and vitamin K supplements prescribed as needed. Temperature and white blood cell counts should be followed. Since lowered resistance to infection is seen in many alcoholics, vigorous workup of fever persisting beyond detoxification periods is indicated.[13]

Since many patients seen for substance abuse have grossly inadequate nutritional status,[14] a comprehensive evaluation of vitamin deficiency states should be performed and specific deficiencies corrected.

Since patients may forget or distort intake amounts or may not be aware of the composition of purchased "street" samples, the first focus of physical examination is the identification of acute overdose or withdrawal patterns.

4. Intoxication and Withdrawal

Signs of alcohol intoxication (see Table 17-1) include slurred speech, incoordination, and nystagmus. Tachycardia, elevated systolic blood pressure, orthostatic hypotension, hand or facial tremulousness, nausea, and vomiting are characteristic of early

Table 17-1. Signs and Symptoms of Intoxication, Overdose, and Withdrawal States

Drug	Intoxication	Overdose	Withdrawal
Alcohol	Slurred speech; incoordination; unsteady gait; nystagmus; flushed facies; irritability; mood lability; decreased attention	Relatively uncommon; shallow coma with frequent aspiration	Nausea; vomiting; hand or facial tremors; tachycardia; elevated blood pressure; sweating; anxiety; irritability
Opioids	Miosis, lethargy, sedation, decreased attention span	Pinpoint pupils; depressed respiration; coma; occasionally, pulmonary edema	Lacrimation; rhinorrhea; dilated pupils; pilo-erection; diarrhea; tachycardia; fever; mild hypertension; insomnia
CNS Depressants (other than alcohol, including glutethimide, ethchlorvynol, meprobamate, chloral hydrate, methaqualone, barbiturates, and benzodiazepines)	Slurred speech; incoordination; unsteady gait; impaired attention and memory	General: Coma with depressed respiration; nystagmus; small, reactive pupils Gluthetimide: cyclic coma and wakefulness Benzodiazepines: coma extremely rare, usually implies mixed-substance ingestion Methaqualone: more intact pain sensation and gag reflex	Nausea; vomiting; coarse tremors of the hands or face; tachycardia; elevated blood pressure; weakness; anxiety; irritability
PCP or similar agent	Vertical or horizontal nystagmus: increased blood pressure and heart rate; diminished responsivity to pain dysarthria; ataxia, psychomotor agitation; emotional lability; grandiosity; synsthesias	Ataxia; muscle rigidity; hypothermia; elevated blood pressure, pulse; delirium; convulsions; coma	
Cannabis	Tachycardia; injected conjunctivae; dry oral mucosae; euphoria or apathy; sensation of slowed time and increased perception; increased appetite; recent memory failures	Delusional thinking, frequently of paranoid nature	Controversial: Case reports of anxiety, irritability, sweating, chills, insomnia, anorexia, and tremulousness occurring within 48 hrs of cessation following regular, heavy use of high-potency THC preparations
Hallucinogens	False experiences of visual, auditory, or other sensory modal-	Dilated pupils; tachycardia; sweating; blurred vision; incoordination;	

(continued)

Table 17-1. (*Continued*)

Drug	Intoxication	Overdose	Withdrawal
	ity; macropsia or micropsia; synesthesia; variable mood changes—euphoria, lability, or dysphoric states; depersonalization; derealization	tremors; marked ideas of reference	
Inhalants	Very variable: intoxication may be similar to alcohol, with exaggerated euphoria, or may produce hallucinations, or delusions; effects peak and dissipate rapidly	Occasionally, arrhythmias occur with rapidly repeated doses	
CNS stimulants including cocaine, amphetamine, and other sympathomimetic amines	Tachycardia; pupillary dilation; elevated blood pressure and pulse rate; psychomotor agitation; nausea; vomiting; elation, hypervigilance	Delirium; delusional disorders, with ideas of reference; aggressiveness, hostility; occasionally, generalized convulsions, hyperthermia, arrhythmias	Irritable or depressed mood; fatigue; disturbed sleep with increased dreaming

withdrawal. Barbiturate and other CNS sedatives produce similar intoxication and withdrawal patterns.

Signals of opioid withdrawal include dilated pupils, tachycardia, hypertension, diarrhea, piloerection, lacrimation, rhinorrhea, sweating, and fever, whereas overdose signs include pinpoint pupils, depressed respiration, and coma.

Phencyclidine intoxication often include marked psychomotor agitation, anxiety, emotional lability, and synesthesias. Ataxia, vertical and horizontal nystagmus, decreased pain sensitivity, and increased pulse and blood pressure are commonly reported.

Cannabis intoxication signs include reddened conjunctivae, dry mouth, and tachycardia.

Intoxication with central nervous system stimulants produces pupillary dilatation, tachycardia, and elevated blood pressure. Withdrawal states include irritability, fatigue, and disrupted sleep cycle.

5. Laboratory Confirmation of Diagnosis

Even if the history of recent drug ingestion is reported with complete candor, laboratory identification of drug intake is necessary. Supposedly identical "street" samples have, on analysis, varied tremendously in combination, quantity, and quality of active components. Adulterants are rarely known to the purchaser. Further, developed tolerance to many drug effects may mislead an examiner viewing the patient following recent use. Quantitative laboratory serum and urine drug analyses can help prevent serious clinical errors. For example, failure to uncover chronic benzodiazepine use can lead to confusion when late-onset withdrawal symptoms occur. Again, PCP is a common "additive" to THC preparations, and its ingestion can lead to a cycle of episodic emotional and behavioral lability alternating with clearing (possibly as a result of intermittent, uneven intestinal absorption). If not anticipated by quantitative laboratory analysis, such cycles can easily be misunderstood by clinical staff. More ominous is underestimation of acute toxic or withdrawal potentials because of clinical "guesstimates" of the amount or potency of samples recently used. Sequential quantitative analyses allow for a meaningful correlation of mood or behavioral changes with drug effects as evaluation progresses. This can be critical when one is attempting to differentiate autonomous from substance-induced affective syndromes ("organic affective syndromes"). In those patients already on psychotropic medications, quantitative serum analysis can be crucial; for example, concomitant use of certain illicit drugs can alter the serum level of tricyclic antidepressants by more than 200%.[15]

5.1. Testing Methodology

Clinicians can now choose among methodologically different drug analysis procedures. Thin-layer chromatography (TLC) "drug screens" have been widely used and can rapidly provide important, basic information about substances recently ingested in large amounts. The procedure utilizes thin-layer plate migration patterns to identify substances. However, it is the least sensitive of the available analytical methods, and it may fail to detect drug levels that can still produce significant psychiatric symptomatology. Also, most TLC procedures fail to detect THC, PCP, and LSD.

5.2. Radioimmunoassay and Enzyme Immunoassay

The specificity of the immunoassays is considered far less than that of GC and GC–MS. This can be an advantage in some cases, however, because interaction with drug plus metabolites in a sample by the immunoassay system increases sensitivity in "total" drug detection. In chromatography a single molecular species is determined. The sensitivity, depending on the particular assay, ranges between micrograms and picograms. The EIA system is very popular and commonly used because no extraction or centrifugation is required, and the system lends itself for easy automation. Although an EIA screen is more costly than TLC, toxicological screens using EIA are much more sensitive for most drugs and are more likely to detect lower level of drug use. However, EIA screens yielding one or many positives should be confirmed by GC–MS.

Greatly improved sensitivity and specificity can be gained by using enzyme immunoassay, or radioimmunoassay techniques. These systems use specific substance antibody preparations to identify accurately drugs in serum or urine samples. Such screens will identify accurately the long-term, low-dose substance use patterns often important in psychiatric evaluations (see Table 17-2). However, the most sensitive and

Table 17-2. Sensitivity of Assays (μg/ml)

Drug	Enzyme immunoassay	TLC	GC–MS
Opiates	0.30	1.00	0.025
Methadone	0.30	1.00	0.025
Amphetamine	1.00	1.00	0.025
Barbiturates	1.00	1.00	0.025
Cocaine	1.00	1.00	0.050
Benzodiazepines	0.5	1.00	0.050
PCP	0.08	NA[a]	0.010
THC	0.02	NA[a]	0.005
Propoxyphene	1.00	1.00	0.025
Methaqualone	0.30	1.00	0.025

[a]Not applicable.

specific analytic method utilizes gas chromatography and mass spectrometry procedures; such systems can accurately identify specific substances present in samples in nanogram ranges.[16]

Many clinicians prefer routinely obtaining serum samples for drug analysis. Blood levels most accurately correlate with observed mood or behavioral drug effects, and serum samples are preferable whenever specific, very recent use is reported or suspected. Blood is the sample of choice for forensic testing or proving a person was "under the influence" at a specified time. However, urine samples can also provide accurate records of historical or recent use if sample collection is properly supervised to prevent "trading" or dilution of samples.

First morning voided samples are acceptable for follow-up drug screen checks and to evaluate patients who have left the grounds on pass or have had visitors.

6. Psychiatric Evaluation

A comprehensive assessment for autonomous psychiatric syndrome should be completed in every patient presenting with a history of substance abuse. This population apparently represents a high-risk group for certain syndromes. Multiple studies suggest point prevalence ranges for major depressive or anxiety syndromes alone at between 10% and 50%.[17–19]

Several authors suggest that predominant stimulant abusers are overrepresented in the group diagnoses as major depressive episode (unipolar plus bipolar).[20] However, important subgroup variations also occur. Some clinicians feel that heavy cocaine abusers are overrepresented in patients eventually diagnosed as bipolar disorder. Patients abusing opiates show very high rates of major depression following detoxification (possibly as high as 25% point prevalence for heroin users and 60% for methadone users).[5]

In similar fashion, some reports claim that alcoholic populations show higher than average prevalence of generalized anxiety disorder, panic disorder, and phobic disorders.[20]

The actual rate of major depressive disorder among alcoholics is more controversial. Estimates of prevalence range from below 10% to above 60%.[17,18,19,21,22] Such variance likely results from the different rating instruments and diagnostic criteria used to make this diagnosis and also from issues of diagnostic interview timing. If interviews are completed during or very soon following alcohol detoxification, a high number of patients will report multiple depressive symptoms, including insomnia, anorexia, anergia, and depressed mood. Examinations conducted 2 to 4 weeks later will differ substantially. In one study, utilizing strict RDC criteria, patients were examined between 3 and 4 weeks following completed detoxification: the point prevalence of major depression was only 7%.[23]

In summary, a number of depressive symptoms are common to both alcoholism and major depression. In the majority of patients interviewed during or closely following detoxification, depressive complaints represent a transient alcohol-induced organic affective syndrome. Diagnosis of an autonomous major depressive episode should only be made in those patients who meet strict criteria and who have attained a minimum of 3 weeks of sobriety.

7. Diagnostic Laboratory Tests in Substance Abusers

Certain laboratory tests can serve as important adjunctive aids in the psychiatric evaluations of patients presenting with substance abuse. However, special considerations are necessary to correctly choose, schedule, and interpret the tests in this special population.

The dexamethasone suppression test (DST), described in detail elsewhere, has been widely accepted as an aid in the diagnosis of major depressive illness.[24,25] As discussed above, major depression occurs frequently among substance abusers; its correct diagnosis and treatment can be crucial to the patients' sustained recovery. Since correct interpretation of the DST, therefore, can be a very important part of the patients' workup, clinicians need to be aware of the reasons for false-positive or false-negative results.

If the substance-abusing patient's history or quantitative laboratory analysis reveals recent barbiturate, phenytoin, or carbamazepine use, a false-positive DST may result. This apparently occurs because of induction of corticosteroid metabolism, producing rapid clearing of the dexamethasone test dose.[26] Conversely, use or abuse of even topical steroid compounds can produce a false-negative DST.

Among alcoholic patients, some reports suggested unacceptably high false-positive DST rates.[27] However, such findings may result from inadequate patient screening or improper test scheduling. First, DST studies performed during or soon following detoxification from alcohol may produce false-positive results.[24,26,28] This is most likely related to the altered physiological state of withdrawal itself rather than the benzodiazepine regimens frequently used during detoxification.[29,30]

False-positive DST results can also occur in alcoholic patients with clinically significant liver disease manifested by hepatomegaly, elevated bilirubin, or elevated liver enzyme levels.[24]

To summarize, the DST appears to maintain clinically useful specificity levels for major depression in alcoholics if (1) patients with significant liver disease are excluded and (2) the DST is properly scheduled—a minimum of 3 weeks following completed alcohol detoxification.[23,31,32]

Following similar guidelines of patient screening and test scheduling, investigators report acceptable sensitivity and specificity levels for DST use in diagnosing major depressive illness among polysubstance- and opiate-abusing patient groups.[33]

Abnormal daily cortisol secretory patterns occur in a subgroup of patients with major depression.[34,35] The diurnal cortisol test measures serum cortisol at several points in a 24-hr cycle. Loss of the normal diurnal pattern or persistant hypersecretory states can identify substance-abusing patients with autonomous major depressive episodes. However, we presently lack clear sensitivity and specificity levels regarding the diagnostic use of the diurnal cortisol test among substance-abusing populations. As discussed previously in regard to the dexamethasone suppression test, use or abuse of exogenous steroid compounds can interfere with interpretation of the diurnal cortisol study.

The TRH infusion study is another important diagnostic aid in the evaluation for major affective syndromes.[36–39] A diminished, or "blunted," TSH response following intravenous TRH infusion is seen in a subgroup of patients with unipolar depression and in mania. However, TRH interpretation is problematic in certain substance-abusing patients. A blunted TSH response reportedly can occur in abstinent alcoholics independent of the level of depressive symptoms.[24,40] The exact reason for this is unclear. Although it is conceivable it represents a "trait" marker, for example, of alcoholics at increased risk for depressive episodes, it may also be a direct persistent drug effect of alcohol on the HPT axis at the hypothalamic or pituitary levels.

Among other patient groups, certain screening should be done. Recent exposure to lithium, thyroid extracts, or neuroleptics will interfere with TRH interpretation and must be ruled out by drug history and quantitative drug screens.[36]

The TRH infusion remains useful as a sensitive screen for subclinical hypothyroidism, a condition with symptoms that can closely mimic major depression.[41]

Measurement of platelet MAO activity level offers further aid in the evaluation for major depression. Platelet MAO activity has been reported to be low in patients with bipolar depression.[42] Two other studies primarily investigated as potential state markers for major depressive episodes are interesting as potential "vulnerability" trait markers. Studies have suggested that both decreased platelet MAO activity levels and decreased platelet serotonin (5-HT) transport rates correlate with personality traits of impulsivity, risk-taking and sensation-seeking behaviors, and possibly with increased rates of alcohol and other drug abuse.[43,44] Although still controversial, development of accurate markers for such traits could help identify individuals at higher risk for developing serious substance abuse patterns. The findings in unipolar depression are less clear, although a subgroup of patients with "atypical" features may demonstrate elevated platelet MAO activity.[45,46]

Measurement of 24-hr urinary MHPG may not help identify substance-abusing patients with autonomous major depression but may demonstrate groups who will respond preferentially to selected antidepressent medications: patients with low urinary MHPG levels may respond preferentially to agents with predominant noradrenergic activity.[47,48]

8. Evaluation of the Outpatient

Outpatient evaluations should include all the components of the comprehensive evaluation outlined above. A careful review of substance use history, accurate definition of medical histories, and sequential ratings of psychiatric symptoms should be completed. Ideally, the outpatient clinical setting will allow easy utilization of physical examination, and laboratory diagnostic procedures. Accurate, quantitative laboratory identification of recent substance use is even more important when beginning an outpatient versus inpatient evaluation. Testing results may by themselves cause a reevaluation and an admission to a hospital.

Frequently, individuals will request "bypassing" any recommended inpatient phase of evaluation or treatment. Occasionally, a highly motivated patient can be successfully treated on an outpatient basis. However, many patients report numerous prior unsuccessful outpatient attempts to alter their substance use patterns and require the intensive "break in the cycle" an inpatient setting provides. As noted previously, an inpatient setting not only also allows the very efficient coordination of all evaluation components and reduces the risk of drug-related death but also frequently provides a critical brief, intensive introduction to new peer groups and group aftercare programs.

Some clinicians use parameters such as "dependency rating scores" when deciding on inpatient treatment. For example, certain groups utilize minimum scores obtained by adding the axis IV level (stressor level) and axis V level (level of functioning) ratings to decide on the need for inpatient treatment. The presence of current medical conditions or a concurrent axis I psychiatric diagnosis usually makes inpatient treatment preferable.

It is critical to obtain information from secondary informants such as spouse and family members when evaluating an outpatient. It is usually a mistake to continue outpatient treatment attempts unless regular laboratory confirmation of abstinence is available and unless objective family reports of behaviors and mood states are regularly obtained.

9. Evaluation of the Adolescent

The evaluation of adolescent substance abusers introduces certain unique features. First, experimentation with drugs is so common in this age group that even regular users often initially insist that their use pattern is "normal." Families also often mistakenly assume that regular heavy use is a normal, developmental "stage." Adolescent substance use is the major cause of death, disability, school and family problems, and failure to develop as an adult organism. Therefore, evaluators must clearly state that unless interrupted, adolescent use is dangerous and frequently progresses to escalating serious abuse patterns with severe consequences.

Second, adolescents are usually seen in the earlier stages of abuse patterns. Therefore, the "danger signals" are different. Evaluators should focus on signals such as early tolerance development, preoccupation with use, solitary use, or use in school rather than looking for episodes of overt withdrawal.

Comprehensive psychiatric evaluation is mandatory in this patient group. Some clinical surveys suggest high prevalence rates of unipolar depression (up to 15%) and residual attention deficit disorder/hyperactivity syndrome (up to 20%) in this population.

Evaluation of school performance is also critical, as learning disabilities are reported in greater than 50% of these patients. Input from the school on recent performance or disruption in school activities should be obtained.

Truly comprehensive drug use histories are important, as polysubstance abuse patterns are the rule. Although alcohol and marijuana abuse is most common, many adolescents incorporate hallucinogens, other sedatives, and stimulants (increasingly including cocaine) in their use pattern.

Although medical and neurological examinations should be completed, many adolescents react to stern warnings about potential future physical complications as "scare tactics." Therefore, this information should be presented in a straightforward, factual manner. Serious family system disruptions frequently coexist with the adolescent's substance abuse pattern. Family assessment should be routinely completed, and, as discussed below, active family involvement in the evaluation process must be sought. It goes without saying that the most sensitive and specific testing is necessary by the psychiatrist as well as the pediatrician at annual physical examination time to make an early and accurate detection and successful intervention.

10. Evaluation of the Codependents

There are several important reasons to actively involve family members, or "codependents," in the evaluation and treatment processes. First, the input, advice, and active encouragement of spouse or other family members is often critical in convincing the patient to finally break his/her cycle of substance use. Second, other family members may themselves be abusing legal or illicit substances—an intolerable situation for the person leaving treatment to face when he/she returns home. More commonly, there is a critical need to educate codependents about the natural progression of chemical dependency and to explain that their family member's treatment will need to continue long after the inpatient phase. Family therapists stress the need to interrupt family cycles of "enabling," e.g., protecting the patient from the interpersonal or financial consequences of his/her drug use. Codependents should be encouraged to enter self-help groups designed specifically for their needs, such as Alanon or Alateen.

Family members frequently need education, support, and specific behavioral change directives as much as the patient does. Early and active involvement of codependents in the evaluation stage not only produces more comprehensive evaluations but can lead to tremendous clinical gains as treatment continues.

References

1. Senay EC: *Substance Abuse Disorders in Clinical Practice*. Boston, John Wright PSG Inc, 1983.

2. Single E, Kandel D, Faust L: Patterns of multiple drug use in high school. *J Health Soc Behav* 15:344–357, 1974.

3. Hamburg B, Kraemer H, Jahnke W: A hierarchy of drug use in adolescence; behavioral and attitudinal correlates of substantial drug use. *Am J Psychiatry* 132:1155–1163, 1975.

4. Nelson D: *Frequently Seen Stages in Adolescent Chemical Use.* Minneapolis, CompCare Publications, 1978.

5. Wikler A: *Opioid Dependence: Mechanisms and Treatment.* New York, Plenum Press, 1980.

6. Louria DB, Hensle T, Rose F: The major medical complications of heroin addiction. *Ann Intern Med* 67:1–22, 1967.

7. Geelhoed GW, Joseph WL: Surgical sequalae of drug abuse. *Surg Gynecol Obstet* 139:749–755, 1974.

8. Reichman LB, Felton CP, Edsall J: Drug dependence, a possible new risk factor for tuberculosis. *Arch Intern Med* 139:337–339, 1979.

9. Becker CE: Medical complications of drug abuse. *Adv Intern Med* 24:183–202, 1979.

10. Gold MS: *800-Cocaine.* New York, Bantam Books, 1984.

11. Delaney P, Estes M: Intracranial hemorrhage with amphetamine abuse. *Neurology* (Minneap) 30:1125–1128, 1980.

12. Chillar RK, Jackson AL: Reversible hemiplegia after presumed intracarotid injection of Ritalin. *N Engl J Med* 304:1305, 1981.

13. Greenblatt DJ, Shader RI: Treatment of the alcohol withdrawal syndrome, in Shader RI (ed): *Manual of Psychiatric Therapeutics.* Boston, Little, Brown, 1975, pp 211–235.

14. Korsten MA, Lieber CS: Nutrition in the alcoholic. *Med Clin North Am* 63(5):963–972, 1979.

15. Weller RA, Preskorn SH: Psychotropic drugs and alcohol, pharmacokinetic and pharmacodynamic interactions. *Psychosomatics* 25:301–309, 1984.

16. Verebey K, Martin D, Gold MS: Interpretation of drug abuse testing: Strengths and limitations of current methodology, in Hall R (ed): *Psychiatric Medicine.* New York, Spectrum Publications, 1985.

17. Hamm JE, Major LF, Brown GL: The quantitative measurement of depression and anxiety in male alcoholics. *Am J Psychiatry* 136:580–582, 1979.

18. Winokur G: Family history studies: VIII. Secondary depression is alive and well, and. . . . *Dis Nerv Syst* 33:94–99, 1972.

19. Weissman MM, Pottenger M, Kleber H, et al: Symptom patterns in primary and secondary depression. *Arch Gen Psychiatry* 34:854–862, 1977.

20. Mirin SM (ed): *Substance Abuse and Psychopathology.* Washington, American Psychiatric Press, 1984.

21. Weissman MM, Myers JK: Clinical depression in alcoholism. *Am J Psychiatry* 137:372–373, 1980.

22. Keeler MH, Taylor CI, Miller WC: Are all recently detoxified alcoholics depressed? *Am J Psychiatry* 136:586–588, 1979.

23. Dackis CA, Bailey JB, Pottash ALC, et al: Specificity of the DST and the TRH test for major depression in alcoholics. *Am J Psychiatry* 141:680–683, 1984.

24. Carroll BJ, Feinberg M, Greden JF, et al: A specific laboratory test for the diagnosis of melancholia. *Arch Gen Psychiatry* 38:15–22, 1981.

25. Carroll BJ: The dexamethasone suppression test for melancholia. *Br J Psychiatry* 140:292–304, 1982.

26. Carroll BJ: Use of the dexamethasone suppression test in depression. *J Clin Psychiatry* 43:44–50, 1982.

27. Swartz CM, Dunner FJ: Dexamethasone suppression testing of alcoholics. *Arch Gen Psychiatry* 39:1309–1312, 1982.

28. Newsom G, Murray N: Reversal of dexamethasone suppression test nonsuppression in alcohol abusers. *Am J Psychiatry* 140:353–354, 1983.

29. Langer G, Schonbeck G, Koinig G, et al: Hyperactivity of hypothalamic–pituitary–adrenal axis in endogenous depression. *Lancet* 2:524, 1979.

30. Oyama T, Kimura K, Takazawa T, et al: An objective evaluation of tranquilizers as preanesthetic medication: Effect on adrenocortical function. *Can Anaesth Soc J* 16:209–216, 1969.

31. Lamberts SW, Klijn JG, deJong FH, et al: Hormone secretion in alcohol induced pseudo-Cushing's syndrome. *JAMA* 242:1640–1643, 1979.

32. Noble EP: Ethanol and adrenocortical stimulation in inbred mouse strains, in Mello NK (ed): *Recent Advances in Studies of Alcoholism.* Rockville, National Institute on Alcohol Abuse and Alcoholism, 1971, pp 72–106.

33. Dackis CA, Pottash ALC, Gold MS, et al: The dexamethasone suppression test for major depression among opiate addicts. *Am J Psychiatry* 141:810–811, 1984.
34. Sachar EJ, Hellman L, Roffwarg HP, et al: Disrupted 24 hour patterns of cortisol secretion in psychotic depression. *Arch Gen Psychiatry* 28:19–24, 1973.
35. Asnis GM, Sachar EF, Halbreich U, et al: Cortisol secretion and dexamethasone response in depression. *Am J Psychiatry* 138:1218–1221, 1981.
36. Loosen PT, Prange AJ: Serum thyrotropin response to thyrotropin releasing hormone in psychiatric patients: A review. *Am J Psychiatry* 139:405–416, 1982.
37. Sternbach H, Gerner RH, Gwirtsman HE: The thyrotropin releasing hormone stimulation test: A review. *J Clin Psychiatry* 43.4–6, 1982.
38. Gold MS, Pottash ALC, Ryan N, et al: TRH induced TSH response in unipolar, bipolar and secondary depressions: Possible utility in clinical assessment and differential diagnosis. *Psychoneuroendocrinology* 5:147–155, 1980.
39. Extein I, Pottash ALC, Gold MS, et al: Using the protirelin test to distinguish mania from schizophrenia. *Arch Gen Psychiatry* 39:77–81, 1982.
40. Loosen PT, Prange AJ: Thyroid function in abstinant alcoholics, in Struwe G (ed): *Abstracts of the Third World Congress of Biological Psychiatry,* Tryckeri Ab Orion, Solna, Sweden, 1981, p F283.
41. Gold MS, Pottash ALC, Extein I: Hypothyroidism and depression. *JAMA* 245:1919–1922, 1981.
42. Murphy DL, Weiss R: Reduced monoamine oxidase activity in blood platelets from bipolar depressed patients. *Am J Psychiatry* 128:1351–1357, 1972.
43. Coursey R, Buchsbaum MS: The relationship of platelet MAO activity to psychological variables underlying psychiatric diagnosis, in Houston L, Hannon L (eds): *Biological Markers in Psychiatry and Neurology.* New York, Pergamon Press, 1982, pp 97–109.
44. Garvey MJ, Tuason VB, Hoffman N, et al: Suicide attempters, non-attempters, and neurotransmitters. *Compr Psychiatry* 24:332–336, 1983.
45. Davidson JRT, McLeod MN, Turnbull CD, et al: Platelet monoamine oxidase activity and the classification of depression. *Arch Gen Psychiatry* 37:771–773, 1980.
46. Fieve RR, Kumbaraci T, Kassir S, et al: Platelet monoamine oxidase activity in affective disorder. *Biol Psychiatry* 15:473–478, 1980.
47. Maas JW, Kocsis JH, Bowden CL, et al: Pre-treatment neurotransmitter metabolites and response to imipramine or amitriptyline treatment. *Psychol Med* 12:37–43, 1982.
48. Hollister LE, Davis KL, Berger PA: Subtypes of depression based on excretion of MHPG and response to nortriptyline. Arch Gen Psychiatry 37:1107–1110, 1980.

The Assessment of Anorexia and Bulimia

William S. Rea, M.D., and Mark S. Gold, M.D.

1. Introduction

The serious psychiatric illness involving seemingly willful self-starvation and overexercise coupled with distortions of body image that constitutes anorexia nervosa was apparently once not so common as it is today. The syndrome was first clinically described by Gull in 1873.[1] At that time it was approached as a psychiatric oddity and curiosity. In the ensuing 100 years, the syndrome has been more completely characterized and investigated, and its prevalence and incidence have been shown to be much higher than could have been anticipated at that time.[2] In fact, recent estimates of incidence suggest that one out of every 200 girls between the ages of 13 and 19 in a highly industrialized western nation will experience symptoms of anorexia nervosa.[3] Although most other authors suggest an incidence somewhat lower than this, it is still recognized by both physicians and popular press as being an illness that strikes with increasing frequency. This condition has been examined and explained on medical, psychological, familial, and cultural bases; the explanations, although plausible and intriguing and leading to valuable methods of treatment and amelioration, have not led to a cure or a method of prevention for this debilitating and often fatal disease. In this, it shares many common features with drug addiction.

2. Diagnosis

The first prerequisite to clarifying the nature of the illness is to simply define what the illness is. To this end, the third edition of the *Diagnostic and Statistical Manual of Mental Disorders*[4] suggests five necessary criteria to make this diagnosis. Of the criteria, two are psychological, one behavioral, one an objective measure, and the last a criterion of exclusion. The anorectic shows an intense fear of becoming obese, which

William S. Rea, M.D. • Lake Hospital of the Palm Beaches, Lake Worth, Florida 33460, and Fair Oaks Hospital at Boca/Delray, Delray Beach, Florida 33445.   *Mark S. Gold, M.D.* • Research Facilities, Fair Oaks Hospital, Summit, New Jersey 07901, and Fair Oaks Hospital at Boca/Delray, Delray Beach, Florida 33445.

has little or no relationship to the actual degree of weight that the patient has. In addition, he or she shows a disturbance of body image toward feeling more obese than other observers would claim. The patient, in addition, refuses to maintain a body weight above a minimum normal weight for her age or height. Measurably, the anorexic shows a weight loss of at least 25% of the original body weight. If the anorectic is under 18 years of age and therefore expected to be still growing, the weight loss from her original weight plus the projected weight gain expected from growth charts may be combined to make the 25%. Finally, there must be no known physical illness that would account for the weight loss.

The diagnostic criteria for bulimia[4] require recurrent episodes of binge eating, awareness that the eating pattern is abnormal, and depressed mood or self-deprecatory thoughts following eating binges. In addition, the patient must show at least three of the following five symptoms: (1) consumption of high-caloric easily ingested food; (2) inconspicuous eating during a binge; (3) termination of binge eating by abdominal pain, sleep, social interruption, or self-induced vomiting; (4) repeated attempts to lose weight by severely restrictive diets, self-induced vomiting, or use of cathartics or diuretics; and (5) frequent weight fluctuations greater than 10 lb.

In addition, to satisfy the diagnosis of bulimia, the patient must not suffer from anorexia nervosa. It is evident from these criteria that anorectic patients may be divided into those who suffer from bulimiclike episodes and those who do not.

From these diagnostic criteria, it is clear that to make a diagnosis of anorexia nervosa or bulimia does not require extensive laboratory testing. This is not to say, however, that laboratory investigation is not critical in evaluating the current status of the patient's illness and suggesting various forms of treatment. Anorexia nervosa involves some disturbances of neuroendocrine function on what is likely to be a primary basis as well as multiple complications and neuroendocrine effects secondary to starvation. It is essential in both of these illnesses to evaluate fully the functioning of the patient's homeostatic chemical systems in order to improve prognosis and suggest necessary treatment.

It is well known on the basis of experimentation in lower primates and other animals that both feeding and satiety are governed by centers in the lateral hypothalamus and the ventromedial hypothalamus.[5,6] Roughly speaking, the lateral hypothalamus seems to be responsible for feeding, and the ventromedial hypothalamus is responsible for satiety. Although this is an oversimplification, all current research has confirmed the importance of both of these areas in the regulation of eating. To date, at least ten neurotransmitters have been implicated as having some impact on the regulation of feeding in lower animals.[6] It is conceivable that each or any of these neurotransmitters will prove seminal in the dysregulation of appetite and satiety seen in anorexia nervosa and bulimia. At this point, however, no single neurotransmitter abnormality has been implicated as causative in the production of these syndromes. For this reason, current laboratory investigation of anorexia nervosa is by and large descriptive rather than explanatory of the biochemical disturbances that may be involved. This chapter, therefore, takes the form of describing some of the major disruptions of neurohormonal regulation involved in these illnesses.

Given the complexity and depth of research currently focused on this illness, this chapter is not meant to be exhaustive in its review of the syndrome. The reader is instead referred to several excellent reviews recently published for further description of areas of interest.[7-9]

3. Endocrine Findings

3.1. Hypothalamic–Pituitary–Thyroid Axis

Some of the original research on the chemical disturbances involved in anorexia nervosa was prompted by the clinical similarity between anorexia nervosa and hyperthyroidism. Both illnesses may show in their extreme course severe emaciation and hyperactive behavior. It was initially hoped that anorexia nervosa would prove to be a variant of hyperthyroidism, leading to a relatively definitive surgical or medical treatment for this illness. Unfortunately, this did not prove to be the case, and, in fact, the disruption of thyroid function seen in this illness bears little resemblance to that of hyperthyroidism.

Simple measurement of thyroxine (T_4) levels has revealed a general tendency for levels to be at or near the low end of the normal range.[10-13] This was true not only during the acute stages of the illness but at times after several weeks of weight gain.[12] This was, of course, a marked difference from the findings in hyperthyroidism.

Triiodothyronine (T_3) levels are highly reduced in anorexia nervosa.[11,14,15] The reduction is often as much as 40%.[11] The reduction in T_3 levels is accompanied by an increase in the levels of the inactive form, reverse T_3.[14] It is of interest that these findings of thyroid dysfunction are completely reversed to normal by weight gain.[12] It is also critical to observe that these same findings occur in starvation from other causes.[16-18]

The low resting levels of T_3 and low normal levels of T_4 are not accompanied by elevated levels of thyroid-stimulating hormones (TSH), which, on the contrary, are in normal limits.[12,13] These findings are not related to body weight.[12] This serves as further corroboration that the thyroid changes seen in anorexia nervosa are not caused by a primary failure of the thyroid gland.

In an attempt to further elucidate the functioning of the hypothalamic–pituitary–thyroid axis in anorexia nervosa, anorectic patients were injected with standardized quantities of thyrotropin-releasing hormone (TRH); TRH is the mediator going from the hypothalamus to the pituitary that leads to release of TSH. Administration of this hormone intravenously leads to a release of TSH in measurable quantities in normal subjects. In a group of subjects with major depressive disorder, intravenous administration of TRH leads to a blunted release of TSH.[18] In patients with hypothyroidism, administration of TRH leads to an augmented response of TSH. When anorectic patients are given an injection of TRH, in most studies they produce a normal amount of TSH.[12,20,24] However, several investigators have seen a delayed peak of TSH response to TRH in anorexia nervosa.[23,24] This response is also seen with simple starvation.[19,25]

In sum, it seems likely that the alterations in thyroid function seen in anorexia nervosa are primarily caused by adjustments of thyroid function in response to simple weight loss and do not represent an etiologic disturbance.

3.2. Hypothalamic–Pituitary–Adrenal Axis

Morning plasma cortisol levels have generally been found to be elevated in patients with anorexia nervosa.[10,13,26] The diurnal variation of the plasma cortisol is flattened.[27] Cortisol metabolic studies have shown an increased half-life of cortisol in the body, with a decreased metabolic clearance rate,[27] which parallels that found in malnutrition from other causes.[28] It is of note that in anorexia nervosa added triiodothyronine (T_3) normalizes the cortisol half-life.[27] From this finding, it is evident that alterations in the regulation of the adrenal gland are at least partially mediated by associated changes in thyroid regulation.

In normal subjects, ingestion of 1 mg of dexamethasone at midnight leads to suppression of cortisol secretion for the ensuing 24 hr.[29] In both anorexia nervosa[30,31] and malnutrition from other causes,[28,32] the dexamethasone suppression test is positive for the early release of cortisol despite the presence of dexamethasone. ACTH stimulation tests show a normal to hyperactive adrenal response.[33,34]

Investigation of the cortisol production rate in anorectics shows a rate that is within the normal range.[27] However, if the rate is calculated relative to body size as compared with normals, the cortisol production rate is increased in anorectics.[27] In malnutrition from other causes, the cortisol production rate is somewhat reduced.[28] The 24-hr excretion of urinary free cortisol is also increased in anorexia.[27,35]

As can be seen from the above results, the alterations in cortisol metabolism, specifically urinary free cortisol and cortisol production rate, cannot be entirely ascribed to malnutrition However, some of the changes in cortisol metabolism, including the increased cortisol half-life, may be secondary to changes in the thyroid gland with a shift from T_3 to reverse-T_3 production.[27]

Given the well-known linkage of hypothalamic–pituitary–adrenal dysregulation in affective disorder and the association of family affective disorder history in the history of anorectics, it is interesting to conjecture whether anorexia nervosa may be at some point shown to be a variant of mood disorder. Bulimia certainly appears to be related to affective disease in genetics and response to tricyclics.

3.3. Gonadotropin Regulation

Early investigation of gonadotropins in anorexia nervosa was prompted by the readily apparent association of amenorrhea with this clinical syndrome. In fact, as many as 24% of anorectics show signs of amenorrhea before the onset of any significant weight loss.[36] Amenorrhea may be the most persistent symptom of anorexia nervosa even after recovery of all other symptomatology to normal.[7,25] Amenorrhea may be accounted for on at least four separate bases in anorexia nervosa: (1) primary hypothalamic–pituitary dysregulation; (2) dysregulation of gonadotropins secondary to emotional distress; (3) dysregulation of gonadotropins secondary to self-induced hyperactivity; (4) low levels of gonadotropins secondary to malnutrition.

Initial studies show low resting levels of estradiol not associated with hot flashes.[37] Both luteinizing hormone (LH) and follicle-stimulating hormone (FSH) are reported to be low in anorexia nervosa. Proportional deficiencies of LH are reported to be much greater than that of FSH.[13,33] Both LH and FSH levels were reported in several studies to return to normal with weight gain.[38,39] However, in weight gain where amenorrhea persists, the LH levels remain abnormal.[39,40]

In addition to resting LH and RH levels, 24-hr patterns of secretion of LH have been studied in anorectics. These studies have revealed a pattern very similar to that found in normal prepubertal girls. The pattern seen is that of low LH levels throughout the entire 24-hr period or by decreased LH secretion during the day and high LH secretion during night.[27,39,41] Amenorrhea caused by gonadal dysgenesis has not been shown to result in this prepubertal type of LH secretion.[42] Again, this prepubertal pattern was found to persist in anorectics who had gained weight but who remained amenorrheic.[39]

Investigation of LH release by administration of luteinizing hormone-releasing hormone (LHRH) in measured quantities has yielded results that are similar to a pattern seen in normal prepubertal girls: LHRH administration results in a somewhat diminished to low normal release of LH and FSH, with a greater decrease in the LH release.[13,43,44] In addition, the peak of LH release may be delayed.[45]

Further evidence of a deficiency of endogenous LHRH secretion in anorexia comes from the observation that repeated administration of LHRH results in a gradual return of the LH response towards normal[46,47] along with institution of a normal ovarian cycle.[47]

As we have seen in other hormonal systems, gonadotropins seem to be influenced by the thyroid changes induced by anorexia. Anorectics show a shift of the androsterone/etiocholanonene (A/E) ratio downward, which is similar to that seen in hypothyroidism. This shift is reversible by ingestion of T_3.[48]

In summary, marked alterations of the gonadotropin regulatory systems are seen in anorexia nervosa. These alterations are not common to all types of amenorrhea, nor are they entirely attributable to triiodothyronine (T_3) deficiency. Although abnormal amounts of exercise may itself produce amenorrhea, it is likely that in anorexia nervosa we are dealing with a complex interchange of physical activity, emotional factors, and primary hypothalamic–pituitary changes that result in a profound change in the regulation of gonadotropins to a pattern similar to that seen in prepubertal girls.

4. Central Catecholamine Regulation

Initial interest in catecholamine regulation in anorexia nervosa was prompted from several sources, including elucidation of monoamine pathways in the control of eating in lower animals and a case report of an anorectic patient who was helped by the adrenergic blocker phenoxybenzamine.[49] Plasma norepinephrine levels in anorectics have been reported to be somewhat low.[50] Investigation of a metabolite of norepinephrine in the urine, 3-methoxy-4-hydroxyphenylglycol (MHPG), has shown lower levels than normal for a 24-hr period.[8,31,50–52] This may indicate a reduced production of norepinephrine centrally for these patients. However, it has been shown that urinary MHPG in anorectics returned to normal with weight gain.[50] Similarly, urinary homovanillic acid (HVA), a dopamine metabolite, was decreased during acute starvation only.[50]

At this time the significance of acute changes in central catecholamine levels is uncertain. These changes may reflect mere acute starvation or may indicate underlying changes similar to those seen in affective disorders.

5. Other Central Nervous System Factors

Growth hormone has been investigated in both anorectics and patients with other types of malnutrition.[26] It is reported that basal GH levels are elevated in both kwashiorkor[53] and marasmus.[54] Basal GH levels have been reported to be elevated in most studies on anorectics,[10,55,56] although they have also been reported to be somewhat decreased.[57] Basal GH levels seem to return to normal with recovery.[55] One study links the normalization to caloric intake rather than absolute weight.[55] In response to administration of L-DOPA, anorectics show a decreased release of growth hormone. This has been reported not to return to normal in some anorectics following weight gain.[46]

In normal subjects, administration of thyrotropin-releasing hormone (TRH) usually results in no change in growth hormone. In anorexia nervosa, however, a release of GH usually occurs after administration of TRH.[58] The significance of this finding is uncertain.

Recent studies have shown an increased cerebrospinal fluid level of opioid activity in patients with anorexia nervosa, leading to conjecture as to the involvement of endorphins on this illness.[59] Further confirmation is necessary before these findings become clear. Vasopressin has also been reported to be abnormally low in anorectics, leading to a partial diabetes insipidus and further complicating the weight loss of these patients.[43] Partial diabetes insipidus has also been reported in patients with weight loss without anorexia nervosa.[37]

6. Complications of Anorexia Nervosa and Bulimia

The drastic reduction in body weight seen in severe anorectics may lead to failure of multiple organ systems. It would not be unusual in any patient who had lost 40% of her body weight to observe malfunctioning of chemical homeostatic, cardiac, renal, gastrointestinal, and neurological systems. However, certain complications occur frequently in anorexia and should be looked for.

Many anorectic patients and bulimics show marked alterations of serum electrolyte levels.[7] This is very likely a result of self-induced emesis, laxative abuse, and diuretic abuse. Some 6% of anorectic inpatients have been reported to have serum potassium levels less than 2.6 mEq/liter.[7] Hyponatremia seems to be relatively uncommon.[60] The alterations in plasma electrolytes can be life threatening and lead to cardiac arrhythmias, renal complications, and general weakness.

In addition to electrolyte disturbances, hematological complications are common.[7] Mild anemia is fairly frequent[33,61] and may be of either normochromic or hypochromic type.[61] White blood count, as well as red blood count, is often decreased,[33,62] and cholesterol levels are often abnormally high.[63] The significance of the elevated cholesterol levels is not immediately apparent.

With the severe malnutrition seen in anorexia, the hyponatremia, the extraordinary demands for physical activity, and the mild anemia often present, it is not surprising that cardiac complications are fairly common. Electrocardiographic changes have been seen in up to 70% of anorectic patients, including sinus bradycardia, nonspecific STT wave changes, T-wave inversion, and AV block.[64,65] Ventricular arrhythmias have been reported in anorectics and may account in part for the high mortality rate seen in this illness.[66]

Convulsions have been reported in approximately one out of every ten anorectics,[67] and nonspecific EEG changes are fairly common.[69] These are likely to be related to changes in serum electrolytes. Computed axial tomographic (CAT) scans have generally been reported either normal or with mild cerebral atrophy, which may or may not be reversible.[69] Peripheral neuropathies seem to be somewhat uncommon, possibly because of the maintenance of vitamin intake despite low caloric intake.[7,69]

Recently, salivary gland enlargement has been reported in anorectic patients.[70] As we can see from this brief interview, the complications of anorexia nervosa may be protean. Garfinkel and Garner[7] exhaustively review the current literature on complications of anorexia.

7. Differential Diagnosis

The differential diagnosis of anorexia nervosa and bulimia is not particularly extensive. Although many chronic medical illnesses including cancer and chronic infections may lead to cachexia and amenorrhea, there are relatively few that lead to a persistent fear of obesity and a disturbance of the body image in that direction. Any investigation of anorexia, therefore, should begin with an in-depth clinical interview with special attention paid to body image and ideal body image. In addition, relatively few medical illnesses lead to hyperactivity of the sort seen in anorexia.

An important differential diagnosis is that of drug abuse and schizophrenia, which can lead to distortions of body image and bizarre eating habits. The schizophrenic, however, will usually evidence other primary signs and symptoms of that disorder including disturbances of reality testing outside the sphere of body image. Drug addiction may be more difficult to diagnose.

It should be noted that various forms of central nervous system insult may masquerade as anorexia nervosa. Tumors of the hypothalamic region have been reported to simulate this disorder,[71,72] as has the lateral hypothalamic syndrome in rats.[73] For this reason it seems prudent to obtain CAT scans or sella turcica skull X rays in the initial workup of any anorectic patients. The proportional costs are low compared with the enormous cost of an undiagnosed craniopharyngioma.

8. Laboratory Testing

It is clear from this chapter than anorexia nervosa and bulimia may lead to disturbances of multiple body systems, either from a primary disruption or from secondary complications. Assuming that the diagnosis of anorexia nervosa has been achieved and is in full accordance with the DSM-III criteria outlined above, and that for that reason purely medical causes of cachexia and anorexia have been eliminated, what laboratory studies are important to undertake in the evaluation of the anorectic?

Initially, in anorexia and bulimia, it is extremely important to obtain base-line evaluation of the patient's physical state in order to determine whether or not acute hospitalization is necessary and in order to plan further therapy. For this reason, a minimal workup would consist of electrocardiogram, complete blood count with differential, chest X ray, liver screen, cholesterol, serum electrolytes, comprehensive vitamin examination, thyroid screen including base-line TSH, comprehensive testing for drug and medication abuse, and, of course, accurate determination of weight. All of these tests should be readily available to most practitioners and may be repeated as often as seems clinically useful.

In addition, in anorexia consideration should be given to a dexamethasone suppression test in order to evaluate dysfunction of the hypothalamic–pituitary–adrenal axis and to an LHRH test or 24-hr LH test to evaluate amenorrhea and gonadal functioning. Finally, although the likelihood of a tumor causing anorecticlike behavior is low, the noninvasiveness of sella turcica views of the skull and CAT scan make both of these procedures advisable in ruling out intracerebral tumors. An EEG will help make a diagnosis of cerebral dysrhythmia, which may support an anticonvulsant trial.

For the physicians of patients with anorexia, the life-threatening nature of the disease and the disease's ability to thwart the clinician make treatment extremely difficult. Finding a causative or exacerbating medical illness to treat is a blessing the clinican can only realize after a complete work-up. Bulimic patients who will be given a tricyclic trial should have a dose-prediction test and regular blood levels to reduce the risks of treatment and maximize benefits.

9. Conclusion

There is a great deal of research currently being conducted on central mechanisms underlying anorexia nervosa, and it is to be hoped that within the next several years testing more specific to this illness may be available. Which eating disorders are strongly related to affective disorders should become evident. At this point, bulimia appears to be the likely candidate. A diagnostic trial with desipramine may be a useful procedure for treating clinicians. Testing that predicts response to antidepressant, anticonvulsant, psychotherapy, and other modalities is needed. At present, emphasis should be placed on reducing misdiagnosis and preventing eating disorders through education and early intervention.

References

1. Gull WW: Anorexia nervosa (apepsia hysterica). *Br Med J* 2:527, 1973.
2. Crisp AH, Palmer RL, Kalney RS: How common is anorexia nervosa? A prevalence study. *Br J Psychiatry* 128:549–558, 1976.
3. Garfield EG: Anorexia nervosa: The enigma of self-starvation. *Curr Contents* 32:3–13, 1984.
4. American Psychiatric Association: *Diagnostic and Statistical Manual of Mental Disorders,* ed 3. Washington, American Psychiatric Association, 1980.

5. Stellar E: Neural basis: Introduction, in Stunkard AJ, Stellar E (eds): *Eating and Its Disorders*. New York, Raven Press, 1984, pp 1–4.
6. Hoebel BG: Neurotransmitters in the control of feeding and its rewards: Monoamines, opiates, and brain–gut peptides, in Stunkard AJ, Stellar E (eds): *Eating and Its Disorders*. New York, Raven Press, 1984, pp 15–38.
7. Garfinkel PE, Garner DM: Anorexia nervosa: A multidimensional perspective. New York, Brunner-Mazel, 1982.
8. Halmi KA: Anorexia nervosa, in Hippius H, Winoker G (eds): *Psychopharmacology: A Biennial Critical Survey*, vol 2. Princeton, Excerpta Medica, 1983, pp 313–320.
9. Halmi KA: Anorexia nervosa, in Hippius H, Winokur G: *Psychopharmacology: A Biennial Critical Survey*, vol 2. Princeton, Excerpta Medica, 1983, pp 313–320.
10. Hurd HP, Palumbo PJ, Gharib H: Hypothalamic–endocrine dysfunction in anorexia nervosa. *Mayo Clin Proc* 52:711, 1977.
11. Miyai K, Yamamoto T, Azukizawa M, et al: Serum thyroid hormones and thyrotropin in anorexia nervosa. *J Clin Endocrinol Metab* 40:334–338, 1975.
12. Wakeling A, DeSouza VFA, Gore MBR, et al: Amenorrhea, body weight and serum hormone concentrations, with particular reference to prolactin and thyroid hormones in anorexia nervosa. *Psychol Med* 9:265–272, 1979.
13. Brown GM, Garfinkel PE, Jeuniewic N, et al: Endocrine profiles in anorexia nervosa, in Vigersky RA (ed): *Anorexia Nervosa*. New York, Raven Press, 1977, pp 123–135.
14. Burman KD, Vigersky RA, Loriaux DL, et al: Investigations concerning thyroxine deiodinative pathways in patients with anorexia nervosa, in Vigersky RA (ed): *Anorexia Nervosa*. New York, Raven Press, 1977, pp 255–261.
15. Moshang T, Parks JS, Baker L, et al: Low serum triiodothyronine in patients with anorexia nervosa. *J Clin Endocrinol Metab* 40:470–473, 1975.
16. Schussler GC and Orlando J: Fasting decreases triiodothyronine receptor capacity. *Science* 199:686–687, 1975.
17. Vagenakis AG, Burger A, Portney GJ: Conversion of peripheral thyroxine metabolism from activating to inactivating pathways during complete fasting. *J Clin Endocrinol Metab* 41:191–194, 1975.
18. Portney GI, O'Brien JT, Bush J, et al: The effect of starvation on the concentrating and binding of thyroxine and triiodothyronine in serum and on the response to TRH. *J Clin Endocrinol Metab* 39:191–194, 1974.
19. Extein I, Pottash ALC, Gold MS: The thyrotropin-releasing hormone test in the diagnosis of unipolar depression. *Psychiatry Res* 5:311–316, 1981.
20. Aro O, Lamberg BA, Pelkonen R: Dysfunction of the hypothalamic–pituitary axis in anorexia nervosa. *N Engl J Med* 292:594–595, 1975.
21. Lundberg PO, Walinder J, Werner I, et al: Effects of thyrotropin-releasing hormone on plasma levels of TSH, FSH, LH and GH in anorexia nervosa. *Eur J Clin Invest* 2:150–153, 1972.
22. Vigersky RA, Loriaux DL: Anorexia nervosa as a model of hypothalamic dysfunction, in Vigarsky RA: *Anorexia nervosa*. New York, Raven Press, 1977, pp 109–121.
23. Gold MS, Pottash AL, Martin DM, et al: Thyroid stimulating hormone and growth hormone responses to thyrotropin releasing hormone in anorexia nervosa. *Int J Psychiatry Med* 10:51–57, 1980.
24. Casper RL, Forhman LA: Delayed TSH release in anorexia nervosa following injection of thyrotropin releasing hormone (TRH). *Psychoneuroendocrinology* 7:59–68, 1982.
25. Garfinkel PE: Anorexia nervosa: An overview of hypothalamic–pituitary function, in Brown GM, Koslow SH, Reichlin S (eds): *Neuroendocrinology and Psychiatric Disorder*. New York, Raven Press, 1984, pp 301–314.
26. Alvarez LC, Dimas CO, Castro A, et al: Growth hormone in malnutrition. *J Clin Endocrinol Metab* 34:400–409, 1972.
27. Boyar RM, Hellman LD, Roffwarg HP, et al: Cortisol secretion and metabolism in anorexia nervosa. *N Engl J Med* 296:190–193, 1977.
28. Smith SR, Bledsoe T, Chetri MK: Cortisol metabolism and the pituitary–adrenal axis in adults with protein–calorie malnutrition. *J Clin Endocrinol Metab* 40:43–52, 1975.
29. Carroll BJ, Curtis GC, Mendels J: Neuroendocrine regulation in depression: I. Limbic system–adrenocortical dysfunction. *Arch Gen Psychiatry* 33:1039–1044, 1978.

30. Doerr P, Fichter M, Pirke KM, et al: Relations between weight gain and hypothalamic pituitary adrenal function in patients with anorexia nervosa. *J Steroid Biochem* 13:529–537, 1980.
31. Gerner RH, Swirtsman HE: Abnormalities of dexamethasone suppression test and urinary MHPG in anorexia nervosa. *Am J Psychiatry* 138:650–653, 1981.
32. Rao KS, Srikantia SG, Gopalan G: Plasma cortisol levels in protein–calorie malnutrition. *Arch Dis Child* 43:365–367, 1968.
33. Warren MP, Vande Wiele RL: Clinical and metabolic features of anorexia nervosa. *Am J Obstet Gynecol* 117:435–449, 1973.
34. Danowski TS, Livstone E, Gonzales AR, et al: Fractional and partial hypopituitarism in anorexia nervosa. *Hormones* 3:105–118, 1972.
35. Walsh BT, Katz JL, Levin J, et al: Adrenal activity in anorexia nervosa. *Psychosom Med* 40:499–506, 1978.
36. Fries H: Studies on secondary amenorrhea, anorectic behavior, and body image perception: Importance for the early recognition of anorexia nervosa, in Vigersley R (ed): *Anorexia Nervosa.* New York, Raven Press, 1977, pp 163–176.
37. Vigersky RA, Anderson AE, Thompson RH, et al: Hypothalamic dysfunction and secondary amenorrhea associated with simple weight loss. *N Engl J Med* 297:1141–1145, 1977.
38. Pirke KM, Fichter MM, Lund R, et al: Twenty-four hour sleep–wake pattern of plasma LH in patients with anorexia nervosa. *Acta Endocrinol (Kbh)* 92:193–204, 1979.
39. Katz JL, Boyar RM, Roffwarg H, et al: Weight and circadian luteinizing hormone secretory pattern in anorexia nervosa. *Psychosom Med* 40:549–567, 1978.
40. Gold MS, Pottash AC, Martin D, et al: The 24-hour LH test in the diagnosis and assessment of response to treatment of patients with anorexia nervosa. *Int J Psychiatry Med* 11:245–250, 1981.
41. Boyar RM, Katz J, Finkelstein JW, et al: Anorexia nervosa: Immaturity of the 24-hour luteinizing hormone secretory pattern. *N Engl J Med* 291:861–865, 1974.
42. Boyar RM, Finkelstein JW, Roffwarg H, et al: 24-Hour luteinizing hormone and follicle-stimulating hormone secretory patterns in gonadal dysgenesis. *J Clin Endocrinol Metab* 37:521–525, 1973.
43. Mecklenburg RS, Loriaux DL, Thompson RH, et al: Hypothalamic dysfunction in patients with anorexia nervosa. *Medicine* 53:147–159, 1974.
44. Isaacs AJ, Leslie RD, Gomez J, et al: The effect of weight gain on gonadotropins and prolactin in anorexia nervosa. *Acta Endocrinol (Kbh)* 94:145–150, 1980.
45. Vigersky RA, Loriaux DL, Andersen AE: Delayed pituitary hormone response to LRF and TRF in patients with anorexia nervosa and with secondary amenorrhea associated with simple weight loss. *J Clin Endocrinol Metab* 43:893–900, 1976.
46. Sherman BM, Halmi KA: Effect of nutritional rehabilitation on hypothalamic–pituitary function in anorexia nervosa, in Vigersky RA (ed): *Anorexia Nervosa.* New York, Raven Press, 1977, pp 211–223.
47. Nillius SJ, Wide L: The pituitary responsiveness to acute and chronic administration of gonadotropin-releasing hormone in acute and recovery stages of anorexia nervosa, in Vigersky RA (ed): *Anorexia Nervosa.* New York, Raven Press, 1977, pp 225–241.
48. Bradlow HL. Boyar RM, O'Connor J, et al: Hypothyroid-like alterations in testosterone metabolism in anorexia nervosa. *J Clin Endocrinol Metab* 43:571–574, 1976.
49. Redmond DE, Swann A, Heninger GR: Phenoxybenzamine in anorexia nervosa. *Lancet* 2:307, 1976.
50. Gross HA, Lake CR, Ebert MH, et al: Catecholamine metabolism in primary anorexia nervosa. *J Clin Endocrinol Metab* 49:805–809, 1979.
51. Abraham SF, Beumont PJ, Cobbin DM: Catecholamine metabolism and body weight in anorexia nervosa. *Br J Psychiatry* 138:244–247, 1981.
52. Halmi KA, Dekirmenjian H, Davis JM, et al: Catecholamine metabolism in anorexia nervosa. *Arch Gen Psychiatry* 35:458–460, 1978.
53. Pimstone BL, Wittman W, Hansen JD, et al: Growth hormone and kwashiorkor. *Lancet* 2:770–780, 1966.
54. Pimstone BL, Barbezat G, Hansen JD, et al: Growth hormone and protein–calorie malnutrition: Impaired suppression during induced hyperglycemia. *Lancet* 2:1333–1334, 1967.
55. Garfinkel PE, Brown GM, Moldofsky H, et al: Hypothalamic–pituitary function in anorexia nervosa. *Arch Gen Psychiatry* 32:739–744, 1975.
56. Casper RC, Davis JM, Pandey GN: The effect of nutritional status and weight changes on hypothalamic

function tests in anorexia nervosa, in Vigersky RA (ed): *Anorexia Nervosa.* New York, Raven Press, 1977, pp 137–147.

57. Halmi KA, Sherman BM: Prediction of treatment response in anorexia nervosa, in Obiols J, Ballus C, Gonzalez Monclus E, et al (eds): *Biological Psychiatry Today.* Amsterdam, Elsevier/North-Holland Biomedical Press, 1979, pp 609–614.

58. Gold MS, Pottash ALC, Sweeney DR, et al: Further evidence of hypothalamic–pituitary dysfunction in anorexia nervosa. *Am J Psychiatry* 137:101–102, 1980.

59. Kaye WH, Pikar D, Naber D, et al: Cerebrospinal fluid opioid activity in anorexia nervosa. *Am J Psychiatry* 139:643–645, 1982.

60. Warren SE, Steinberg SM. Acid–base and electrolyte disturbances in anorexia nervosa. *Am J Psychiatry* 136:415–418, 1979.

61. Berkman JM: Anorexia nervosa, anterior-pituitary insufficiency, Simmonds' cachexia and Sheehan's disease; including some observations on disturbances in water metabolism associated with starvation. *Postgrad Med J* 3:237–246, 1948.

62. Rieger W, Brady JP, Weisberg E: Hematologic changes in anorexia nervosa. *Am J Psychiatry* 135:984–985, 1978.

63. Klinefelter HF: Hypercholesterolemia in anorexia nervosa. *J Clin Endocrinol* 25:1520–1521, 1965.

64. Silverman JA: Anorexia nervosa: Clinical and metabolic observations in a successful treatment plan, in Vigersky R (ed): *Anorexia Nervosa.* New York, Raven Press, 1977, pp 331–339.

65. Brotman AW, Stern TA: Case report of cardiovascular abnormalities in anorexia nervosa. *Am J Psychiatry* 140:1227–1228, 1983.

66. Bruch H: Death in anorexia nervosa. *Psychosom Med* 33:135–144, 1971.

67. Crisp AH: The possible significance of some behavioral correlates of weight and carbohydrate intake. *J Psychosom Res* 11:117–131, 1967.

68. Crisp AH, Fenton GW, Scotton L: A controlled study of the EEG in anorexia nervosa. *Br J Psychiatry* 114:1149–1160, 1968.

69. Nussbaum M, Shenker IR, Mar J, et al: Cerebral atrophy in anorexia nervosa. *J Pediatr* 96:867–869, 1980.

70. Walsh BT, Croft CB, Katz JL: Anorexia nervosa and salivary gland enlargement. *Int J Psychiatry Med* 11:255–261, 1981.

71. Goldney RD: Craniopharyngioma simulating anorexia nervosa. *J Nerv Ment Dis* 166:135–138, 1978.

72. Weller RA, Weller EB: Anorexia nervosa in a patient with an infiltrating tumor of the hypothalamus. *Am J Psychiatry* 139:824–825, 1982.

73. Levitt DR. Teitelbaum P: Somnolence, akinesia and sensory activation of motivated behavior in the lateral hypothalamic syndrome. *Proc Natl Acad Sci USA* 72:2819–2823, 1975.

The Clinical and Laboratory Evaluation of Dementia

R. Michael Allen, M.D. and Mark S. Gold, M.D.

1. Introduction

One of the most important aspects of any discussion about the evaluation and diagnosis of a mental disorder is an agreed-on definition that limits the scope of the investigation. For the purposes of this discussion, the term dementia is used in the more neurological sense as an objective cognitive dysfunction without regard to reversibility or structural involvement. Thus, the more psychiatric term delirium would be included as a reversible dementia. Part of the reasoning for this usage includes the fact that correlation of structural change with degree and persistence of a cognitive deficit is poor and a general bias on the author's part against using outcome as part of the diagnostic criteria for a particular disorder.

This discussion is limited largely to the evaluation of dementia in the elderly population, as it is in this group that the differential of functional versus organic etiology is most crucial and difficult. However, because some causes of dementia are not age related, brief mention is made of dementing illnesses in younger patients. An exhaustive discussion of the etiology and clinical features of the dementias is beyond the scope of this discussion, and the reader is referred to any of the numerous standard textbooks on the subject.

The main purpose of this treatise is to review and examine the new and fascinating world of biological testing in psychiatry and neurology and point out the pitfalls awaiting the unwary from the standpoint of both omission and commission.

2. Epidemiology

It is important to keep some general epidemiologic statistics in mind when approaching the diagnostic evaluation of the cognitively impaired patient. For example, it

---

R. Michael Allen, M.D. • Neuropsychiatric Evaluation Unit, Psychiatric Institute of Fort Worth, Fort Worth, Texas 76104, and Department of Psychiatry, University of Texas Southwestern Medical School, Dallas, Texas 75235.   *Mark S. Gold, M.D.* • Research Facilities, Fair Oaks Hospital, Summit, New Jersey 07901, and Fair Oaks Hospital at Boca/Delray, Delray Beach, Florida 33445.

is a common misconception among both lay people and many non-behaviorally-oriented physicians that most old people become senile if they live long enough, and senility, or more correctly senile dementia Alzheimer's type (SDAT), is too quickly diagnosed in the elderly patient with resulting inappropriate placement in an institution such as a nursing home or state hospital long-term-care unit. Although no truly accurate statistics are available, best estimates place the prevalence of psychiatric illness in the population over 65 at 15% and the incidence of dementia at 6%.[1] Only 5% of the elderly require institutional-level care.[2] One should keep in mind that major depressive illness is the most common major psychiatric illness in the population as a whole (some estimates of life prevalence are as high as 30%), and greater than 50% of first-episode depressions occur in women over the age of 50 and in men over the age of 55.[3] Thus, the risk of a depressive illness is just as high if not higher than that of dementia. The proportion of patients presenting with dementia who actually are suffering from depressive or other psychogenic pseudodementia is not known but may be as high as 11%.[4] It has been estimated that up to 15% of elderly depressed patients have reversible causes for their problems, with drug toxicity, adverse drug interactions, and metabolic disorders leading the list.

3. Etiology

The most common cause of true dementia in the elderly is SDAT. Other causes include multi-infarct dementia (MID), which may account for 5% of dementias in the elderly, and Binswanger's disease, which is a lacunar type of subcortical dementia associated with subcortical microhemorrhages and hypertension. Rare causes of chronic dementias in the elderly include Huntington's, Jakob–Creutzfelt, Pick's, and Parkinson's diseases. Other causes of subchronic dementias include nutritional deficiencies (especially B_{12} and folate), hypothyroidism, substance abuse, especially alcohol and over-the-counter (OTC) remedies, trauma, and various metabolic problems such as hypoadrenalism, renal failure, and cardiovascular, respiratory, and collagen diseases. An area that is now being investigated intensively includes the sleep disorders, especially obstructive sleep apnea, as a cause of potentially reversible dementia. The main cause of presenile dementia is the Alzheimer's type, with Huntington's disease, Pick's disease, and Jakob–Creutzfeld disease being rarely responsible. In younger patients, the main causes of dementia include alcoholism, drug abuse (especially chronic stimulants), trauma, infection, and seizure disorders as well as metabolic causes, especially diabetes and renal failure.

4. Clinical Evaluation

The most important part of any clinical evaluation for suspected dementia is a complete history, physical examination, and mental status examination. Critical information such as type of onset (abrupt versus insidious), history of drug use or abuse, concurrent medical illnesses and medications, family history of mental illness, previous psychiatric history, current psychosocial stressors, a behavioral history from spouse, family, or friends, and a complete review of systems directs one to the appropriate workup. Obviously, the mental status examination is one of the most important aspects of the initial evaluation of the demented patient. There are several structured mental status tests available to the researcher and clinician, with the Mini-Mental State[5] being the most practical screening test. Detailed organic mental status examinations are documented by Taylor[6] and Strub and Black.[7] The physical examination is vital in determining physical signs of etiologic physical ailments as well as defining neurological impairment including "soft" signs of cortical release such as the palmomental, grasp, and Meyerson's signs.

Despite the clinician's vigilance in being aware of the possible causes of reversible cognitive deficits, including history and physical and mental status examinations, many cases of reversible dementias can be missed. Thus, the need for more sophisticated laboratory, electrophysiological, neuropsychological, and radiologic tools is clear.

5. Differential Diagnosis

The differential diagnosis of dementia versus pseudodementia is one of the most critical issues in neuropsychiatry today. There have been many attempts to define clinical diagnostic signs to facilitate this differential. The most notable are the cardinal signs proposed by Wells.[8] He proposed that the most important signs of pseudodementia were excessive dependency, subjective distress, and preoccupation with the cognitive deficit, abrupt onset, preserved attention, poor effort on exam performance with "I don't know" answers being typical, and incongruence between cognitive and behavioral performance. Kiloh[9] was one of the first to note the strong association of major affective disorder with pseudodementia. In addition, a recent report has noted that a previous history of depression is also a useful clinically differentiating factor.[10] More recently, it has become clear that the so-called cardinal signs of pseudodementia are much more valuable in diagnosing patients in whom they are present but that their absence is less helpful in ruling out a diagnosis of pseudodementia.[11] Some investigators go so far as to deny the existence of pseudodementia as a discrete clinical entity.[12] Perhaps the best approach is to drop the term pseudodementia and simply call these entities reversible functional cognitive deficits.

6. Clinical Laboratory Investigation of Dementia

The laboratory evaluation of dementia is not very complex, although it must be complete. The routine screening tests that are usually given to newly admitted patients to screen for metabolic, hematologic, and infectious disease are clearly indicated. With current state-of-the-art laboratory techniques, it is economical to assay for most of the clinically relevant chemicals and enzymes that are involved in maintaining normal metabolic balance. Thus, a routine SMA-22, which includes the electrolytes, glucose, calcium, phosphorus, iron, major cardiac, muscle, and liver enzymes, lipids, and renal function indicators, is extremely helpful as a metabolic screening device. The RPR and

FTA (fluorescent treponemal antibody test) are useful but not diagnostic for central nervous system (CNS) syphilis, and when there is doubt, a cerebral spinal fluid (CSF) VDRL is necessary for a definitive diagnosis.[13] The routine urinalysis is also helpful in detecting the occult urinary tract infection (UTI) that is associated with acute dementias as well as other chronic metabolic problems. The routine hemogram is a *sine qua non*, as many elderly patients suffer from anemias, chronic lymphocytic leukemia, and nutritional deficits that are reflected in the peripheral blood.

In addition to the above routine screening tests, special chemistries are indicated to evaluate the nutritional status, possible environmental toxin exposure such as heavy metals and insecticides, and drug abuse status. A serum B_{12} and folate determination is essential in the evaluation of the demented patient, as functional-appearing psychiatric symptoms as well as dementia may appear before one sees an overt anemia. Other water-soluble vitamin determinations provide a good assessment of the patient's nutritional status, e.g., ascorbate, B_6, zinc, and thiamin. For completeness, one can assay for amino acids that are involved in neurotransmitter synthesis such as tyrosine and L-tryptophan. Deficiencies in thiamin and ascorbate have been correlated with SDAT but have only been hypothesized to be causative.[14] For a complete discussion of nutritional factors and their evaluation, please refer to Chapter 9 in this volume.

A thorough metabolic screening is also indicated in the evaluation of the demented patient. A thyroid profile including a TSH, RT_3U, T_3 RIA, T_4 RIA, and perhaps a free T_4 is necessary to rule out myxedema. Base-line and 4 p.m. cortisol determinations are useful in assessing the adequacy of adrenal function. Fasting and 4 p.m. glucose determinations are indicated in patients with any suggestion of diabetes, and a full glucose tolerance test may be indicated.

A urinalysis for comprehensive drug screen is mandatory for the detection of drug abuse and misuse in the elderly. Many patients, not just the elderly, use a plethora of over-the-counter (OTC) drugs, which have numerous toxic effects with overdose or chronic use. When questioned about medication use, they often do not tell the examiner about them because they do not consider them to be medications. The same applies to megadose vitamin intake, which can cause severe derangements (especially the lipid-soluble ones and pyridoxine). Many OTC drugs for gastrointestinal, upper respiratory tract, and sleep disturbances have significant amounts of both antihistamines and anticholinergic agents, which are extremely psychotoxic to the elderly. Finally, the incidence of alcohol and drug abuse—especially benzodiazepines, stimulants, and even opiates—in the elderly is probably underestimated. In younger patients, drugs of abuse including stimulants, marijuana, opiates, phencyclidine, and OTC sedatives and antihistamines are leading causes of confusional states. Also, a thorough drug screen will often detect those patients who are taking a plethora of prescription drugs that they do not remember or have simply continued old prescriptions along with their new ones without consulting their physician. One must keep in mind that the traditional model of the elderly patient having one primary-care physician is fast disappearing, and these patients may see several doctors including those in the so-called "minor emergency centers" and receive multiple medications for the same chief complaint, resulting in serious toxic accumulation and drug interactions. Also, they may receive drugs with known toxic interactions because none of the many physicians they see is aware of what the others have prescribed.

7. Neuroradiologic Diagnosis

New neuroradiologic or, perhaps better stated, neuroimaging techniques have expanded the horizons of the investigations of the structural and metabolic status of the brain. Formerly, one had to depend on skull films, crude tomographic techniques, static isotope brain scans, pneumoencephalograms, and ultimately invasive cerebral arteriograms to completely evaluate the brain. Although the cerebral arteriogram remains the gold standard for the evaluation of masses, vascular insufficiency, and specific vascular lesions, newer noninvasive techniques have been developed that offer much information with little or no risk to the patient. The first and most widely used technique is the computerized axial tomography (CT) scan. This instrument has been most useful in the evaluation of cerebral atrophy and ventricular size and thus is quite useful in the diagnosis of conditions such as Pick's disease, Huntington's disease, normopressure hydrocephalus, mass lesions, cerebral infarcts, and traumatic insults to the brain. Unfortunately, the degree of cortical atrophy in older patients does not correlate well with the degree of cognitive impairment in Alzheimer's disease until the atrophy becomes extreme. Thus, patients with significant atrophy may not be demented, and patients with no atrophy may be quite demented.

Newer imaging techniques that are destined to give more information about the metabolic function of the brain include the xenon-133 cerebral blood flow scan, which can also be computerized,[15] and the positron emission tomogram (PET), which directly measures glucose utilization by the brain.[16] Although the xenon scan is becoming more of a practical possibility for clinical use, the PET scan is prohibitively expensive and will likely remain limited to research centers. Nuclear magnetic resonance imaging is soon to be approved for clinical use and may supplant the CT and xenon scans. This technique has many advantages in that it involves no ionizing radiation, gives extremely high resolution, and, when the technology develops (more powerful magnets and computer software), will be able to supplant the PET scanner for metabolic studies.[17] The final technique for imaging the CNS is the SPECT or single photon emission computerized tomogram, which involves the administration of α-emitting radiolabeled ligands but will allow for *in vivo* receptor binding studies as well as substrate utilization studies at a much lower cost than the PET or NMR.[18]

At the present time, the main radiologic investigation of dementia involves the CT scan to assess structural integrity of the brain and should be considered a routine part of the dementia workup. Older techniques such as the RISA (isotope cisternography) scan may still have some use in the diagnosis of normopressure hydrocephalus (NPH) when the CT scan is negative or equivocal and in the presence of good clinical evidence.

8. Electrophysiological Evaluation

The most sensitive screening test for brain dysfunction is the scalp electroencephalogram (EEG). Unfortunately, although it is quite sensitive to abnormal brain function, its specificity and diagnostic power are low. Unless there are focal abnormalities, the most information that one can obtain is that the brain is dysfunctional (generalized slowing). In the absence of medications or a clear history of substance abuse or particular metabolic derangement, the EEG only confirms the need for further testing. There are four syndromes in which the EEG may be diagnostic: Jakob–Creutzfelt disease, the epilepsies, Dawson's encephalitis, and some types of trauma. However, the EEG is a critical part of the evaluation of the demented patient because of its sensitivity in detecting metabolic or electrical abnormalities.[19] A more useful test for the subcortical dementias that may slip by the routine EEG is the P-300 auditory evoked response test, which is now more available as a routine clinical tool.[20] It is a simple, noninvasive test that requires sophisticated equipment. The BEAM (brain electrical activity mapping) technique is just now being introduced into clinical practice and may prove to be useful if the extreme expense of setting up the system can be overcome. The BEAM essentially gives a three-dimensional EEG view of the brain and in some studies has been correlated with functional as well as organic disorders.[21]

9. Special Diagnostic Procedures

It is in the area of neuroendocrine, metabolite excretion, and sleep studies that the most progress in using biological markers to diagnose major affective illnesses has been made in the last 10 years. Since affective disorders are the main cause of the pseudodementia syndrome in the elderly and are among the most easily treated conditions in psychiatry, it is imperative that the diagnosis of these disorders not be missed in the patient presenting with a cognitive disturbance. As has been noted above, clinical features, neuroradiologic, and even neurophysiological studies are not always diagnostic in differentiating "functional" from "organic" illness. Thus, the potential usefulness of the above special studies has to be carefully evaluated. Each type of study is presented below with reference to its usefulness.

The main neuroendocrine studies that have been shown to be roughly equivalent to commonly used diagnostic procedures in general medicine in terms of sensitivity and specificity in the diagnosis of major affective disorders are the dexamethasone suppression test (DST) and the thyrotropin-releasing hormone infusion test (TRH). When properly used in the evaluation of suspected affectively ill patients, these tests show a high degree of sensitivity (DST 40–60%,[22] TRH 30–70%,[23]) and specificity (DST 85+%,[22] TRH 90%[23]) for the confirmation of major dperessive illness. Although there has recently been a flood of reports questioning the utility of the DST in detecting endogenous or melancholic depression,[24-26] many of these reports have simply confirmed what Carroll and others have stated previously, that the DST is not useful as a general screening test for depression.[27] In the nonelderly population, it seems clear that significant weight loss, alcoholism, and chronic or acute serious medical illness give a high incidence of DST nonsupression.[28,29]

Of more concern in this discussion are the recent reports that the incidence of DST nonsuppression in demented elderly patients is as high as or higher than those with documented depression who are not demented.[30,31] The problem with these studies is that the patients with dementia for the most part had advanced Alzheimer's disease, which is a chronic, debilitating condition. Other studies have shown that in the early stages of SDAT, when the differentiation of depressive pseudodementia is critical, the incidence of DST nonsuppression is not significantly different from controls.[32] Thus, although one should be cautious in its application, the DST is likely to have significant usefulness in the early differentiation of dementia from pseudodementia. As is the case in all age groups, the presence of a positive result yields the most significant information, and a negative result does not rule out the presence of affective illness.

No one has proposed that the decision to treat or not to treat a presumed depressive illness should be based on the outcome of a laboratory test, but it has been established that when the DST is positive, a return to normal suppression indicates that the treatment is effective and that a recurrence of nonsuppression after cessation of treatment is a strong predictor of imminent relapse.[33] This pattern would presumably hold true for the elderly patient, as the truly demented patient would probably not revert to normal suppression with antidepressant treatment in the first place, although there are no data to substantiate this supposition.

The TRH test is of limited usefulness in the differential diagnosis of depression versus dementia in the elderly. The typical pattern of a blunted ΔTSH_{max} response is common in males above the age of 60 and does not correlate with depression. In females the finding is not as consistent, and the test may have limited usefulness.[34] The one disorder that the TRH test can pick up that may be a cause of occult depressive symptoms and presumably pseudodementia is grade III hypothyroidism, in which one sees an augmented TSH response to TRH with all base-line studies including the TSH being normal[35] and often an elevated titer of antithyroid antibodies (both thyroglobulin and microsomal). Thus, if clinically indicated, i.e., the patient has complaints of anergy and a general "failure to thrive," the TRH infusion test may be indicated in the workup of dementia.

Urine collection for the determination of urinary MHPG is not very useful in the diagnosis of depression in the elderly, or in younger patients for that matter, as the usual findings vary within the normal range. However, once the diagnosis of depression has been made clinically or by previous neuroendocrinologic testing, the results of the urinary MHPG tests may prove quite useful in deciding with what antidepressant to begin treatment.[36] To be a useful and valid test, however, the patients must be on a low-monoamine diet and participate in no vigorous physical activities for at least 3 days prior to the collection of the urines. Although there is some controversy about the usefulness of this test in the selection of an antidepressant drug, it seems clear that low urinary excretion of MHPG (<1900 $\mu g/24$ hr) is quite predictive of a good response to the noradrenergic-type antidepressants such as desipramine, nortriptyline, or maprotyline.[37] The early studies of the excretion patterns of MHPG failed to demonstrate that the age of the patient affected the results.[38]

One procedure that is certainly not new and is apparently not utilized to a great extent in routine psychiatric practice now is the amobarbital interview. It is a time-tested, safe procedure that has been reported to be quite useful in the differentiation of functional versus organic symptomatology in both conversion disorders and suspected pseudodementias. Simply put, if one administers a sufficient dose of sodium amobarbital (50–400 mg) intravenously to induce a twilight state (indicating mild cortical inhibition), one expects the demented patient's cognitive state to deteriorate; the pseudodemented patient will often improve.[39,40]

10. Sleep Studies

All-night sleep studies have been a valuable tool for research into the accurate diagnosis of major depression with endogenous or melancholic features. The classic finding in depression has been decreased rapid eye movement (REM) latency.[41] There has been some question about how useful this measurement would be in the diagnosis of depression in the elderly, as REM latency decreases with age. Also, the question arises as to how useful it is in the differentiation of depressive pseudodementia versus dementia. Recently, it has been determined that if one uses the norms from age- and sex-matched healthy controls, the usefulness of shortened REM latency holds up. Likewise, although patients with advanced SDAT have shortened REM latency, in the early stages of the disease, when the diagnosis is most critical, there is no significant difference between these patients and controls.[42]

Another area of potential importance in the use of the sleep lab is in the diagnosis of primary sleep disturbance as a cause of reversible dementias. Perhaps the most important such problem is sleep apnea. Both obstructive and central sleep apnea can cause significant cognitive and functional deficits. The obstructive type is well known in its association with hypertension, hypersomnolence, and decreased mental acuity.[43] Likewise, it is easily treated with surgery, weight loss, and sometimes with protriptyline. If detected and treated early enough, permanent cognitive disturbances may be prevented.

11. Neuropsychological Evaluation

The development over the past 15 years of reliable neuropsychological testing techniques for the diagnosis of both global and localized cognitive and neurological deficits has opened new horizons in the practice of neurology and more recently in psychiatry. Not only can these testing methods localize areas of specific neurological deficit in previously neurologically silent areas, but now some progress has been made in localizing emotional and psychopathological states and processes to various areas of the brain. The two most widely used tests are the original battery devised by Halstead and Reitan[44] and the recently modified Luria neuropsychological battery as elaborated by Golden and his group at the University of Nebraska.[45] The reliability and specificity of these tests in differentiating dementia from pseudodementia have been questioned, although each of the opposing camps (Reitan and Golden) claim high degrees of reliability. In the author's clinical experience, the Luria–Nebraska battery appears to be more useful in patients with significant psychiatric illness, especially depression and mania, whereas the Reitan–Halstead battery appears to be more specific in localizing structural lesions in brain-damaged patients. Thus, if one is to rely on neuropsychological testing for the diagnosis of neurological and psychiatric disease, it is wise to utilize an eclectic neuropsychologist who is not wedded to any particular system for every circumstance.

12. Conclusion

Although there have been numerous attempts to define those clinical symptoms and signs that distinguish dementia from so-called functional psychiatric illnesses presenting as dementias, these efforts have attained less than total reliability. It has been pointed out that the only way to be quite certain about the diagnosis is by applying the best treatment method for the suspected psychiatric problem, be that electroconvulsive treatment or psychotropic drugs.[11] Likewise, the usefulness of some of the newer diagnostic procedures has been problematic in certain conditions that are peculiar to the aged population. However, the conscientious application of the principles of good medical judgment and practice and the judicious use of some of the new technological tools that are being developed enable one to be reasonably sure of the diagnosis. Some of the newer biological tests can help the clinician make the best initial choice of therapy for the patient with reversible cognitive deficits while following the patient's chemical as well as clinical progress in treatment. The importance of the accurate diagnosis of cognitive problems in the elderly cannot be overemphasized, as the proportion of the population over 65 is increasing steadily and will mushroom in 25 more years as the postwar baby boom generation enters this time in life. The economic burden of supporting or providing custodial care for elderly patients who in reality have treatable causes of cognitive disability will be unacceptable, and unpleasant social consequences might result for all elderly.

References

1. Cohen GD: Senile dementia of the alzheimer's type (SDAT)—nature of the disorder, in Crook T, Gershon S (eds): *Strategies for the Development of an Effective Treatment for Senile Dementia*. New Canaan, CT Powly Associates, 1981, pp 1–16.
2. Terry RD: Dementia, a brief and selective review. *Arch Neurol* 33:1–4, 1976.
3. Geriatric psychiatry, in Kaplan HI, Sadock BJ (eds) *Modern Synopsis of Comprehensive Textbook of Psychiatry III*. Baltimore, Williams & Wilkins, 1981, pp 1017–1022.
4. Smith JS, Kiloh LG, Ratnavale GS, et al: The investigation of dementia. *Med J Aust* 2:403–405, 1976.
5. Felstein MF, Felstein SE, McHugh PR: "Mini-Mental State": A practical method for grading the cognitive state of patients for the clinician. *J Psychiatr Res* 12:189–198, 1975.
6. Taylor MA: *The Neuropsychiatric Mental Status Exam*. New York, S P Medical and Scientific Books, 1981.
7. Strub RL, Black WF: *The Mental Status Exam in Neurology*. Philadelphia, FA Davis, 1977.
8. Wells CE: Pseudodementia. *Am J Psychiatry* 136:895–900, 1978.
9. Kiloh CG: Pseudodementia. *Acta Psychiatr Scand* 37:336–351, 1961.
10. Rabins PV, Altaf M, Nestadt G: Criteria for diagnosing reversible dementia caused by depression: Validation by a 2-year followup. *Br J Psychiatry* 144:488–492, 1984.
11. Allen RM: Pseudodementia and ECT. *Biol Psychiatry* 17:1435–1443, 1982.
12. Schraberg D: The myth of pseudodementia and the aging brain. *Am J Psychiatry* 135:601–603, 1978.
13. Adams RD, Victor M: *Principles of Neurology*. New York, McGraw-Hill, 1977, p 645.
14. Spector R, Cancilla P, Dimasio A: Is idiopathic dementia a regional vitamin deficiency state: *Med Hypotheses* 5:763–767, 1979.
15. Risberg J: Regional cerebral blood flow measurements by 133-xenon inhalation: Methodology and applications in neuropsychology and psychiatry. *Brain Lang* 9:9–34, 1980.
16. Bunney WE, Garland G, Buchsbaum M: Advances in the use of visual imaging: Techniques in mental illness. *Psychiatr Ann* 13:420–426, 1983.
17. Erkinhuntti T, Sipponen JT, et al: Cerebral NMR and CT imaging in dementia. *J Comput Assist Tomogr* 8:614–618, 1984.
18. Kuhl DE: Quantifying local cerebral blood flow by N-isopropyl-*p*-[123]iodoamphetamine (IMP) tomography. *J Nucl Med* 23:196–203, 1982.

19. Johanson G, Hagberg B, Gustafson L, et al: EEG and cognitive impairment in presenile dementia. *Acta Neurol Scand* 59:225–240, 1979.
20. Pfefferbaum A, Wenegrat BG, Ford JM, et al: Clinical application of the P_3 component of event-related potentials II. Dementia, depression, and schizophrenia. *Electroencephalogr Clin Neurophysiol* 59:104–124, 1984.
21. Morisha JM, Duffy FH, Wyatt RJ: Brain electrical activity mapping (BEAM) in schizophrenic patients. *Arch Gen Psychiatry* 40:719–728, 1983.
22. Carroll BJ, Feinberg M, Greden JF, et al: A specific laboratory test for the diagnosis of melancholia: Standardization, validation, and clinical utility. *Arch Gen Psychiatry* 38:15–22, 1981.
23. Extein I, Pottash ALC, Gold MS: TRH test in depression. *N Engl J Med* 302:923–924, 1980.
24. Dewan MJ, Pandurangi AK, Boucher ML, et al: Abnormal dexamethasone suppression test results in chronic schizophrenic patients. *Am J Psychiatry* 139:1501–1503, 1982.
25. Ensel TR, Kalin NH, Guttmacher LB, et al: The dexamethasone suppression test in patients with primary obsessive compulsive disorder. *Psychiatry Res* 6:153–160, 1982.
26. Peselow ED, Goldring A, Fieve RR, et al: The dexamethasone suppression test in depressed outpatients and normal control subjects. *Am J Psychiatry* 140:245–247, 1983.
27. Carroll BJ: Use of the dexamethasone suppression test in depression. *J Clin Psychiatry* 43:44–50, 1982.
28. Kline MD, Beeber AR: Weight loss and the dexamethasone suppression test. *Arch Gen Psychiatry* 49:1034–1035, 1983.
29. Newsom G, Murray N: Reversal of dexamethasone suppression and non suppression in alcohol abusers. *Am J Psychiatry* 140:353–354, 1983.
30. Spar JE, Gerner R: Does the dexamethasone suppression test distinguish dementia from depression? *Am J Psychiatry* 139:238–240, 1982.
31. Raskind M, Peskind E, Rivard M-F, et al: Dexamethasone suppression test and cortisol circadian rhythm in primary degenerative dementia. *Am J Psychiatry* 139:1468–1471, 1982.
32. Castro P, Lemaire M, Toscana-Aguilar M, et al: Depression, dementia, and the dexamethasone test. *Am J Psychiatry* 140:10, 1983.
33. Greden JF, Albala AA, Haskett RF, et al: Normalization of the dexamethasone suppression test: A laboratory index of recovery from endogenous depression. *Biol Psychiatry* 15:449–458, 1980.
34. Snyder PJ, Utiger RD: Thyrotropin response to thyrotropin-releasing hormone in normal females over 40. *J Clin Endocrinol Metab* 34:1096–1098, 1972.
35. Gold MS, Pottash ALC, Extein I: "Symptomless" autoimmune thyroiditis in depression. *Psychiatry Res* 6:261–269, 1982.
36. Cobbin DM, Requin-Blow B, Williams LR, et al: Urinary MHPG levels and tricyclic antidepressant selection in clinical practice. *Arch Gen Psychiatry* 36:1111–1115, 1979.
37. Rosenbaum AH, Schatzberg AF, Maruta T, et al: MHPG as a predictor of antidepressant response of imipramine and maprotyline. *Am J Psychiatry* 137:1090–1093, 1980.
38. Maas JW, Fawcett J, Dekirmenjian H: 3-Methoxy-4-hydroxyphenylglycol (MHPG) excretion in depressive states. *Arch Gen Psychiatry* 19:129–134, 1968.
39. Weinstein EA, Kahn RS, Sugerman LA, et al: The diagnostic use of amobarbital sodium (Amytal sodium) in brain disease. *Am J Psychiatry* 109:889–895, 1953.
40. Dyskin MW, Chang SS, Casper RC, et al: Barbiturate facilitated interviewing: A review. *Biol Psychiatry* 14:421–432, 1979.
41. Coble P, Foster FG, Kupfer DJ: Electroencephalographic sleep diagnosis of primary depression. *Arch Gen Psychiatry* 33:1124–1127, 1976.
42. Vitiello MV, Bokan JA, Kukull WA, et al: Rapid eye movement sleep measures of Alzheimer's-type dementia patients and optimally healthy aged individuals. *Biol Psychiatry* 19:721–734, 1984.
43. Schmidt HS: Sleep disorders: The new nosology, in *Psychiatry Clinical Update*. Kalamazoo, Upjohn, 1982, pp 6–9.
44. Reitan R, Davidson L (eds): *Clinical Neuropsychology: Current Status and Applications*. New York, John Wiley & Sons, 1974.
45. Golden CJ, Hammeke TA, Purisch AD: *The Luria–Nebraska Neuropsychological Battery*. Los Angeles, Western Psychological Services, 1980.

Index